Meetings between experts

MEETINGS
BETWEEN EXPERTS
An approach to sharing ideas
in medical consultations

by David Tuckett, Mary Boulton,
Coral Olson, and Anthony Williams

TAVISTOCK PUBLICATIONS

London and New York

First published in 1985 by
Tavistock Publications Ltd
11 New Fetter Lane,
London EC4P 4EE

Published in the USA by
Tavistock Publications Ltd
in association with Methuen, Inc.
29 West 35th Street, New York NY 10001

Printed in Great Britain by
Richard Clay, The Chaucer Press,
Bungay, Suffolk

British Library Cataloguing in Publication Data

Meetings between experts : an approach to
sharing ideas in medical consultations.
1. Physician and patient   2. Physicians
(General practice)
I. Tuckett, David
610.69′6   R727.3

ISBN 0-422-79650-6
ISBN 0-422-79660-3(pbk.)

*Library of Congress Cataloging in Publication
Data*

Main entry under title:
Meetings between experts: an approach to
sharing ideas in medical consultations.
Includes bibliographies and indexes.
1. Physician and patient.   2. Medical history
taking.   3. Patient education.
4. Interpersonal communication.
5. Family medicine.   I. Tuckett, David.
[DNLM: 1. Physician-Patient Relations.
2. Referral and Consultation. W 64 M495]
R727.3.M44 1985   610.69′6   85-12576

ISBN 0-422-79650-6
ISBN 0-422-79660-3 (pbk.)

CONTENTS

ACKNOWLEDGEMENTS

The research study on which the ideas in this book are based was conducted between 1977 and 1983 while the authors were members of the Health Education Studies Unit, Hughes Hall, University of Cambridge. Data was collected between April 1979 and May 1980 and earlier reports to the Health Education Council were published in a limited way in 1980, 1981, and 1982.

The first author wishes particularly to acknowledge the support of the King Edward's Hospital Fund for London whose grant to him made the writing of this book possible. Thanks are also due to George Brown and Peter Higgins for their support and constructive comments on earlier drafts of the text and to Lesley Barnes and Fanny Tuckett for their encouragement and tolerance throughout the project.

The study would have been impossible without the help and co-operation we received from the general practitioners, reception staff, and patients whom we studied. To protect their confidential relationship we will not name them individually. Many other physicians gave us help, encouragement, and advice at various stages of the project. Among them were: Dr Neville Barley, Dr Marie Campkin, Dr Hugh Cornford, Dr Alan Maryon Davis, Dr Chris Donovan, Dr Andrew Elder, Dr Paul Freeling, Dr Gerry Griffin, Professor Brian Jarman, Dr Derek Lambert, Dr Bill Marson, Dr Roger Neighbour, Dr Jack Norrell, Dr Lotte Newman, Dr Chris Page, Dr Bernard Reiss, Dr Piers Ricordon, Dr Norma Rink, Dr Jane Robson, Dr Theo Schofield, Dr Gordon Sharpe, Dr Peter Tomson, Dr Tom Williamson, Dr John Woodall, Dr John Woodward, and Dr Luke Zander.

The Health Education Studies Unit was financed by the Health Education Council and housed both at the HEC offices in London and at Hughes Hall, Cambridge. Thanks are due both to the Council and Staff of the HEC and to the President and Fellows of Hughes Hall for making us welcome. We are also especially grateful to the Chairman and members of the Unit's Academic Advisory Committee who assisted with comments and advice throughout the life of the project. The members of the committee were: Mrs Ena Abrahams, Professor Dick D'Aeth, Professor George W. Brown, Dr David Bruce, Professor Sir John Butterfield, Mr Jim Davies, Professor John Davis, Professor Paul Hirst (Chairman), Professor Peter Kelly, Dr Brian Lloyd, Dr Bernard Reiss, Dr Martin Richards, Mr Ian Sutherland, and Dr Keith Tones.

At the Health Education Council we should especially like to thank Ian Sutherland, Don Freeman, and Jo Walker as well as David Sharp and all the HEC library staff. Jim Davies, Rosemary Bond, Pieris Elinas, Jane Gardiner, Simon Nation, Kathryn McMullin, Ken Paternoster, Sarah Rayman, and Cathy Stopes-Roe all helped us at different times as members of the Health Education Studies Unit. Pat Deleulemeester typed a great deal of an early manuscript onto a word processor. We would also like to acknowledge our debt to Dr Judy Bailey and the staff of the Cambridge University Computing Service and to the British Library Lending and Reference Divisions.

David Tuckett
Mary Boulton
Coral Olson
Anthony Williams

London, February 1985

PART 1

Introduction

CHAPTER 1

Sharing ideas and its importance in medical consultations

The meetings between doctors and patients, which we will refer to as medical consultations, are frequent and regular occurrences throughout the developed world. In the UK alone, for example, there are upwards of half a million such meetings every working day. The aim of this book is to explore a little-discussed aspect of these rather frequent occurrences: namely, the extent to which ideas are shared in them. In particular, our interest is in how far what is said in consultations can help patients to an understanding of what is happening to them. The concern is partly specific to the interests of the medical sociologist and medical educator – techniques of communication and explanation are relatively neglected areas of medical education and ones to which social scientists can make a contribution (Walton *et al.* 1980). But wider and more fundamental issues are also relevant. A consideration of the exchange of ideas between a doctor and a patient, or the lack of it, raises important issues about a doctor's and a patient's relative autonomy and authority; the extent to which it is possible for patients to evaluate scientific and technical advice; or, more generally, the limits constraining ordinary citizens from participating in the determination of public policy based on scientific and professional advice.

The 'Competence gap'

One approach to the question of how far ideas can be shared in a medical consultation (or analogously in other meetings between technical experts and their clients) has been to assume, more or less, that there is a competence gap between doctor and patient which makes shared understanding impossible. Indeed, one distinguished analyst, Talcott Parsons, has gone so far as to base his theory of the social organization of medical practice on the assumption that, in most instances, patients could not be expected to consent to medical examination or treatment on the basis of understanding its medical merits (1). Rather, he suggested, consent was routinely obtained through affective and institutional means. Put simply, patients would agree to the demands and suggestions of their doctors not because they understood the need for them, but because they had faith in the doctor as a person and as a representative of his profession. Such faith, he considered, was constructed by means of various common beliefs about the way doctors and patients should behave rather than by means of any understanding of the processes of making a diagnosis or deciding on a suitable treatment (Parsons 1951: 441).

The notion of a competence gap is one that cannot be ignored when trying to understand what is said in medical consultations and how they are conducted. The extent to which the gap is an unbridgeable chasm, however, deserves more examination than Parsons or many of his critics have been able to give. After all, there would be very little point in consulting many kinds of expert if it was not the case that in some sense they possessed specialist expertise. To some extent all experts may carry conviction by creating feelings of deference or by utilizing the mantles of tradition and institutional power. However, a moment's reflection also suggests that most experts must also regularly have to communicate their specialist assessment and advice and to translate it in such a way that at least the essence of their ideas can be comprehended correctly by an individual not privy to their expert knowledge. It seems likely that being able to share expert understanding may be an essential requirement of the specialist. Certainly, in the scientific and technical environment of the modern world, the impossibility of expertise in every area means that reliance on specialist expertise makes its communication a daily problem in many fields. It would seem that at least to some degree specialist knowledge is shared successfully between experts on a daily basis. For instance, physicians of one specialty obtain advice from colleagues from another; army commanders consult meteorologists or psychologists; pupils learn from teachers and parents; architects rely on structural engineers; and businesspeople, cabinet ministers, and government servants consult a range of experts from physicists and physicians to computer scientists and lawyers. At least in some of these cases it is inconceivable that the expert operates solely by manipulating affects. Information is also shared. Individuals with different models of understanding and different degrees of background knowledge have to succeed in communicating, if only to a degree and not without difficulty. One reason for success is likely to be that the expert being consulted will not try to communicate nor succeed in communicating every fine detail of his assessment and reasoning. He will concentrate on making clear his recommendations and providing sufficient reasoning in their support to convince his client of their veracity and to enable him to choose a course of action.

If communication is to a degree possible between experts in some areas of the modern world why not between doctors (with one sort of expertise) and patients (with another)? The central question we shall address, therefore, is whether it is really the case that there is something so different and so difficult about medical consultations that a process of communicating and translating specialist knowledge, at least to the degree of success achieved between other experts, is impossible.

Emotions and social conflict

Several among those who have discussed the sharing of information in medical consultations (like Parsons) would appear to argue that the situation of medical practice is different. Two particular sources of communication difficulty have been isolated: these are the specific emotional content and context of medical work and the social (particularly the conflictual) nature of patient–professional relationships.

The argument about the emotional content and context of medical work and the limits it places on sharing understanding is fairly straightforward. The idea is that doctors deal with situations of potential misfortune: death, disability, trauma, pain, depression, anxiety, etc. Every patient will die eventually and any patient may proceed to disability or death sooner rather than later. Moreover, in the mind of doctor and patient the outcome of misfortune is frequently uncertain creating an emotionally loaded situation. Patients (and perhaps also doctors) have a need to defend against misfortune and uncertainty and the accompanying feelings of helplessness. The defences they employ include the idealization or denigration of each other or recourse to magical and omnipotent thinking. Raised emotions and the defensive responses generated by them are not conducive, it is thought, to 'rational' communication and shared understanding (for example, Parsons 1951: 442).

The argument that communication to achieve a shared understanding is pro-hibited, or made nearly impossible, by the social nature of doctor–patient rela-tionships may be less immediately plausible than the previous argument about emotions, at least to someone not trained as a social scientist. In essence, the argu-ment is that medical consultations take place in the context of a power struggle between patients and doctors who have mutually contradictory interests. The control of information is part of this conflict. 'The professional', wrote one exponent of this view, 'is jealous of his prerogative to diagnose and forecast illness, holding it tightly to himself. But while he does not want anyone else to give information to the patient, neither is he himself inclined to do so' (Freidson 1970b: 143). The claim to a monopoly of expertise and knowledge has been one of the foundations of the professional's claim to a privileged social and economic status and not one, it is argued, that will be given up lightly. Moreover, a degree of mystification and admiration in the client, along with a devaluation of lay knowledge, is sometimes thought to bolster professional power. Further, knowledge can be used by each participant in the consultation to control the other: a doctor can use it to ease his work as by shortening the length of time he is in contact with a patient (Lorber 1975); a patient can use it to attain an end such as a desired prescription (Stimson and Webb 1975). Some authors have described in detail the way doctors and patients 'negotiate' verbally with each other (Stimson and Webb 1975; Bloor 1976; West 1976). Others have argued that the setting itself and the way it is organized func-tion to control and limit the verbal interaction (Rosengren and De Vault 1964; Sharrock 1979). The point is that in these ways both doctors and patients may limit what they say more in the interest of achieving their aim than in helping the other to understand their point of view.

A further aspect of the social nature of consultations is that in different societies there may be legal constraints which inhibit communication. For example, in the US anxiety about litigation and the intrinsic uncertainty of medical knowledge may keep a doctor from telling a patient what he thinks is wrong. He might subsequently be proved incorrect and be sued. In the UK, on the other hand, the legal system may inhibit communication in a different way. A successful prosecution for not giving information is much less likely than in the US (Robertson 1981) and this may may act as a disincentive to communication. Finally, another influence of social factors on the consultation process derives from differences in the social status of doctors and patients. Such differences may encourage attitudes of deference or superiority that inhibit communication.

If the emotional and social conflicts just mentioned are the routine and overriding feature of medical consultations the barriers they are likely to present to a process of sharing understanding between individuals of different competence may indeed be formidable. It may be, however, that the emotional issues are neither so demanding nor the social ones so widespread as the authors of these viewpoints have assumed. One influence upon the emotional constraints operating in a consultation is likely to be the nature of the illness from which a patient suffers. To the extent to which the illnesses dealt with in consultations are mainly experienced as life-threatening, disabling, and disfiguring or difficult to diagnose and predict, one might expect emotions to be overwhelming and 'rational' discourse to be most difficult – although discourse and understanding could also be seen as containing and reducing anxieties. However, many of the illnesses seen in contemporary western medical consultations are not of this extreme kind. Clinically urgent and acutely frightening diseases are the exceptions and, over time, even the most severe illness (if the patient survives) tends to lead to many years of more routine consultations (Szasz and Hollender 1956; Tuckett 1976: 229). Similarly, the social dimension of doctor–patient relationships may not always militate against sharing information. It is an open question in many situations whether doctors' motives are always or even solely concerned with enhanced socio-economic status or whether the battle for control in the consulting room is as 'hot' as some writers have suggested. It is possible to imagine that some doctors at least could be pursuing a goal such as achieving well-informed and autonomous patients. In fact, whatever the emotional difficulties, social conflicts or competence gaps in medical consultations, some attempt to share information is probably routine. Giving advice and providing instructions are an integral part of daily medical work as is the provision of verbal reassurance. More interesting, therefore, than the question of whether it is possible to share understanding is the question of how difficult it is to achieve this task and what priority should be given to it.

The importance of sharing ideas

The proposition that sharing ideas with patients should have an important priority among the tasks a physician sets himself is one that may have gained ground in recent years. Five strands of argument point in this direction.

First, one set of arguments is based on the recognition that attending to the provision of information, reassurance and understanding are intrinsic and very important parts of therapy. The view has been argued in different ways. Balint (1964) focused on the ways a doctor can use contact with himself as therapeutic. Egbert *et al.* (1964) and Skipper and Leonard (1968) have demonstrated how providing information as part of surgical treatment speeds recovery and improves outcome. Joyce *et al.* (1969) has argued that 'often' communication is virtually the only form of treatment there is and Lever (1977) has countered the criticism that medical care is ineffective by arguing that the effects of reassurance as one traditional form of therapy have not been properly included in the balance sheet.

These arguments remind the physician that he is heir to a long tradition of healing. In recent years western general practitioners have been trained to think of their diagnostic activities as first and foremost preliminaries to treatments which are 'effective' rather than symbolic and so in part they often must be. But everyday western medical practice also includes the traditional healer's task of reducing a patient's anxiety and uncertainty by containing it within a structure of explanation that provides reassurance. The healer is likely to give information to the patient not only about what he suffers, but at the same time about how it came about, what is to blame, what will happen, and what should be done. The latter may often involve investigation, intervention, or expiation depending on the social and cultural context. In the process the healer assigns meaning and significance to an illness event and helps to organize and render comprehensible the experience. Although what a western doctor thinks and says may be couched in terms of physiological processes rather than as social causation, by analogy with the healer's activities it can nonetheless function to sort out and invest with cultural meaning a patient's illness experience and to contain personal and corporate anxiety (Kleinman, Eisenberg, and Good 1978; Zola 1973; Horton 1967). It is, therefore, part of a process of structuring and reconstituting aspects of an illness experience which, as in the traditional setting, can be communicated both in verbal discourse and through ritual and therapeutic processes which draw attention to cultural principles and moral issues. Information, in this context, can be provided to a patient in the idiom of lay theories of illness and its causation or in the language of biomedical models of pathology. The objective is that the patient's anxiety and uncertainty about the significance of his symptoms be contained within a reassuring explanatory framework.

Based on these arguments we might expect some consultations to be ones in which sharing information with patients, as a way of trying to structure and render more tolerable their experience, would be a priority activity. Among these consultations might be ones in which patients were prepared for hospital treatment, those in which the main issue was the need to help the patient to recognize he did not have a serious illness and those in which the patient and his family needed to come to terms with his misfortune.

A second set of arguments for giving information in consultations is based on the recognition that the patient's co-operation in carrying out advice cannot be taken for granted. As a former president of the American Medical Association observed, the patient's co-operation 'depends on whether or not he understands the need for the measures advised' (Ernstene 1957: 1111). By contrast, a limited explanation or none at all leaves 'many questions unanswered in the patient's mind and seldom convinces him of the harmlessness of his symptoms' (Ernstene 1957: 1111).

It is recognized that many patients ignore a doctor's advice and this fact has received increasing attention in recent years. In various studies it has been suggested that between 10 per cent and 90 per cent of patients, with an average of 50 per cent, do not take their prescribed treatment correctly (Ley 1976; Blackwell 1976; Ley 1979; Haynes, Taylor, and Sackett 1979: 11). In the UK it is estimated that the hoarded or wasted drugs that are the result of this 'noncompliance' cost well in excess of £300 million per year (Walton *et al.* 1980). In these circumstances doctors have been advised that 'Once a decision has been taken to prescribe a drug, time should be spent in explaining what the drug is intended to do, what likely symptoms the patient may experience...and the time sequences of the drug's actions...' (Cormack 1981: 181)

The need to provide information for the purpose of persuading patients to co-operate with what their doctors think is best also arises from the extension of modern medical treatment in terms of both time and space (Rosengren and Lefton 1969: 125; Tuckett 1976: 229). Intervention is now likely to embrace an individual's feelings and habits as well as his environment and to extend over longer periods of time. Some indication can be found in the clinical literature directed at primary care physicians who are advised by their colleagues of the need to explain or, as one author put it, to provide 'corrective advice' to patients (Oliver 1981), about a whole series of 'health education' topics. Doctors have been advised to educate their patients about smoking, diet, exercise, and alcohol risks (for instance Smail 1982; Russell *et al.* 1979; Walt 1971; Pike 1969; Fowler 1982). Failure to follow such advice is probably even more widespread than failure to take medication (Haynes, Taylor, and Sackett 1979).

In the context of evidence about how patients do not follow advice, providing them with information is seen as an important priority for two reasons: information is necessary to know what to do (Svarstad 1974; Ley 1979); and it may help to motivate a patient to do what he is advised (Fletcher 1973; Svarstad 1974; Becker and Maiman 1975).

Information given to help a patient to co-operate can be regarded as information given with the aim of persuading the patient. In the sense that the patient is expected to adopt the doctor's view of the problem and to follow his advice unequivocally this aim of giving information inevitably implies a high degree of professional control of the patient.

The third argument for giving priority to the task of sharing information in consultations derives from the recognition that the outcome of medical treatment is multi-dimensional and also often a subjective matter (Tuckett 1976: 28). Imagine the case of a man who believes himself thoroughly fit but finds, after a medical examination required in connection with a life insurance proposal, that his blood pressure is raised above the limit most doctors consider puts him 'at risk'. His doctor advises him that he should take more exercise, cut down or cut out alcohol and cigarettes, alter his diet, and try to relax more. At the same time he provides beta-blocking drugs (designed to bring down his blood pressure) and suggests to the patient he attend for a regular check-up. The man in this situation not only has to adjust emotionally to the fact that although he feels perfectly well he has a theoretically greater risk of having a stroke or heart attack than if he did not have high blood pressure. He also has to experience the implications of the advice he has been offered. Changes in habit may affect his social, occupational, or married life. Taking the drugs may give him side effects from headaches to impotence (with further consequences). And all this because he 'might' at some future time have problems if he ignores the advice now. What is best for him?

Within the limits imposed by the patient's condition and the intervention and help that is available, some authors have argued that the patient's best interests cannot be served unless some effort at least is made to explore whether the patient himself has a view of the priorities. To ignore the patient can seem paternalistic. As Szasz and Hollender (1956: 568) put it 'Do we take a patient's word for it? Or do we place ourselves into the traditional parental role of 'knowing what is best' for our patients?'

As medical interventions have been extended in an attempt to treat a wider range of chronic and longstanding problems by more intrusive means, the problem of assessing the best interests of a patient has become more complex. As a cost of long-term treatment, such as in the case of a man with raised blood pressure, a patient may be required to 'put up' with 'minor' physical side effects, to accept a self-image which includes an ongoing dependency on treatment, and to accept social consequences such as disruptions to social drinking or eating routines. To make matters more problematic in some cases (as in the treatment of high blood pressure) such modifications may be necessary not because of symptoms of which the patient is aware but because of symptoms which he may not get. Hart (1976) has argued how in circumstances such as these consultations must be concerned with a great deal more than diagnosis. A diagnosis, he argued, is only the first stage in a communication process in which a plan of action must be elaborated. He considered that in drawing up the plan patients' social and personal circumstances must be considered realistically and they must be given 'the opportunity to share in decisions that must ultimately become their own' (Hart, 1976: 12). Although a joint approach by doctor and patient may be unfamiliar to some doctors and many patients, Hart argues that 'a successful shift away from dogma and ex-officio authority' is necessary and 'depends on the creation of a new implied contract between care-giver and care-receiver, and an altogether higher level of understanding on both sides to that which we have been accustomed' (Hart 1976: 13).

One group of workers have developed a special approach to motivating their patients based on the experience of working in a clinic in which patients often did not follow the advice they were given (Lazare, Eisenthal, and Wasseman 1975). The essence of their idea is similar to that of Hart's: physicians should pay attention to the patient's wishes. However, these authors have actually experimented with an approach in which the requests patients have for a particular treatment approach and the goals towards which they are striving are carefully ascertained by the physician. Lazare and his colleagues have found that knowing a patient's ideas helps the doctor to make a diagnosis. But it also opens a discussion through which the physician can consider the relevance of the patient's approach, can produce reasons for and against different approaches, and can facilitate the patient to exercise his or her 'right to evaluate and ultimately accept or reject any treatment proposal' (Lazare, Eisenthal, and Wasserman 1975: 554). The idea is that doubts and theories that a patient may have are better discussed in the consulting room and modifications to the advice agreed, than left to undermine and frustrate everything afterwards. Similar ideas have been advanced by other physicians including Slack (1977) who has stated that he believes much failure to follow treatment-advice may be caused by the implicit assertion that doctors know best and should be in charge. He argues that 'communication between patients and doctors should not be used to persuade patients to do what physicians want them to do; rather it should be used to outline the possible plans of action so that patients can decide clinical matters for themselves' (Slack 1977: 240). Indicating that not every patient may want to assume this role and should not be made to do so he argues that consultations must be re-orientated so that doctors 'recognize the right of patients to make their own medical decisions and help them to do so' (Slack 1977: 240).

Views such as these see the aim of giving information as to facilitate a patient in making difficult choices. If treatment is to be jointly planned or negotiated sharing information is necessary to help the patient exercise his autonomy and follow an agreed plan. The doctor may well have a view about what he would do himself and may try to influence the patient accordingly but the ethos with which he would approach giving his views would be of a different order to that implicit if persuasion was the aim. The doctor would be trying to help the patient to clarify his values and to indicate which choices might be appropriate to them. As an analogy one might think of the way information is given in a consumer magazine as opposed to the way it would be given by the manufacturer. Certainly, information given to help patients to make their own decisions demands a particular context for the consultation. The doctor will want to spend time to discover and agree with the patient the purpose of the consultation, the problem for which he seeks help, the patient's ideas about it, and the implications of different solutions for the patient's life. To achieve this the doctor will have to seek the patient's views as well as to make his own (technical) judgements about the options. Sharing information becomes a process in which both a doctor's and a patient's ideas are relevant.

Mahler (1975) and Kickbusch (1981) have applied this line of argument to the health care system as a whole. They were concerned with the fact that all health care systems face a resource crisis in which the escalating costs of care are forcing a consideration of priorities. Mahler suggests that in selecting on what to concentrate it is essential that policy makers accept that the final decisions be made by society at large and not only by concerned and interested professionals. To achieve this end he advocates a drive for a larger population participation and an informed public debate in which everyone can join. Arguing along similar lines, Kickbusch emphasizes the importance of recognizing the existence of lay competence to judge priorities at both individual and social levels.

So far we have turned to medical writers in order to explore some of the reasons they have advanced for making an exchange of ideas a high priority at the heart of the consultation. A fourth line of argument, however, derives from the view of the consultation that emerges in the writing of social scientists. Several social scientists have based their ideas on the fact that for a consultation to occur at all patients must decide to seek a doctor's advice. Moreover, there is evidence that individuals will usually have experienced their symptoms for some time before seeking help and do not, on average, seek help for many of the symptoms they experience. Attention has been drawn, therefore, to the ways in which people cope and to the knowledge that they must draw on to do so. How individuals as members of social groups routinely attempt to make sense of and experience their symptoms has been described by many authors (for example, Freidson 1961; Zola 1973; Dingwall 1976; Mckinlay 1973; Robinson 1971; Stimson and Webb 1975). Individuals attempt remedies of different kinds. They consult friends, relatives, workmates, chemists, and clergymen and live within a 'lay-referral' system. There are many sources to help in giving meaning to experience. They can listen to radio, watch television (not necessarily 'medical' programmes), read books and magazines, and examine what is written on old medicine bottles. They can also learn by swapping stories about doctors on the bus, in the launderette, picking up their children from school, or even in the doctor's waiting-room. In all these ways they learn the meaning of symptoms and develop ideas about, for example, what to put or not to put in their tea (and other remedies) and how to get advice and from whom. They also learn about what help may be required, try out proprietary medicines or old prescriptions, and think of their troubles by identifying them with those of others who seem to have what they see as the same symptoms. They gain knowledge about how to present themselves to a doctor, what to say and not say, etc.

After the consultation what has been said in it is likely to be remembered, inter-preted and evaluated within the context of the same round of discussions, influences and ideas. In short, according to this view, the consultation is one event, usually a rather short one, within an ongoing process of making sense, evaluating and acting on symptoms. This intellectual activity, it can be argued, is probably essen-tial to the survival of many modern medical systems. It provides the filter through which people come to care and through which they attune themselves to the doc-tor's concerns and ideas. Its low cost as a source of health care advice is now recognized by national governments as evidenced by their current preoccupation with 'self-care'. For the present discussion, however, the important point about the existence of a lay framework of health beliefs is that it indicates that it is very simplistic to conceive of consultations as meetings between one person who has ideas and another who does not. The patient entering the consultation brings his own social world with him in the shape of beliefs and ideas. The doctor, also, has his ideas and theories. A consultation, therefore, can be considered as a meeting between systems of belief and ideas. From this point of view several authors have argued that a priority activity for consultations is the task of allowing an exchange or sharing of these systems of belief (Tuckett 1976: 20; Kleinman, Eisenberg, and Good 1978; Tuckett 1978; Katon and Kleinman 1981; Good and Good 1981). With-out such a process there can be no certainty that the consultation can be 'suc-cessful' and a great risk of talking and acting at cross-purposes.

Finally, a fifth set of arguments has its origins in contemporary society, specifically in what may be termed consumer or patient movements. The past decade has seen an explosion of lay interest in detailed medical arguments. Books such as *Our Bodies Our Selves* (Phillips and Rakusen 1978), originally published in the US by a femin-ist group in Boston, have informed women in particular about many detailed aspects of medical theory, therapy and policy. Such books which have achieved wide cir-culation, are more searching and questioning than the traditional encyclopedias of health and medicine, and are not deferential. They have often been written by or with the help of physicians and have an explicit policy of trying to increase the patient's authority in the consultation. Specialties such as obstetric care have, perhaps, been most affected: demands being made to take account of patients' inten-tions to control their own bodies and the decisions that affect them. More generally, consumer and patient rights groups have grown in membership and influence. They have tended to voice the need for more information, more discussion and more patient influence in consultations (Haug and Lavin 1979). Such developments have probably been uneven between countries, social classes, genders, and regions. Some argue that influences of this kind are small and affect only a minority of people. None the less, where they occur they are a source of pressure to make sharing information a central part of the medical consultation.

Sharing ideas in general practice consultations

To summarize the various arguments which have been reviewed, there appear to be a number of reasons for believing that attempts to originate a process of sharing ideas in a medical consultation might be advantageous – at least in many of them. At the same time there are also powerful arguments about the likely difficulties and about the limited extent to which giving information takes place.

To try to explore the issues that have been raised and particularly to examine the extent to which ideas are shared in medical consultations it seems necessary to have available some evidence about several issues: what ideas are mentioned by the doctor to the patient and vice versa; how far these ideas are mutually explored and elaborated; and how far patients subsequently share an understanding with their doctors. However, empirical studies which provide evidence about the success or otherwise of efforts to share ideas in medical consultations are notably absent. As we shall discuss in more detail in the next chapter, research on consultations and their outcomes has been almost exclusively preoccupied with matters of style: it has been about how patients and doctors 'related' to each other as opposed to what they said. In so far as the latter has been investigated it has been by means of small case studies, employing no formal measurement or statistical analysis, or by larger 'quantitative' studies. The latter have usually limited themselves to counting units of information (summing ideas almost indiscriminately) without conceiving explicitly what informing a doctor (if one is a patient) or a patient (if one is a doctor) might be about. Most studies of the cognitive outcome of consultations have been conducted in a similar fashion and have been limited to counting the number of statements a patient can remember. Because of this emphasis in past research there is little secure knowledge about the extent to which ideas are shared in consultations or the process through which problems may arise. There is, therefore, little evidence about how far the competence gap is bridged or how far emotional and social conflicts prohibit sharing ideas in day-to-day medical practice.

During the course of this book each of the aspects of trying to share ideas in consultations will be addressed by describing the observations made about them in a series of over one thousand UK general practice consultations. These observations have led to some suggestions for both doctors and patients which have been used in an educational programme with them. In the course of describing this programme and its effects some of the reasons why doctors and patients behaved in the way they did when observed should become clearer.

For a number of reasons, although the conclusions ought to be applicable to many other medical consultations, it has been general practice consultations (the principal component of primary care in the UK) which have been chosen for study. First, within most official health care systems general practice consultations (or equivalent meetings with internists, pediatricians or gynaecologists in countries such as the USA) are by far the most numerous – most of the half million or more consultations taking place in the UK every working day are of this type. For most patients the general practice consultation is their main and perhaps only experience of a medical consultation. They think of their GP as *the doctor.* Second, general practice consultations are the ones in which it is argued by the doctors themselves that communication is often central. Ideas must be exchanged with the patient before the doctor can identify the appropriate problem with which to help (Horder *et al.* 1972; Browne and Freeling 1976). Beyond this it has been argued by the Royal College of General Practitioners that a main reason for a patient's visit to a general practitioner is often to obtain information: 'to *learn* the significance of his symptoms or the advisability of a course of action' (Royal College of General Practitioners 1976). Finally, the importance of the primary care consultation in the minds of health care planners, after a period of possible decline, is being greatly emphasized. In the UK the general practice consultation is the pivot around which the health service functions. Patients almost always see their GP before gaining access to other forms of care. In other countries it may be a pediatrician, family practitioner, internist or gynaecologist who plays the general practitioner's role. It is none the less this role as personal doctor, gate-keeper, informer and stimulus to 'lay competence' and 'self-reliance' that many governments see as the crucial one for containing medical costs and providing health care for the year 2000 (World Health Organisation 1978; Commission of the European Communities 1980; Mahler 1981).

Summary

The aim of this book is to explore the extent to which ideas can be shared in medical consultations. It has been argued that sharing ideas between a doctor and a patient is difficult because of their differences in technical competence and the special emotional and social dimensions of medical practice. However, the extent to which these factors are prohibitive is likely to depend on the prevalence of emotional and social conflicts as central features of ordinary medical consultations and on the efforts that are made to overcome the difficulties caused by them. Among the arguments that have been made for making such efforts a priority activity are those that say that giving information is often the only available help in a consultation, that patients need information to follow advice, that information is needed to assist a patient to make difficult choices, that patients already act as experts in their own self-care and have to be considered as individuals who interpret and make sense of what happens to them, and that there is a demand for more information from patients influenced by the consumer movement in health care. To explore the process of sharing information in contemporary medical consultations a study of more than one thousand primary care consultations was planned.

CHAPTER 2

A study of general practice consultations and their outcomes

The study we conducted examined those aspects of communication between doctors and their patients to which we have just drawn attention: what ideas are mentioned by the doctor to the patient and vice versa; how far these ideas are mutually explored and elaborated; and how far patients successfully share their doctor's understanding. For this purpose a series of consultations taking place in the UK during normal surgery hours was observed and a sample of the patients in them were subsequently interviewed in their homes. Altogether 108 surgery sessions comprising 1,470 consultations were tape-recorded and analysed (1). Of those individuals taking part in the consultations 328 were interviewed in their homes within a few days after the consultation. In future we shall refer to the research interview as 'the interview' and to the tape-recorded consultation as 'the consultation'. Data from the interview (also tape-recorded) and the corresponding consultation made it possible to examine the consultation process and its outcomes and it is this that we have mainly relied upon to draw conclusions.

Theory and method in consultation research

One feature of writing about medical consultations and their outcomes is that there is a gap between the concerns of those who have explored and developed ideas about the processes in consultations ('developmental research') and those who have conducted what will be called 'quantitative' studies (2) designed to examine the effects of consultation processes on outcomes in a precise way.

'Developmental' research has been thoroughly preoccupied with the content of the ideas doctors and patients exchange with one another (3). It has considered intensively such matters as the negotiation that goes on between doctors and patients, their attempts to control one other, the conflicts in their perceptions of each other's roles, the place of belief and linguistic systems in creating communication problems and the careful attempts of patients to make sense of their symptoms and experiences before and after consultations. Originating largely from the work of social scientists, such studies have usually involved an investigator observing a number of consultations and, perhaps, talking to patients or doctors about them before or after. Typically, the observations stimulate theories which are closely 'fitted'

(Bulmer 1979) to the data by means of extracts from consultation or interview data chosen to illustrate ideas. Because of the close and flexible relationship between theory and data in this kind of work it has been particularly useful as a way of introducing new perspectives. The studies have mainly been conducted with a view to developing and refining concepts and theories rather than to seek to support or quantify their applicability. Consequently, observations have not been attempted in a way that is easy to repeat nor in a manner amenable to statistical analysis. It is, therefore, inevitable that there is sometimes doubt about the frequency or typicality of observed behaviour. This has led some observers to cast doubts on the validity of conclusions generalized from such studies. For example Sharrock (1979) and Hughes (1982) have queried how far earlier case study approaches to the struggle for control in consultations are supported by their data or generalizable to other situations.

Studies using quantitative methods, which might make it possible to overcome some of these difficulties by allowing a statistical analysis of the frequency of hypothesized consultation processes and their relation to outcomes, however, have been problematic in a different way (Tuckett and Williams 1984). Essentially they have focused on quite different issues. Rather than being concerned with the content of the ideas doctors and patients exchange with each other, they have focused, almost exclusively, on various aspects of the style of the relationship between doctors and patients. They have examined, for example, whether participants were friendly, attentive, understanding, amusing, antagonistic, instructive, controlling, expressive, encouraging, relaxed, responsive, prescriptive, acquiescent, precise and organized in their statements, and have tried to relate these to aspects of outcome. These studies have informed us that doctors talk more towards the end of consultations, ask more questions, and show less tension than do patients (Freemon *et al.* 1971). They also rarely ask patients for suggestions (Freemon *et al.* 1971). Research has also indicated that doctors who behave as if they like their patients (Larsen and Smith 1981), those who allow them to tell their story in their own words (Stiles *et al.* 1979), and those who give more objective information about their problems (Stiles *et al.* 1979) achieve more satisfied patients. It has also been claimed that when doctors structure and package their advice in an organized and clear manner patients are able to remember more of what they were told (Ley *et al.* 1973, 1976).

The contrasting emphases and methods of research approaches have had different effects on medical educators. Judging by the frequency of citations to it quantitative research such as that of Ley and his colleagues has been influential. Medical educators have understood it to justify making a series of recommendations to doctors about the style they should adopt in consultations. It is suggested they should be friendly and caring towards their patients, look interested, and be clear and precise when giving information (for example, Walton *et al.* 1980). By contrast, the findings of developmental research, emphasizing the interpretive and negotiating features of the way patients behave in consultations, appears to have been less noticed. The conclusions for practice that might be based on it, for example that doctors should pay careful attention to the detail of what patients say and treat as problematic their reasons for coming for help, have been cited by very few.

On those occasions when the content of the ideas exchanged in consultations has been examined in quantitative studies it has frequently been in a fixed and restricted way. How many statements of information a doctor makes have been counted and the number of statements a patient can remember has been summed. The time for which a doctor spoke has been recorded and even the number of words he has used have been summated – all to provide some indication of how much information a patient has been given. What ideas have been communicated by doctors and patients or how they have been understood, however, have received almost no attention (4).

In the few instances where the information doctors have given to patients has been considered in quantitative research *ad hoc* or common sense definitions appear to have been used to identify it. Investigators have not recognized that before a statement can be counted as more or less informative the various purposes for informing patients have to be considered. For example, several purposes for giving information were identified in the previous chapter. How informative a doctor has been may depend on which purpose for giving information one has in mind. Without a clear idea of what the purpose of giving information might be, it is hard, not only to know how informative a doctor has been, but also to know how to evaluate the conclusions of research studies. For example, if we are unsure of the significance or value of the information they have received, how do we know what patients gain by remembering more information statements than others or by being given more information than is given to members of other social classes? Similarly, what does it mean when investigators inform us that patients have forgotten a half, a quarter or a tenth of the statements the doctors made?

One reason why it may have been difficult for research workers to use less *ad hoc* and so more conceptualized definitions of 'information' or 'understanding' is because little detailed attention has been paid to the clinical value of giving information, if indeed giving information is a value at all. Although some doctors (like those mentioned in the last chapter) have advocated particular topics as important very few seem to have given much systematic consideration to the objectives of giving information to patients. Certainly, there is little consensus in the medical literature about what to tell patients or why one should do so. Nor has there been much discussion of the level of patient understanding at which one should aim (5). For some doctors even the vague idea that giving information ought to be part of consultations and a 'good thing' is controversial. In many postgraduate discussions the focus is likely to be on the ethics of the 'white lie': leading to a debate about what *not* to tell rather than vice versa.

Recourse to clinical textbooks also provides little guidance for either the aspiring doctor or research worker. One finds no significant mention of what, when or why to inform patients in the current editions of *Hutchinson's Clinical Methods* (Mason and Swash 1980), *Davidson's Principles and Practice of Medicine* (MacLeod 1977) or the *Cecil and Loeb Textbook of Medicine* (Beeson and McDermott 1975): three of the most widely used British and American medical school textbooks. Postgraduate texts otherwise greatly concerned with communication in medicine were no greater help. For example, the issues of what and how to explain were not the subject of a specific section in the widely used general practice training document *The Future General Practitioner* (Horder *et al.* 1972). Indeed, in that document a doctor's ability to give information or to explain is not mentioned as one of the eleven broad goals for a trainee general practitioner nor does it feature as one of the eight steps of the consultation. Trainees are, however, advised to convey their intentions, plans and the likely outcomes to the patient 'in a kind of mirror-image of history-taking' (Horder *et al.* 1972: 17). Reviewing the literature in earlier decades, Ernstene (1957) and Fletcher (1973) reached similar conclusions. Strikingly Fletcher also reported he could find no significant mention of communication and information-giving in the report of the Royal Commission on Medical Education (Royal Commission on Medical Education 1968).

Given the absence of criteria on which to determine what is medical information a similar situation confronts both research workers and physicians. The physician cannot begin to evaluate whether he or his colleagues have given information appropriately and the research worker cannot evaluate whether information has been shared unless some criteria are invented: implicitly if an *ad hoc* approach is used, explicitly if concepts are developed. The implicit assumption in much of the work so far mentioned has been the empiricist one that all talk in consultations is equivalent in importance. However, this empiricist assumption that differences in the lengths of time for which someone speaks, or in the number of words or statements he uses, indicate whether a doctor is being more or less informative (or the similar assumption that communication is more successful if patients remember or understand more points) leads to serious problems when one has to try to interpret the conclusions achieved with these methods. For example, when a patient is found to forget a proportion of the information given, how do we know that what is forgotten is of importance? Daily experience tells us that a person may forget a great deal and still feel he has retained the main points of what 'really' mattered. Empiricist methodology provides no guidance for considering these implications. Again, when an investigator links the proportion of information retained by a patient to his subsequent understanding or behaviour, empiricist methods (even assuming the jargon and clarity of what doctors say is considered) make it impossible to know whether a patient is ignorant of information because he failed to appreciate it or because the doctor failed to give it. Without attending to content it is impossible to assess a patient's understanding or evaluation of what he has been informed, except in the most general way. Yet, as Svarstad (1974) has demonstrated in the specific case of instructing patients how to take medicines, only by looking at the content of what doctors say can one exclude the possibility that in many cases patient ignorance of drug regimens may be caused by the fact that the relevant information was never given.

To summarize this brief review of consultation research, those developing theories about communication in consultations have rarely tested their ideas quantitatively. Those attempting quantitative studies, on the other hand, have produced questionable results and have not used (or perhaps have not been aware of) the ideas generated in case studies and other developmental research. Hence, there is little secure evidence about the value of trying to share ideas in consultations or what one might expect patients to be able to understand. There is also no secure knowledge about the impact on consultation processes and outcomes if patients present their ideas or try to negotiate these with doctors.

If a more substantial and balanced picture of the process of giving information to patients is to be attempted, one way of achieving it might be to bring together some of the features of past research in both the developmental and quantitative traditions. To draw more precise conclusions about the potential consequences of efforts by doctors and patients to achieve some degree of shared understanding by a process of mutually exploring each other's ideas the obvious requirement is that readers be satisfied about the way the different phenomena to be observed are defined and be informed about the relative frequencies of different types of behaviour and its outcome. To state that patients do not usually understand the information their doctors give them and to draw inferences about it, one needs to have working definitions of the concepts of 'understanding' and 'information' which are clear and so open to misinterpretation to the smallest possible extent. One also needs to know how to recognize, when interviewing patients or observing consultations, when a patient is 'understanding' or being given 'information' in the previously defined sense. Moreover, unless all understanding or information is assumed equivalent, as in the approaches we have reviewed, one also needs to have some way of distinguishing when more or less of each is present.

A rating scale approach

The study was designed in the context of the difficulties in interpreting the results of previous consultation research. The first task, therefore, was to try to find measures of different aspects of the likely processes involved in sharing understanding. This was attempted by trying to ensure a close relationship between theoretical ideas and the events which could be observed in the consultation. A second task was to ensure that any examples used to illustrate judgements and results would be representative of the consultations studied.

To systematize and quantify observations so that a statistical analysis would be possible, a series of conceptually defined and reliable rating scales were developed according to the general principles described by Brown and Rutter (1966). Starting with ideas derived from the literature and pilot observations, concepts relevant to likely processes of sharing ideas in consultations were generated. These concepts were then gradually refined in the course of making rating judgements about different aspects of consultations or their outcomes.

Rating scales have the advantage that they make explicit the frame of reference and rules of inference for categorizing and hence quantifying observations. The scales were used to observe how much information patients were given or how far they could understand what they were told, etc. To do this it was necessary to know exactly what would be meant by giving information or achieving a correct understanding and to define this in such a way as to create categories that could distinguish worthwhile differences. For example, whether patients were provided with information about a doctor's reasoning was assessed by a four-point scale distinguishing if it was 'elaborate', 'moderately elaborate', 'minimal', or not present at all. To be applied reliably (that is for two or more independent observers to arrive at the same judgement) it was essential that each scale, or certainly each scale component, examined one thing at a time. For instance, it is much easier for two people to agree whether or not a doctor has given an 'elaborate' amount of reasoning if it has previously been agreed what topic the doctor was explaining and also that there were different types of supporting arguments which would be considered separately.

To develop each rating scale it was first defined in principle so that a frame of reference could be created. A series of 'worked' scale point examples were then used to make detailed judgements. Such scale point examples (using case material) laid down criteria about what should be examined in what order, the steps of inference that should be followed, and the decisions to be taken if a rater felt an example was at the margin. The different scales and some details of the process will be described in some of the succeeding chapters and in the accompanying notes. The development of each rating scale involved a process of clarifying each rater's understanding of the theoretical frame of reference and their relationship to individual observations (6). Raters had to have a similar understanding of concepts and criteria to achieve their task reliably. Inevitably, they also often had somewhat different perspectives during developmental work. The concepts that emerged from the development of agreed rating scales, therefore, were probably much more specific to theoretical concerns and precisely fitted to observations than those at the start of work.

The reliability with which raters could agree on observations, using the scales, was tested on a random sample of cases (concurrently with the process of rating) by arranging for two investigators to make each rating without reference to each other (7). The results achieved by the two raters were then compared and are reported in detail in the notes to relevant chapters. In general, they provided satisfactory evidence that independent observers, trained to use the scales, can agree their observations.

The use of rating scales has the advantage that every consultation was analysed and summarized, from the various points of view, in a standardized way. This fact has then been used to try to overcome the more obvious problems of 'selecting' examples that has been a limitation of developmental research. By randomly selecting consultations classified by rating scales as equivalent, case examples can be used which are statistically representative of the sample. Throughout the text of this book, therefore, when it has been necessary to illustrate rating scales, arguments or conclusions with case material, the consultations (or patients) used for this purpose have normally been selected at random (8). Choosing examples at random rather than to aid exposition will mean that some examples are neither as clear nor as convincing as would be possible.

Methods of interview

If conceptual difficulties have been one important source of confusion in consultation research, other more operational problems have also been apparent. The two main sources of data in any study of consultation processes and their outcomes are the consultation itself and the account given by patients about it afterward. By tape-recording the entire consultation, we were able to ensure that all audible events, at least, were available for analysis (9). Obtaining a complete record of the patients' accounts, however, was more complicated. A technique had to be employed to discover what patients could report.

The commonest methods used to discover what patients remember and understand following their consultations, have been mailed questionnaires (for instance, Ley *et al.* 1976) or highly structured 'schedule' interviews (for instance, Ley *et al.* 1973). The essence of both is that they restrict the questions that can be asked and the answers that can be given. In this way the methods are highly economical: staff are easily trained to use them and are given little opportunity to introduce their own prejudices. The debatable aspect of the questionnaire or the schedule is validity. On the one hand, the schedule approach can be considered highly standardized: those administering questionnaires or interviews and those coding replies are tightly restricted as to what they can ask. In this way, it may be argued, each respondent is given the same chance to provide the same information and replies are, therefore, comparable. On the other hand, given that the research situation is one which respondents experience subjectively, a schedule or questionnaire approach can be standardized only in a superficial way. If research workers do not take steps to indicate and explore the meaning of questions or to clarify with respondents their answers, it is respondents who are left to interpret and supply meaning idiosyncratically or in culturally patterned ways (Strauss and Schatzman 1960; Cicourel 1964; Richardson, Dohrenwend, and Klein 1965; Brown and Rutter 1966). If personally or culturally variable matters are the subject of inquiry, difficulties of interpretation are most likely. To study the outcome of medical consultations, therefore, and to collect data about a patient's memory, understanding and evaluation of what took place (a circumstance in which data is personally and culturally variable) it may not be suitable to adopt a schedule, questionnaire or other highly structured approach.

Ley *at al.* (1973) used the schedule interview technique of 'free recall' to determine the proportion of statements made by doctors which patients could remember. Patients were asked 'What did the doctor say to you about the reasons for seeing him?' after which interviewers were not permitted to probe in any detail (10). The investigation found that half the statements made by the doctor were not recalled. But did patients forget what the doctor said or, alternatively did they misunderstand that investigators wanted to know about all the statements doctors had made, on any topic? The question may have prompted patients to think the investigator was literally interested only in those statements made about the patient's reasons for coming – bearing in mind that the investigators who conducted this research have also frequently reported that patients remember more 'diagnostic' than 'treatment' information (Ley 1979).

An alternative method for establishing patients' accounts of what they were told was used by Joyce *et al.* (1969). These authors explored patient recall by asking two interviewers to ask questions in their own way. Interestingly, they reported that one interviewer consistently found patients to recall 75 per cent more than the other investigator. More than anything else this finding impressed on us the need to adopt an interview method which would permit careful attention to be paid to the way patients understand the questions they are being asked.

Consideration of work such as that reported by Ley and Joyce indicated the potential drawbacks both of scheduled and unstructured approaches – particularly as it seemed the difficulties would multiply when research was concerned more with a patient's understanding and evaluation of what he was told and less with simple recall. We decided, therefore, to develop a standardized non-schedule interview (Richardson, Dohrenwend, and Klein 1965; Brown and Rutter 1966; Brown and Harris 1978). The approach, to be described in detail in Part 4, provides the flexibility to probe a patient's meaning systematically and to ensure questions and answers are mutually understood. Rating scales were used to standardize the information obtained, to guide the interviewer in his questioning, and to determine the reliability of judgements.

Generalizing observations

Another set of problems in consultation research are those connected with 'external validity' – how far conclusions based on observing a sample of consultations can be generalized. Two important matters in this respect are the problems that can be caused by the way a sample is selected and those that are created by 'obtrusive effects'. The sampling method that is adopted to select consultations for study is one influence determining how representative conclusions are likely to be. The steps taken to guard against the obtrusiveness of the investigation (and those taken to estimate the effect) are another factor determining the external validity of conclusions. If observation 'changes' important aspects of what is being observed the status of observations for drawing wider conclusions is uncertain.

As we have already indicated, the context of consultation research suggested to us that the first priority of our study should be to develop internally valid and, therefore, easily interpretable measures. Less resources, therefore, were devoted to considering how far observations were likely to be generalizable, whether due to sampling error or to the consequences of being obtrusive. None the less, attention was paid to methods of sampling and to the effects of observing consultations.

The sample of doctors

In many previous studies of consultations the doctors involved usually worked in or near the university in which research was being conducted or had personal contact with the research workers. The studies were mainly exploratory and a series of consecutive consultations was usually recorded and studied without much selection (11).

Before selecting doctors for the present investigation the results of pilot work analysing the consultations of twenty-five doctors, chosen in a similar manner to that in most earlier studies, were considered. Using preliminary measures a minority of doctors were found to give elaborate explanations to patients and an even smaller number were considered to explore patients' ideas and models of explanation. Such findings on a representative sample might have made it possible to generalize about how little explanation or interest in patients' ideas could be noticed and might have called attention to this lack. However, a sample of that kind would have minimized the opportunity to distinguish consultations in which there were elaborate explanations or thorough attempts to explore patients' ideas and inhibited research efforts to explore the consequences of these activities. It was decided, therefore, that one aim when selecting a sample would be to try to maximize the chance of finding doctors who gave elaborate explanations or explored patients' ideas. At the same time there was a need to retain a representative sample as far as possible. The compromise was to ask two groups of doctors to participate: a Study group of doctors reputed to be interested in communication and patient education who might therefore be the most likely to adopt the relevant behaviours; and a Comparison group who might provide some indication of the behaviour fairly typical of UK general practitioners.

Given available resources we estimated it would be possible to study the consultations of sixteen doctors altogether (12): of whom eight would be in the Study group and eight in the Comparison group. To reduce the investigators' travelling time, selection was restricted to doctors working within a 100-mile radius of London.

The study group of eight doctors was selected by choosing doctors with formal responsibility for teaching about consultation skills. To qualify for these responsibilities they would have, in some way, to have developed a reputation for being 'good communicators'. They were all doctors who had attended a lengthy and prestigious (if controversial) course which emphasized consultation skills. They were senior general practitioners with university undergraduate or postgraduate teaching appointments. Several had contributed to policy decisions on medical education or preventive health care. Some had published and conducted research. From a social and geographical perspective they worked in varied settings: three of the doctors worked in inner-city practices, one in an outer-city residential district, one in a rural village in a commuter area, one in a provincial town in a rural area, and two in commuter suburbs fifteen to twenty miles from the City of London. They included two women. All eight doctors whom we approached agreed to take part in the study.

The eight doctors in the Comparison group were chosen at random, one for each member of the Study group, from the names of doctors working in geographically adjoining practices, excluding those reputed to work very short hours, to have a small list of patients, or to be in ill health. The Comparison group of doctors, like those in the Study group, all worked in the National Health Service. Six of the eight doctors whom we first approached agreed to participate. The other two were substitutes for the two that refused (13). One of the doctors was a woman. The doctors in both groups were ethnically white.

The characteristics of doctors in the Comparison group differed, on average and as intended, from those in the Study group (*Table 2.1*). They did not have university or vocational trainer appointments to the extent of those in the Study group, although one was a postgraduate 'trainer' and one had applied for such a position. The exact ages of doctors was not determined but the Comparison group doctors were drawn from a wider range of age-groups than those in the Study group: they included among their number a doctor in his late sixties in semi-retirement and a newly qualified member of the Royal College of General Practitioners in his early thirties. However, doctors in the Comparison group also differed, on average, from doctors nationally (*Table 2.1*). More of the doctors in the Comparison group were members of the Royal College of General Practitioners than general practitioners nationally. Because Comparison group doctors were more qualified in this way than general practitioners as a whole (perhaps an indicator of how progressive a general practitioner may be) it might be argued that they were more willing to explain to patients and to explore their views than general practitioners nationally. We shall return to such questions of generalization in the final chapter.

Sampling consultations for detailed study
Each of the sixteen doctors was asked to designate two calendar weeks during which about six full surgeries were tape-recorded. Further surgeries were tentatively arranged within these weeks in case of problems (14). Patients were warned on

Table 2.1 *A comparison between some characteristics of doctors in the study and comparison groups with general practitioners nationally*

	study group (%)		comparison group (%)		national figures[1] (%)
*sex**					
female	2	(25)	1	(13)	15
male	6	(75)	7	(87)	85
country of qualification+					
GB/	7	(88)	8	(100)	80
Eire/ NI	0		0		8
Asia/	0		0		8
other	1	(13)	0		3
qualification+					
licentiate	0		3	(38)	22
degree	8	(100)	5	(62)	78
trainer+	8	(100)	1	(13)	7
*number of partners**					
0	0		1	(13)	17
1	1	(13)	0		20
3+	7	(87)	7	(87)	39
MRCGP or FRCGP+					
yes	8	(100)	5	(63)	17

1 National figures are derived from Cartwright and Anderson
   (1981) pages 204 (+) and 206 (*).

arrival at the surgery (either by a notice or by the doctor's receptionist) that a Cambridge University study was being conducted with the eventual purpose of helping the doctor to understand more about his communication skills. They were informed that for this purpose tape-recording of all the doctor's consultations at that surgery was in progress but that they could opt out by asking the doctor to turn off the microphone. In this way, 108 surgeries were recorded containing 1,470 consultations. Of these consultations, 18 were of a patient whose consultation had been recorded on an earlier occasion and in 106 there was a patient who asked the doctor not to make a recording (15). In a further 44 consultations a recording was made but was subsequently recognized to be inaudible. Eventually 1,302 consultations were available for study (97 per cent of those recorded, 90 per cent of all those in the 108 surgeries) (16).

By their nature as part of a system of providing primary care, general practice consultations deal with a varied set of problems and issues. The patients attending any general practice surgery are inevitably at different stages of care. A very small number of patients will be seeing the particular doctor for the first time, a larger but still relatively small proportion will be coming with apparently 'new' problems, a much greater proportion will be coming with a new episode of an 'old' problem, and still more will be visiting to report progress about an ongoing episode. Moreover, some patients will not be presenting problems because they want diagnosis or treatment in the usual sense. For instance, they may be presenting their problem only because they need a certificate to tell their employer they are legitimately absent or to obtain some other kind of certification (for example, in connection with disability). Other patients may be visiting the doctor solely because he controls a particular resource, such as vaccination or contraception.

It was readily apparent in the pilot work that not all consultations were equally suitable for studying those aspects of communication in which we had declared an interest. In some of the consultations little exchange of information occurred. They were over in one or two minutes. In such consultations, and also in some of those of more average length there was little speaking. This was noticeable if patients were coming back to see a doctor about some problem about which he had already made up his mind (17); if the issues were mostly of an administrative nature (18); or if patients presented symptoms of sore throat, spots, and colds and doctors chose to give prescriptions without exploring matters in much detail (19). In such consultations the incidence of patients' presenting ideas or seeking to clarify what doctors said and of doctors providing information or seeking to clarify what patients said, was very low. We cannot say whether the lack of conversation meant that a shared understanding had already been achieved. But the behaviour of both doctors and patients did not indicate there was anything problematic to discuss (20). What was certain, if the aim was to explore the process and effect of spoken words, was that these were not consultations which it would be useful to study.

Bearing these points in mind, the study was designed so that after a brief analysis of every consultation recorded it would be possible to concentrate attention on those consultations in which more was said. This was done by defining consultations which were mainly of an administrative nature, those in which coughs and cold were presented and simply given a prescription, and consultations in which little new was decided, as ones we would not study in detail provided that in the consultations there was no apparent modification in diagnosis, treatment, or the way the doctor thought about the implications of the illness (21,22).

Taking advantage of the technical opportunity provided by using a radio-microphone (allowing investigators to listen to and briefly to analyse consultations unobtrusively as they took place) 619 consultations fulfilling the above criteria (48 per cent of the 1,302 recorded) were selected. Choice was restricted to those consultations involving a single adult or an adult bringing a child (23). The patients (or parents) taking part in the selected consultations were invited to allow an interviewer to call at their home in the next few working days. Of those invited for interview, 214 (34 per cent) either said they could not manage it or subsequently proved unable to do so. The remaining 405 consultations were available for detailed study and provide the main sample from which conclusions are drawn.

To allow some opportunity for a formal comparison between the 405 consultations and all those tape-recorded and so to make possible a check on the influence of the methods of selection for detailed study, a group of 69 consultations, a 5 per cent but otherwise unselected sample of the 1,302 consultations, was also chosen for detailed study (24). Also to explore the further potential influence of the effect of patients being unable to take part in an interview, another 51 consultations (a 25 per cent sample of those in this category) were also analysed.

Despite their relatively restricted selection, patients in the '405 sample' undoubtedly presented a very broad spectrum of problems. Comparing those in the 405 sample with those in the 5 per cent sample it can be seen from *Table 2.2* that they were broadly comparable. The consultations in the 405 sample were sometimes very short (about two minutes) and sometimes very long (over thirty minutes). They included patients seeing the doctor for the first time and patients who had seen the doctor all their lives. They included patients with entirely new problems and those whose problem had been under treatment for a long while. They differed because in all the consultations in the 405 sample something 'new'

Table 2.2 *Some characteristics of patients in the main sample and 5 per cent sample*

	main sample (%)	5 per cent sample (%)
length of consultation		
< 4 minutes	46 (11)	18 (26)
4 to 6 mins	146 (36)	18 (26)
6 to 9 mins	103 (25)	15 (22)
9 to 20 mins	74 (18)	16 (23)
> 20	36 (9)	2 (3)
patient's gender		
female	269 (66)	37 (54)
male	136 (34)	32 (46)
type of consultation		
adult	338 (84)	63 (92)
child	67 (17)	6 (8)

Table 2.2 (*cont.*):

knowledge of doctor

seen before	355 (88)	62 (90)
not seen before	48 (12)	7 (10)

type of visit
new problem, or

change of diagnosis	169 (42)	24 (35)
old problem	236 (58)	45 (65)

significance of
   diagnosis

significant	121 (30)	22 (32)
not significant	248 (61)	35 (51)
not clear	36 (9)	12 (17)

ICCHP diagnosis[1]

infections (I)	49 (12)	10 (15)
neoplasms (II)	7 (2)	1 (1)
endocrine (III)	9 (2)	2 (3)
psychiatric (V)	40 (10)	7 (10)
eye and ear (VI)	32 (8)	2 (3)
cardiovascular (VII)	14 (4)	8 (12)
respiratory (VIII)	46 (11)	7 (10)
digestive (IX)	23 (6)	8 (12)
urinary and menstrual		
(X)	23 (6)	2 (3)
skin (XII)	23 (6)	4 (6)
muscular-skeletal		
(XIII)	43 (11)	3 (4)
ill defined (XVI)	14 (3)	4 (6)
injuries (XVII)	45 (11)	2 (3)
social/normalize	32 (8)	9 (13)
other	5 (1)	0

1 The diagnoses given to patients were coded into the above
   categories by means of the International Classification
   of Health Problems in Primary Care (WONCA 1979).

happened and there was some discussion of it. To give a more detailed idea the brief details of five randomly selected cases from the 405 sample are in *Table 2.3*.

Table 2.3 *Five random cases*

Mr Austin (1048)

A fifty-four year-old railway supervisor attending the doctor to discover the results of a blood test taken in a consultation two weeks ago. He had attended his doctor on that occasion with a very painful foot which he had suspected was gout. The doctor had also thought this and prescribed treatment for that condition, which the patient had never suffered from before. In the tape-recorded consultation the doctor reported that the blood test showed slightly raised uric acid levels indicating gout and explained various aspects of the condition, said to be like arthritis. He then gave the patient some detailed information about using the tablets prescribed, on his own initiative, whenever he gets pain in future. Such tablets could 'nip the problem in the bud'. At the moment the condition was mild and they would only have to consider other treatment if the painful episodes become more frequent. No other measures were discussed and no aspects of the patient's behaviour were mentioned. The consultation lasted just over sixteen minutes.

Mr Bright (1770)

A thirty-two year old personnel manager who visited his doctor following the advice of his works doctor that he see a specialist. He had been having elbow trouble for four months. His doctor had refused to refer him without seeing him and the consultation took place in the context of his doctor asserting his authority. The doctor diagnosed tennis elbow and gave the patient the choice of referral or a cortisone injection on the spot. The patient opted for the latter. He was given it and advised not to play squash for two weeks, then to decide if it was better. If he wanted he could return to report progress and to have another injection. The consultation lasted just under seven minutes.

Mrs Crouch (1796)

A sixty-four year-old married to a retired insurance agent returning to the doctor after a previous visit (three weeks ago) and still complaining of a blocked nose. The doctor explained to her that she appeared to have a deviated septum and (chronic) sinus trouble. He arranged for a referral to an ENT specialist so she could have her nose 'washed out'. The patient's past depressive state was alluded to indirectly by both parties while discussing how depressed her symptoms make her, but there was no discussion or exchange of view on this topic. The consultation lasted just over three minutes.

Mr Dance (2339)

A forty-one year-old Ghanaian accountancy trainee returning to discuss the swelling in his left foot which began when he bought a new pair of shoes. His doctor reported the result of an X-ray suggesting that the problem was tubercular in origin but also mentioned that blood tests had proved inconclusive and puzzling. The question was whether TB was active at present. He referred the patient to a specialist chest hospital for further investigation. All this was mentioned to the patient. The consultation lasted nearly six and a half minutes.

Miss Ellsberg (2374)
A thirty-two year-old bank cashier with a long and severe history of asthma and eczema which had become greatly exacerbated following her quite recent broken engagement. The patient was under numerous hospitals and specialists and taking many types of medication. On this occasion she visited the doctor to complain of a rash on her head which was getting worse–both itchy and painful. Her doctor diagnosed these symptoms as a side effect of her hospital doctors' attempts to reduce her steroids. He tried to clarify her medication and to establish what the different specialists (who do not keep him informed) were doing. The consultation lasted just over seven minutes.

The interview sample
We have mentioned that interviews with selected patients, conducted in their homes shortly after their consultation (25), provided the essential data to determine how they understood and evaluated the information their doctor gave them. In addition, these interviews provided the opportunity to obtain background data about each patient and to discover some of their attitudes and ideas about the consultation process. Unfortunately, although the intention (as mentioned earlier) was to analyse the understanding and evaluation of their consultations achieved by all 405 patients who agreed to be interviewed, this subsequently proved impossible. For a variety of technical reasons only demographic and other background data were available in the case of 77 patients (26). In the chapters that follow, therefore, a sample of the remaining 328 patients only will be used when describing the relationship between consultation processes and patients' understanding and evaluation of what doctors told them (27).

The effects of observation
Given that we considered it was not ethically acceptable to study consultations without the knowledge of doctors and patients (28), it was impossible to study the effect of our observations by utilizing an experimental design to compare consultations that had been observed with those that had not. In these circumstances the best the research worker can do is first, to minimize any potentially damaging obtrusive effects, and second, to find ways of estimating the effect of his presence, albeit that without an experimental design such estimates cannot be conclusive.

To minimize potentially obtrusive effects three steps were taken. First, doctors were studied in normal surgery hours as they saw their usual volume of patients. It was reasoned that to change their behaviour thoroughly and in a consistent way (over the ninety or so consecutive consultations they conducted while recording was carried out) doctors would have required such an incredible capacity for dissembling that it would be inconceivable, even if any saw any point in doing so. Second, and as mentioned, to record consultations in as minimally intrusive way as possible, a radio-microphone and a tape-recorder in another room were used. This meant patients could see no revolving spools or cassettes. Third, the research was introduced to both doctors and patients in a way which it was hoped would allow the research to benefit from such obtrusive effects as there were. Doctors were told some of our ideas about what constituted information and the topics on which we thought they could give information were mentioned. They also knew of the intention to interview patients afterward and to assess their understanding (although they did not know which patients would be selected for interview). In this way if doctors were out to please investigators it was reasoned that this would encourage them to inform and so ensure that more rather than less information was available to study. Patients were informed about the study in the same way as (in many of the practices) they were regularly informed about other intrusions into their consultations – for postgraduate and undergraduate training, visits by overseas doctors, etc.

To estimate the obtrusive effects of these procedures some patients and doctors were asked about their reactions directly (29). The recording of what doctors and patients said to each other in the consultations was also searched for clues about the effects of the study and inquiries were made from the doctor's reception staff about possible variations in such matters as the comparative length of 'normal' and 'recorded' surgeries. In pilot work recording went on in one surgery for several months. This gave the opportunity to see if, as time passed, anything seemed to change. None of these estimates and inquiries have given us cause to be concerned about the validity of the main conclusions to be reported, although by saying this we are not arguing that observations had no effects in other ways (30).

Summary

Past 'quantitative' research on medical consultations has been notable for an absence of theory when deciding on what aspects of the consultation process to observe. Little attention has been paid to studying what ideas are mentioned by doctors or patients and to what extent. 'Developmental' research, on the other hand, has been difficult to interpret because statistical relationships are not available and the representativeness of case examples is unclear. A study of 1,302 consultations conducted by 16 doctors was devised to allow a systematic and quantitative analysis, using a rating scale approach, of the ideas patients and doctors mentioned to each other and the outcome in terms of patients' understanding. From the 1,302 consultations a random sample of 69 and a specially selected sample of 405 were chosen for detailed study. Three hundred and twenty-eight patients taking part in the latter consultations were also interviewed after their consultation was over.

PART 2

The doctor's part

CHAPTER 3

The problem of information

In this chapter and the next we shall mainly be concerned with the efforts doctors made to share information, whether by informing patients about their ideas or by encouraging them to tell them what they thought. However, before it was possible to examine the information doctors shared with their patients (or indeed the topics on which they sought to help their patients to elaborate their ideas), it was first necessary to develop some frame of reference on which to base observations. As an alternative to the methods adopted in the studies mentioned in the last chapter the principle of our approach has been to examine everything a doctor said in a consultation so as to decide if it covered certain key points of particular topics which we will argue are important. For example, one important aim there might be for giving information would be to try to convey to a patient the value of any advice they were offered. By deciding that there were certain key points that needed to be understood if this aim was to be fulfilled how much information a doctor gave could be determined by asking how many of the key points he had covered. A patient told about such key points as how effective the advice was and what is was likely to achieve, for instance, could be considered to have been given 'more' information than one who was told only to take tablets (1).

A method based on the principle just mentioned clarifies what is meant by giving information much more precisely than if statements are counted with only an *ad hoc* definition of what information is. But it also has another advantage. It makes it unnecessary to follow the practice of some studies in which consultations have been divided up into arbitrary statements or time units which are then considered to fulfill only one communicative function at a time. In those studies, for instance, a particular statement could be considered to inform or to instruct or to express affects but not to do more than one of these at once (see for instance, Korsch, Gozzi, and Francis 1968; Roter 1977; Pridham and Hansen 1980). However, in choosing to adopt the principle we have put forward it was necessary first to consider what were the important topics on which a doctor could give information and what were the relevant key points on each topic.

Topics and key points

In the previous chapter we argued that detailed discussions of what to explain to patients (and, therefore, what might be appropriate topics and key points) are very rare in medical literature. Some recent exceptions are the discussions by Fletcher (1973), Kleinman, Eisenberg, and Good (1978) and a working party of the Nuffield Provincial Hospitals Trust (Walton *et al.* 1980). Fletcher and the Nuffield Working Party arrived at very similar conclusions about what a doctor might routinely try to tell patients. Information should concentrate on the investigations to be done, what they involve and what they will show, the diagnosis, the treatment and the likely outcome. Such topics are those which clinicians view as important. However, taking advantage of their experience as social anthropologists and as clinicians Kleinman, Eisenberg, and Good (1978) have argued that lay (or popular) and medical models for explaining illness address similar issues: etiology; the onset of symptoms; pathophysiology; the course of illness (including the type of sick role it implies i.e., acute, chronic, impaired according to perceptions of the severity of a disorder); and treatment.

While systematic discussions of possible topics and key points about which to inform patients are not frequent in the literature it is not unusual to find clinically orientated contributions which mention one thing or another which patients should know. To try to obtain an overview of the information which doctors consider it relevant their patients should know a content analysis was undertaken of two reference handbooks for UK general practitioners: *Practice* (Cormack, Marinker, and Morrell 1976) and *Treatment* (Drury *et al.* 1978). These volumes, updated annually, contain contributions from eminent physicians and general practitioners in Britain and are supposed to indicate the best current practice. In the thousand or so pages of *Practice*, which covered the common conditions of general practice and how they can be recognized, managed and dealt with, there were 53 separate instances in which doctors were advised to give some kind of information about topics as diverse as fluid intake, weight, diet, smoking, medication-taking, coping strategies, posture, clothing, sleeping, help-seeking, bathing, contraception, or baby feeding. In the similar length *Treatment* there were 150 similar references. The majority of these (31 in all) were concerned with advising doctors to 'warn' patients about the dangers of non-compliance or side effects. In both volumes many of the concrete instances in which doctors were advised to give information involved 'correcting' the wrong beliefs patients were anticipated to have. It was stated, for instance, that patients needed to know that 'a raised ESR does not necessarily indicate disease' or that 'tinnitus does not herald a stroke'. Some advice was also directed at discussing the consequences of illness – for example, how to react to an ill child, how to adjust to a new life-style, how to cope with 'inevitable change' in menopause, or how not to blame oneself for getting certain illnesses.

After considering what doctors actually said to patients in the pilot study it was decided that most of the issues mentioned so far could be studied by concentrating on four central topics. These were:

1 the 'diagnostic-significance' of a problem (that is, what caused it, whether it is life-threatening, progressively deteriorating, likely to recur or self-limiting);
2 the appropriate treatment-action to deal with a problem (that is, what treatments or actions are recommended, their value and purpose and how to carry them out);
3 the appropriate preventive measures that may be necessary to forestall or lessen future episodes (that is, what preventive measures are recommended, their value and purpose, how they relate to the original cause of the problem and how to carry them out);
4 the implications or wider social and emotional consequences of problems or their treatment (that is, what social or psychological problems may be experienced and how the patient can be helped to cope).

The diagnostic-significance of a patient's problems seemed particularly relevant in so far as one of the functions of knowing a diagnosis is that it helps to structure a patient's experience of illness and make it more predictable and comprehensible. Knowing the diagnostic-significance of a problem may also be part of giving information when the aim is to persuade a patient to agree with the doctor's advice or to help him make choices. Knowledge of what is wrong and its significance is clearly vital if 'joint-planning' of action is an aim. If on the other hand information is given mainly to persuade patients to follow advice, knowledge of the diagnosis is still important. It can be used to frighten or otherwise to motivate a patient to agree. As health belief theorists have argued, if patients reach 'biomedically inappropriate' conclusions about the severity of their symptoms, this can lead to false conclusions about the significance of what is wrong. A patient might then lapse into unjustified complacency or alternatively he might worry unduly about his state. In consequence he might assess the importance of treatment and prevention incorrectly (Kasl and Cobb 1966; Becker 1974). Whether the aim of giving information is to structure, to persuade or to facilitate choice what matters about the diagnosis given to a patient is the degree of threat it implies and the probability that it is correct. These were key points of information to know about the significance of a diagnosis a doctor may mention.

Treatment- and preventive-action were also clearly important topics. Knowledge of different aspects of treatment contributes to structuring the patient's illness experience, it can be a component in motivating a patient to accept a doctor's advice and is essential data when it is a question of helping patients to make a choice. Providing treatment in western medicine, no less than in traditional healing, can be part of the process by which a patient is given information not only about what he suffers but also about how it came about, what is to blame and what will happen. Telling patients what should be done often involves actions such as investigation, purification or expiation, depending on the social and cultural context. The wrong action from the point of view of the social and cultural framework embraced by the patient could threaten all efforts to structure experience and to reassure.

With regard to giving information for the purpose of persuasion or facilitating choice, health belief theorists have considered it important for patients to understand the purpose of an action (whether it is intended as ameliorative, curative, investigative, or preventive for a given set of symptoms) in order to evaluate it favourably. If, for example, a patient imagines that an action is intended to be curative, when in fact its purpose is investigative or preventive, he may be inclined to doubt its value in his particular case or to expect an outcome which to a doctor is not feasible. Similarly, once the purpose of the action has been understood, in order to evaluate that action favourably it may be necessary to know how effective it is thought to be for achieving the purpose. Mis-attributions of value or effectiveness could be expected to influence a patient's motivation and to lead to over- or under-estimations of treatment and consequently to biomedically ill-informed decisions. Similarly over- or under-emphasis of side effects or other disadvantages of treatment could influence motivation or lead to ill-informed choice.

The growing interest in prevention and anticipatory care evident in some of the clinical literature already mentioned made it worthwhile to separate as different topics treatment of a present episode and preventive action aimed more into the future. The kind of information relevant to the two topics, although similar, might be somewhat different since the justifications for preventive and treatment action are sometimes divergent. None the less in both cases information about what the action was supposed to achieve and its likely effectiveness in doing so was the key information.

The fourth topic – implications – covered the wider social and emotional consequences of illness and its treatment. They have been particularly emphasized by social scientists as a relevant topic for discussion (for example, Tuckett 1976: 26; Kleinman, Eisenberg and Good 1978; and Helman 1978) but are equally an expressed concern of some physicians (Jackson 1978; Horder *et al.* 1972; Balint 1964). Once the problem on which doctor and patient focus in a consultation has been diagnosed and treatment and preventive suggestions determined, various consequences of the illness or of its treatment and prevention become possible: a patient can have feelings about being diagnosed in a particular way or at being treated by a given method. Or the illness or its treatment may have consequences for the patient's social network, his family, his work and his financial prospects. Some examples are: a life-threatening or disabling illness which may require a subjective as well as external adjustment; a chronic 'nuisance' condition which can have far-reaching complications for social and sexual relationships; a visible handicap which can create difficulties in adjusting to a new self-image and problems in social relationships; conditions requiring changes in eating, smoking or drinking habits which can cause mockery or embarrassment among friends and relatives; illness in a relative which can cause feelings of blame, anxiety or disgust. Failure to deal with such social and psychological implications is likely to frustrate efforts to structure a patient's experience or to place barriers to the aim of persuading a patient to follow advice. Integrating social and psychological components into the treatment plan and, therefore, discussion at some length, would be a key element if the aim of a consultation is to facilitate choice (Hart 1976). It seemed important, therefore, to examine how far doctors gave information relevant to implications in their consultations. The key point would be whether any social or psychological consequences were established as a problem and, if so, what was said about trying to cope.

The four topics mentioned (diagnostic-significance; treatment-action; preventive-action; and implications), therefore, provided a frame of reference for considering what information doctors set out to share with their patients. Given the four topics and the key points within them that a doctor might cover, the question of how much (if any) information was given on each could now be asked.

Stating and reasoning

The three aims of giving information to patients that have been discussed seem to imply two rather different, if related, types or levels of explanation: stating and reasoning. To evaluate a situation or to make a choice about an appropriate treatment, for example, it seems necessary to be informed about 1) what the treatment actually is and 2) the rationale behind it – much the same information as is required to evaluate a matter of policy or, indeed, the adequacy of the methods of this study. The two types of information are relevant to each of the topics: 1) what the doctor's view is and 2) the rationale for it. The aim of the former (stating the view) is to clarify, make plain, or interpret what is said. The aim of the latter (the rationale) is to give reasons to justify and support that statement (2).

Even brief consideration of the kind of information doctors might give their patients indicated that sometimes they would want to provide their patients with reasons. Sometimes doctors would want to give information to anticipate the doubts or questions their patients might have about the view expressed to them on one or more of the topics. If, for instance, a doctor felt that prescribing medication was an option for a patient and if he thought giving information would be important to facilitate that patient's choice (or alternatively to persuade him to a particular view), then the doctor could anticipate the patient's questions about the value of medication by setting out his reasons. The patient could be told about the value of treatment, the risks if it were not taken, the possible disadvantages and the reasons against alternative treatments. A patient to whom a doctor made some of these points about the value of treatment proposals could be considered to have been more informed than one not given such information or given only some of it. Similarly, it was possible to imagine that some of the other things doctors said to patients might provide rationales to support their diagnostic-hypotheses or their views about implications. In the latter case, perhaps, one could anticipate a patient's concerns about the effects on aspects of their social and sexual relationships, for example, and spell out some of the reasons why this might or might not be so and how it could be coped with. In the former case, perhaps, a patient with a newly diagnosed duodenal ulcer could be given information relating to the process of making a diagnosis to explain why a doctor thought this was the cause of recurrent pain. Such 'explanations' might be considered relevant, although the context might be different, according to whether a doctor sought to persuade a patient, to facilitate his choices or to structure his experience of illness.

The need to distinguish reasoning from stating types of information was both theoretical and practical. Providing reasons to a patient, as in the examples just mentioned, is quite different to stating a view – although it seems likely that the former would be most confusing without the latter. Stating refers to giving information about the details of the doctor's view on one of the topics. He tells the patient about the diagnostic-significance and implications of his problem and what treatment and preventive actions he recommends. The doctor might explain that the pain in the patient's stomach is a duodenal ulcer which is a troublesome and recurrent condition but not likely to kill (diagnostic-significance). He might tell a patient that eczema is something which a child and his parents will have to adjust to and advise that the parents might want to talk to the child and other relatives about it so as to anticipate difficulties of being termed 'pox-ridden' at school (implications). He might explain that the patient should adjust smoking habits in order to reduce his chance of bronchitis in the future (prevention).

If stating refers to information setting out a view on the topic, reasoning is concerned with explaining the rationale for it. The diagnosis of duodenal ulcer can be supported by explaining that it can be seen on the X-ray taken before and is consistent with the way the patient has described his symptoms. The advice to give up cigarettes can be supported by an explanation of how smoking can increase the frequency and severity of chest complaints and so increase the likelihood of recurrent bronchitis.

Determining how often doctors stated their view on a topic and how often they gave reasons depended, as in the examples just quoted, on drawing up different criteria – hence the need to assess them separately. But the decision to assess them separately was also arrived at because it was clear that an exploration of how far it was possible to use consultations to facilitate choice required an exploration of the reasons that doctors gave and their effect on patient understanding. The method adopted to determine how detailed were the reasons doctors gave to support their views on each topic will be described in the next chapter.

Hitherto, only Svarstad (1974) appears to have examined the rationales doctors offer in consultations. Her efforts, however, were mainly limited to the reasons provided to support the treatment. She decided to explore this by anticipating in each case what a doctor might say. 'For example, if the patient was diagnosed as having hypertension, a thorough explanation might have included discussions of: a) the fact that one can have the condition without being aware of it or without having any symptoms, b) what 'high blood pressure' actually means and does not mean, and c) the long-term benefits of keeping this chronic condition under control (reduced risk of stroke, heart damage, kidney failure and other complications)' (Svarstad 1974: 247). However, because doctors in the consultations she studied did not provide such reasons Svarstad was unable to investigate whether patients provided with such reasons were more likely to take their medication.

Strategies for giving information

So far we have concentrated on the ideas a doctor might choose to try to share with a patient. The chances that these ideas will be understood will of course depend on the way he attempts to communicate with his patient as well as on the patient himself. Three elements of the strategy he might choose to adopt for communicating can be discerned in medical and social science literature. One element places the emphasis on the clarity of the doctor's spoken words. What is thought to matter is his use of language, the sequential organization of what he says, and his use of emphasis and repetition (Ley *et al.* 1973, 1976; Svarstad 1974). A second element places the emphasis on generating a process of mutually sharing each other's spoken ideas by a process of verbal clarification and exchange. What matters is the extent to which the participants in the communication process understand each other (Flavell *et al.* 1968; Katon and Kleinman 1981; Lazare, Eisenthal, and Wasserman 1975; Good and Good 1981; Tuckett 1978; Byrne and Long 1976; Pridham and Hansen 1980; Stiles *et al.* 1979). The third strategy is concerned not with the use of the spoken word to convey ideas but with the use of all body communication systems to generate feelings of mutual understanding and warmth. The emphasis is on non-verbal communication and on the ways the doctor and his advice can appear positive, persuasive, authoritative, helpful, sympathetic and trustworthy (Davis 1968; Korsch, Gozzi, and Francis 1968; Larsen and Smith 1981; Svarstad 1974; Hall, Roter, and Rand 1981). By generating positive feelings of this kind in the communication process what the doctor says is likely to receive a receptive and attentive audience. Until recently research studies focusing on this strategy have been very general and rather difficult to interpret (Svarstad 1974; Tuckett and Williams 1984). However, two recent studies have adopted much more precise and exhaustive efforts to explore the non-verbal elements in doctor-patient communication. Larsen and Smith (1981) examined the postural aspects of non-verbal communication which help to interpret the significance of the physical and postural reactions between doctors and patients that can routinely be observed in a consultation. Hall, Roter, and Rand (1981) examined electronically filtered speech to explore when doctors and patients were angry, anxious, doubtful, etc. Both techniques mean that non-verbal communication can (in principle) be studied separately from verbal content. The postural method requires a video-recording. The filtered speech approach involves removing certain sound frequencies from a tape-recording so that while words are indistinguishable expressive features of speech such as intonation, contour, speed, and rhythm are available to indicate affects (Rogers, Scherer, and Rosenthal 1971).

The present study had as its main aim the study of the ideas which doctors and patients spoke about to each other. Adequate time to devote to the examination of the non-verbal atmosphere created in consultations by means of postural analysis or filtered speech was not available. Attention was, therefore, paid to the two verbal elements of communication strategy: making ideas clear and seeking to encourage a mutual exchange of views.

Being clear

Communicating ideas with clarity was likely to be an aim of any doctor intending to share information for the purposes of persuasion, facilitating choice or structuring a patient's experience. The work of Ley and his colleagues was designed to help doctors in this regard. Summarizing that work, Ley (1979) considered that patients would comprehend and remember information better if it was presented to them in an organized and coherent way. Drawing on learning theory and a series of experiments he and his team conducted in their psychology laboratory, Ley and his colleagues advocate explicit categorization (for example, I am going to tell you what is wrong with you. . . I am now going to talk about what should be done. . .) to help patients process information, attention to the sequence of giving information, repetition of important points, the use of short words and sentences (not jargon), and giving the most important information at the beginning of the consultation. Ley has argued that the use of such techniques is possible and that when employed by doctors they increase the proportion of statements a patient remembers after his consultation by a substantial amount (Ley *et al.* 1973, 1976).

The drawback of Ley's studies just mentioned is that they were designed as experiments in such a way that the actual behaviour adopted by the experimenters – the doctors – was not observed. Doctors first saw a control group of patients and consulted as usual. Then, after learning about Ley's recommendations for clear communication, saw a second, experimental, group of patients. The experimental group patients remembered more and so Ley's suggestions receive some general support. However, since no direct observation of how doctors behaved was attempted, it is difficult to be sure how doctors changed their behaviour and which aspects of it had been influential. This means that doctors trying to put Ley's techniques into practice or research workers trying to determine when doctors are using them have to guess exactly what behaviour is consistent with that Ley recommends. To try to assess how far the information given by doctors was 'clear' in terms of Ley's criteria we decided to examine everything they said but to explore separately the clarity of the way they stated their ideas or gave reasons and to do so within each topic. The way the doctor stated his view of diagnostic-significance or the way he gave reasons for treatment-action was examined for clarity. This was done by attending to factors like the coherence of the phraseology used by the doctor, whether his statements were grammatical, whether he used explicit categories, the extent of jargon, the pace at which a doctor spoke and how audible he seemed to the patient.

Exchanging views

Sharing information with patients in the context of a mutual exchange of views is a *sine qua non* if the aim of giving information is to facilitate choice. The doctor has to know about the patient's aims and ideas and has to work with the patient towards integrating lay and medical theories so that the patient understands the choices facing him. To help patients make their own decisions the doctor will want to give priority to the task of discovering the patient's views and to agreeing the purpose of the consultation, the problem for which the patient seeks help and the implications of the different solutions for the patient's life. How far an exchange of views is an important part of a doctor's strategy, if information is intended to persuade the patient to follow advice or to structure experience, depends on the theory of communication a doctor has. Two schools of thought emphasize the importance for communication of a two-way exchange of ideas. But they do so in rather different ways.

One school of thought is evident in the ideas of Kleinman, Eisenberg, and Good (1978) and Flavell *et al.* (1968). Flavell and his colleagues studied learning in the school situation. They argued that the central educational task was for teachers and pupils to clarify each other's cognitive maps of understanding and to articulate them one to the other. Similarly Kleinman's idea (Kleinman, Eisenberg, and Good 1978; Katon and Kleinman 1981) is that the central issue in the consultation is the transaction between patient's and doctor's explanations of illness. Eliciting the patient's model of explanation is an essential precursor to providing information so that lay and medical ideas are negotiated and integrated.

The second school of thought tends to see the value of exchanging ideas and responding to one another as an aspect of the style a doctor adopts. Instead of focusing on the ideas as such, authors like Byrne and Long (1976), Stiles *et al.* (1979), and Pridham and Hansen (1980) have concerned themselves with the extent to which doctors listen to what patients say and are influenced by it. For example, Byrne and Long (1976) have distinguished between 'doctor-centered' and 'patient-centered' approaches to consulting. A doctor-centered approach is one where the doctor is mainly concerned with gathering information, analysing and probing. Typically, he seldom listens to his patient, seldom waits for him to speak or think, and seldom clarifies or interprets to him. A patient-centered approach is usually more balanced in this respect: in particular the doctor's questions tend to develop from the patient's ideas and answers and any clarifications eventually come back to them. They are concerned with the responsiveness of a doctor to his patient: does he listen, stay attentive, show interest, come back to what the patient has said, phrase questions in terms of what has gone before, and avoid 'negative' behaviours such as interrupting or changing the subject for no apparent reason. Stiles *et al.* (1979) examined similar issues but from the point of view of various linguistic aspects of the way doctors respond to patients and Pridham and Hansen (1980) have extended Byrne and Long's approach. However, methods like these, particularly those of Stiles *et al.* (1979) are, according to Inui *et al.* (1982), difficult to repeat and perhaps without much predictive power.

To assess the extent to which doctors gave information in the context of trying to encourage a mutual exchange of ideas we decided to pay attention exclusively to the doctor's behaviour in relation to the patient's ideas. We explored in turn: doctors' efforts specifically to encourage patients to volunteer and elaborate their ideas; their response to evidence that a patient had ideas; the extent to which reasoning was directly related to patients' ideas; and the extent to which doctors checked their patient's understanding. The latter behaviour, checking a patient's understanding, might possibly be a relatively simple and rather effective way in which a doctor could inform himself about his patient's thinking and the need or otherwise to improve his own efforts at communication. Instead of giving or withholding information and making assumptions about what their patients understand doctors could actually find out. The efficacy of this approach has been demonstrated by Bertakis (1977). In an experimental study he demonstrated that doctors in an experimental group, who were encouraged to ask patients to repeat in their own words the information they had been given and then make corrections to patients' understanding (as they thought necessary), enabled their patients to remember more than those doctors in a comparison group whose patients were not given the opportunity to repeat what they understood.

Summary

The problem of how to recognize the efforts doctors make to share information has been approached in this study by exploring what they said on each of four topics: diagnostic-significance; treatment-action; preventive-action; and implications. Within each topic attention was paid to whether doctors stated their views and gave reasons for them. Rather than dividing consultations into segments, units of time or statements (as in many previous studies) the amount of information given was determined by examining the whole consultation to ask how far key aspects of the topics were stated and how far reasons for the view the doctor took on each topic supported his view. Finally, the strategies doctors adopted in giving information were assessed by examining how far information was given with clarity and how far it was given in the context of trying to encourage a mutual exchange of ideas with a patient. Indicators of the latter were efforts to discover patients' ideas, the reactions doctors had to them when presented, how far reasoning related to patients' ideas and whether doctors checked patients' specific understanding of what they had been told.

CHAPTER 4

The information shared with patients

We have suggested that one condition for studying the extent to which doctors tried to share information is to establish whether they took a view on each of four topics: diagnostic-significance, treatment-action, preventive-action and implications. How far doctors stated their view or gave reasons for it could then be assessed. In deciding on this approach it was expected that sometimes a doctor might give no indication in a consultation that he had a view on one or more of the topics (presumably because he did not consider the topic relevant at that juncture).

The first task, therefore, was to examine consultations to see if a doctor seemed to take a view about diagnostic-significance, treatment- or preventive-action, or implications. One difficulty here was that conceivably a doctor might take a view on one of the these topics which could be guessed only by drawing inferences from his actions. For example, he might refer a patient to hospital without actually saying anything to indicate what was wrong but in doing so imply a broad diagnosis but not state it. Alternatively, there might be no indication, even by action, to enable a guess as to what diagnosis had been made. For each topic, therefore a judgement was made as to whether a doctor had said something to indicate his view (he had stated it), whether he had done something to enable one to infer that view (view taken but not stated) or whether there was no indication of what his view was at all (1).

The first finding, therefore, concerns the frequency with which doctors appeared to have no view at all on different topics. While they seemed to have a view about treatment-action and diagnostic-significance in all or nearly all consultations, they were much less likely to indicate whether prevention was relevant and very unlikely indeed to indicate what they thought about implications (2). Treatment-action occurred in every consultation, a view about diagnostic-significance was evident in nine out of ten (91 per cent), and a view about preventive-action was implied in a third (31 per cent). Implications appeared to be considered in less than one eighth (12 per cent). The last finding was particularly interesting bearing in mind the emphasis on social and psychological consequences in the various writings referred to earlier. Moreover, in the small proportion of cases where implications were considered by the doctor very little was actually said (3). In fact, the rarity with which the topic was mentioned made it impossible to develop reliable measures of the information given concerning it and it has not been possible to explore it further in any part of the study.

Stating views

From the point of view of trying to state views, if they held them, the doctors set out to share information with patients in nearly every consultation. In well over nine out of ten consultations where he seemed to have taken a view on at least one topic, a doctor explicitly stated it to the patient (*Table 4.1*). In fact, doctors were judged to have stated the key points about diagnostic-significance to their patients on more than four-fifths of the occasions when they took such a view (*Table 4.1*). This means they provided the patient both with information about

Table 4.1 *Stating information in 405 consultations*

	information topics			
	diagnostic-significance (%)	*treatment-action* (%)	*preventive-action* (%)	*at least one of the three* (%)
topic mentioned				
yes	369 (91)	405 (100)	124 (31)	405 (100)
no	36 (9)	-	281 (69)	-
topic stated (if mentioned)				
yes	308 (83)	375 (93)	112 (90)	396 (98)
no	61 (17)	30 (7)	12 (10)	9 (2)

the diagnosis and about the chances that this was what was wrong. Mrs Bruce's consultation (2185) was an example. The doctor said to the patient's mother: 'It isn't a corn, its a verruca' and in doing so informed her of the diagnosis in a manner which suggested he was certain. Similarly doctors were judged to state the key points about treatment- and preventive-action on more than nine-tenths of the occasions on which they seemed to have a view. An example, relevant to treatment-action is Mrs Boyd's consultation (2033). Referring to her daughter's foot, her doctor said, 'I think today she does need an antibiotic'.

The reader will have noticed from the two examples that to be considered to state information a doctor did not have to say very much. In Mrs Bruce's consultation what mattered was the diagnostic term and the attitude of certainty. In Mrs Boyd's consultation the name of the type of drug was all the information necessary. The rationale for this approach is that communicating a diagnostic term like that mentioned to Mrs Bruce can be considered an attempt to state to the patient the diagnostic-significance of the condition. From it one can infer whether the trouble is likely to be life-threatening, maiming, stigmatizing or recurrent or whether it is not likely to be of such significance. Similarly, the technical term mentioned to Mrs Boyd can be regarded as conveying the purpose of treatment-action. If (and of course the conditional element is quite crucial) Mrs Bruce and Mrs Boyd know what the terms mean from a medical point of view (and if the doctor uses them correctly) then the doctor will have stated his view. By contrast, Mrs Bannen (1468) attended a consultation in which her doctor made no statement of his views about diagnostic-significance. She had a history of kidney trouble and was complaining of a new episode of pain and sickness. In the consultation, the doctor carried out a urine test but did not say anything directly about what he found. Instead all that he told Mrs Bannen was that 'there is not much wrong in the kidneys at the moment' but that 'you should see a specialist'. Mrs Bannen would know she was going to hospital and might presume (as investigators have done) that the doctor had some diagnostic possibilities in mind. She might assume that the trouble was not her kidneys (he had said they were alright). But, if so, there is little indication of what the problem was. Mrs Bannen's doctor had not stated the diagnostic-significance of the problem. Distinctions between cases like Mrs Bannen's and Mrs Bruce's could be made reliably (4).

Most doctors were judged to have stated their views to patients in so far as to do this they had only to mention diagnostic or treatment terms. In this way the rating scale was simple to use (5) but hopefully not simplistic. The point is that recognizing the ideas doctors might be trying to communicate cannot be divorced from the means they employed to do so. Otherwise lack of skill at communicating, as opposed to not attempting to give information, might be confused. Rating whether views were stated, therefore, was only one part of a two-stage approach. The second part assessed how clearly doctors stated their views and took account of what terms were explained or interpreted to patients.

When the information doctors gave to state a view was considered from the latter perspective it was found that only a minority of consultations contained information stating a doctor's views clearly on the different topics (*Table 4.2*). Doctors informed patients clearly about the key points of diagnostic-significance in one third of consultations and informed them clearly about the purpose of treatment- and preventive-action in two-fifths and a half of consultations respectively (*Table 4.2*). In making these assessments attention was paid to whether the doctor's statements included technical jargon or assumptions which were not clarified or explained. If technical jargon was explained so that its diagnostic-significance, treatment purpose, etc., was made clear, and if this was done in an organized and explicit way, then a doctor's statement was made 'clear'. An example was the information given to Mr Biggs (2300). In this consultation the doctor amplified technical details so as to make their diagnostic-significance clear: he said 'that is a small cyst...it looks awful...but it is not serious...it should give you no trouble at all...it may go away by itself, it may remain but it should not ever give you any trouble'(6). Many cases in which doctors stated their views 'not clearly' were like those of Mrs Bruce (2185) discussed above. She was informed that her daughter

Table 4.2 *Methods of stating information in 405 consultations*

	information topics			
	diagnostic- significance (%)	treatment- action (%)	preventive- action (%)	at least one of the three (%)
proportion stating a topic view				
clearly	120 (33)	176 (43)	66 (52)	251 (62)
not clearly	249 (67)	229 (57)	58 (48)	154 (38)
total	369 (100)	405 (100)	124 (100)	405 (100)

had a verruca but given no further information about the diagnostic-significance of such a term. Most of the cases in which doctors stated their views 'not clearly' were rated in this way because such jargon was not made plain.

Giving reasons

Giving reasons to support their views was quite common among the doctors studied. In just under two-thirds of consultations doctors gave some reasons to support their view of diagnostic-significance and in about a half gave reasons to support their treatment-action advice. Well over a third of those patients given preventive advice were told something about why it was advisable. Moreover, as many as three-quarters of the patients were given reasons supporting a doctor's view on at least one of the three main topics of information (*Table 4.3*).

While giving patients some reasons to support a particular view was a relatively common practice among the doctors studied, most of the explanations offered were fairly parsimonious. This judgement was arrived at after deciding which explanations did more to support a view than others. Two criteria were used to define reasoning as more supportive. First, an explanation was more supportive if doctors gave reasons both to suggest that patients might accept their views and gave reasons why they should reject some alternative view. Second, reasoning which included several kinds of warrant or a description of underlying processes was con-sidered to be more supportive than if one type of warrant was used without a description of processes. Reasoning was judged 'moderately elaborate' if the infor-mation given on a topic met either of these two criteria for being more supportive and 'very elaborate' if it met both. Otherwise, if present at all, it was 'minimal'. The distinctions made by applying these criteria and which will now be illustrated with case examples, could be made in a reliable way (7).

Mrs Andrews' consultation (1634), in which she was told why her shoulder pain was not caused by heart disease, includes an example of reasoning to which we refer as 'moderately elaborate'. The doctor suggested the heart hypothesis was

Table 4.3 *Giving reasons in 405 consultations*

	information topics			
	diagnostic-significance (%)	treatment-action (%)	preventive-action (%)	at least one of the three (%)
topic mentioned				
yes	369 (91)	405 (100)	124 (31)	405 (100)
no	36 (9)	-	281 (69)	-
reasons given (if topic mentioned)				
elaborate	5 (1)	2 (0.5)	0	128 (32)
moderately elaborate	80 (22)	46 (11)	19 (15)	
minimal	134 (36)	142 (35)	33 (27)	177 (44)
none	150 (41)	215 (53)	72 (58)	100 (25)
total	369 (100)	405 (100)	124 (100)	405 (100)

false because 1) the pain was not effort related, and 2) it was only present in one place which was not the site that would be consistent with heart trouble. The first warrant is based on the patient's account of the timing of the pain and the doctor's theoretical knowledge. The latter is based on the patient's account of the site of the pain and the doctor's theoretical knowledge. Data referring to time and site were considered to constitute different kinds of warrant and so the explanation as a whole was considered 'moderately elaborate'. Mrs Allan's consultation (2436) was also an example of 'moderately elaborate' reasoning. In this consultation the doctor provided an extensive description of what happens to the spine when one sleeps on soft, as opposed to firm, beds and he did this as a support for his preventive advice that in future the patient should use a bed board (8).

Two-thirds of the explanations given in support of a doctor's view on a topic did not include arguments backed by several kinds of warrants or a description of underlying processes. They were, therefore, considered less supportive than those just described. They provided 'minimal' support for a doctor's ideas. Usually, they consisted of reasons supporting a diagnostic hypothesis based on a brief reference to laboratory results, physical examinations, or the circumstances in which symptoms arose. The consultation of Mrs Anson (1769) is an example of reasoning assessed as 'minimal'. She was a pregnant woman who had recently passed blood in her stools and was concerned it might indicate damage to her foetus. Her doctor examined her and said 'there is no sign of bleeding coming from the vagina...as long as it is the rectum it does not matter...Oh! I don't mean it does not matter at all, but it is obviously less significant'. Later in the consultation the patient queried 'Nothing to worry about is there?' to which the doctor replied 'No'. Nothing else was said about the diagnostic-significance of her condition. On this topic, therefore, the doctor offered one warrant (by verbalizing his observation that there was no bleeding from the vagina) but provided no description of underlying processes and adduced no evidence to support his view that the foetus was developing normally.

The explanations given to support doctors' views have been described as parsimonious because only in a minority of consultations, about a third of them, was a patient given a 'moderately elaborate' explanation on any topic. A still smaller number of patients, less than two in a hundred, were given 'elaborate' reason-giving on some topic: that is to say they were given a 'moderately elaborate' explanation both of why a doctor's preferred views were worth accepting *and* why other views were not. Perhaps of interest was the fact that doctors gave reasons more on some topics than others. When doctors took a view they gave 'moderately elaborate' support for diagnostic-significance hypotheses in about one in four consultations whereas the frequency for preventive- and treatment-action was about half of this.

As in the case of judging the extent to which doctors stated their views on a topic, assessments of reasoning were made independently of how clearly a doctor was expressing himself. Using the same rationale for assessing whether doctors stated a view clearly, when the clarity of reasoning was examined it was found that only a minority of explanations were 'clear' (*Table 4.4*). In fact, only 35 consultations, less than ten per cent of all those studied in detail, contained reasoning

Table 4.4 *The clarity of reason-giving in 405 consultations*

	information topics			
	diagnostic-significance (%)	treatment-action (%)	preventive-action (%)	at least one of the three (%)
proportion giving moderately elaborate reasons that were:				
clear	32 (38)	26 (54)	12 (63)	35 (41)
possibly clear	33 (39)	15 (31)	5 (26)	30 (35)
not clear	20 (24)	7 (15)	2 (10)	20 (24)
total	85 (100)	48 (100)	19 (100)	85 (100)

in support of at least one topic that was judged both 'moderately elaborate' and 'clear'.

To assess how clearly a doctor gave reasons, the argument supporting his view on each topic was considered in terms of the phraseology used by the doctor, his use of technical jargon, how far he employed explicit categorization and the general organization of what he said. If his argument avoided jargon and was quite easy to reconstruct and to follow it was judged 'clear'. An example was the reasoning provided to Mr Anstey (2286) whose doctor thought that his pain was muscular in origin. The doctor supported this hypothesis by providing a description of how the pain was caused which was an example of 'moderately elaborate' reasoning. He said: '(it) is because you then stretched the muscle, and what has happened is that somehow, perhaps while you were asleep or doing something, you have torn a few muscle fibres there. And so when you do this (demonstrating to the patient) you stretch it and that produces the pain'. This explanation was quite easy to reconstruct (being mentioned in one set of comments) and was relatively free of jargon. Although the use of the term muscle 'fibre' might be considered jargon in some contexts it was decided in this case that a 'common-sense' understanding of the idea was all that would be necessary. If it is the clarity of explanation that determines a patient's understanding then Mr Anstey was expected to understand the reasons why his doctor thought his pain was muscular in origin. Explanations which were judged 'not clear' differed from that given to Mr Anstey in that the doctor might be a great deal more circuitous in his reasoning, might mix his exposition with other comments or with giving advice, or might use jargon which was judged likely to undermine a patient's understanding of his argument (9).

Much more apparent than the potential limitations imposed by considerations of being clear, however, were those deriving from the almost complete absence of explanations giving reasons which linked the doctor's views to the lay health beliefs and explanatory models of his patients (*Table 4.5*). No consultation in the main sample contained an example of a doctor who had both discovered the patient's health beliefs in a detailed way and precisely related these to the explanations he then gave. There was only one example in which a doctor was both extensively informed about a patient's ideas and able to relate his reasoning to this information,

Table 4.5 *Giving reasons in a reactive way in 405 consultations*

	information topics			
	diagnostic-significance (%)	*treatment-action* (%)	*preventive-action* (%)	*at least one of the three* (%)
proportion giving moderately elaborate reasons that were:				
highly reactive	0	0	0	0
moderately reactive	1 (1)	0	0	1 (1)
somewhat reactive	10 (12)	6 (13)	1 (5)	11 (13)
minimally reactive	19 (22)	13 (27)	3 (16)	20 (24)
not reactive	55 (65)	29 (60)	15 (79)	53 (62)
total	85 (100)	48 (100)	19 (100)	85 (100)

although in an imprecise way. In eleven consultations the doctor seemed to have gained some knowledge of certain aspects of a patient's ideas but only briefly related to them in his explanation or alluded to them vaguely in passing (10). Among the consultations studied, therefore, the doctors' efforts to explain their views on key topics did not relate explicitly to the ideas and theories patients themselves possessed.

Similarly, efforts to check patients' understanding – whether their understanding of what doctors thought or why they did so – were very unusual. On only nine occasions were any patients asked both specific and precise questions about their understanding of what the doctor had just said on one of the topics (*Table 4.6*). Mr Christopher's consultation (1870) was an example. He was a man in his late fifties who presented with a pain his leg. His doctor gave him very detailed instructions about posture, bending, and movement which were concluded by a

Table 4.6 *Checking a patient's understanding in 405 consultations*

	information topics			
	diagnostic-significance (%)	treatment-action (%)	preventive-action (%)	at least one of the three (%)
high and moderate	4 (1)	3 (1)	2 (0.5)	9 (2)
low	11 (3)	9 (2)	1 (1)	19 (5)
none	354 (96)	393 (97)	121 (98)	377 (93)
total	369 (100)	405 (100)	405 (100)	405 (100)

check on his understanding: 'Does this all make sense to you? Can you put it all together?' Although in the context this brief question was considered specific (clearly referring to the patient's understanding of the details just given) and precise (because the patient could be in little doubt his understanding was being checked), it was not especially extensive. The doctor did not actually explore how his patient had understood him. More extensive efforts could not be found among any of the consultations studied. Checking of a less extensive kind occurred in fewer than one in ten consultations (11).

To summarize, three aspects of the way doctors tried to share information stand out. First, it seems that every doctor in most consultations attempted to tell patients what was wrong and what should be done and also usually sought to give some reasons for such views. At this level, attempts to share ideas with patients were usual. Second, however, it seems that in conveying their ideas doctors quite often did not exhibit the organizational and linguistic skills that would have made their efforts clear in the manner advocated by medical educators such as Ley. Third, and perhaps most important, the majority of the doctors that were studied appeared to have little or no apparent interest in their patients as subjective, thinking, and sense-making individuals with their own theories and hypotheses. They made no attempt to establish how patients received their ideas and how far they understood them and they did not relate their explanations to those of their patients. In terms of both the communication strategies mentioned in the last chapter, the doctors studied were not likely to be particularly effective.

Three case histories

The pattern of information-giving found in the consultations may be understood more clearly if we add to the statistical findings just mentioned by a close examination of what was actually said in three of the consultations we studied. Each illustrates the way doctors sought to give patients information and also highlights the potential difficulties that arose from the ways they seem to have conceived it appropriate to do so (12).

Mrs Cumberland

The first case is that of Mrs Cumberland (1910). She was in her late twenties and had brought her small child (as the patient) to discover why she had not been sleeping or eating 'properly' for over a month and why she had recently begun to vomit. The consultation began with Mrs Cumberland explaining this to the doctor:

Patient: She's just not eating and she's not sleeping either.
Doctor: How long has this been?
Patient: About a month, nearly.
Doctor: I see. I see, yes. Tell me more about her.
Patient: Well, she's very naughty to start with.
Doctor: Yes go on.
Patient: The other night, it's every half an hour 'Mum, I want a drink' and I give her a drink.
Doctor: Yes and what else.
Patient: She's been sick this last week.
Doctor: In what way has she been sick? Do you mean she's vomited? Yes? At which stage did she vomit?
Patient: Wednesday she was sick an awful lot, and Thursday night she was sick, and yesterday she was sick.
Doctor: Yes. I see. And what else?
Patient: On Friday. (inaudible)

At this point there is an interruption by the child. This seems to have been caused by the doctor's efforts to try to examine her. He then asks Mrs Cumberland 'What is happening in her world?' leading to a diagnosis that she is depressed (13).

Doctor: What's going on in your life, luv?

Patient: Mine, nothing why?

Doctor: You've got the glums?

Patient: No I haven't got the glums. Well she's at school. She's got everything she wants.

Doctor: She's spoilt, too spoilt. Who spoils her?

Patient: My dad, her nan and everyone.

Doctor: Yes, poor girl. (pause – child still crying) Do you get miserable?

Patient: No. I am feeling a bit run down at the moment.

Doctor: What's getting you down? Is it this bag of tricks?

Patient: Mm. (child still screaming)

Doctor: Now. Her tummy's alright (appears to be said while examining the child). She's not exactly wasting away is she?

Patient: No. No.

Doctor: But you're wretched luv?

Patient: Maybe it's because I'm not getting any sleep, I don't...

Doctor: (interrupting but child is still crying) Who else is indoors?

This question leads to some further background exploration after which, provoked by a new outburst of crying from the child, the doctor (based on his knowledge of the patient) wonders if the child is missing her maternal grandfather, who died a year ago after a painful illness (14). After some more discussion, the patient says :

Patient: You know everything seems to be going wrong at the moment.

This leads the doctor to inform her that the child is not, in his view, significantly ill and to a discussion of the help the patient needs.

Doctor: Yes. Well. She's not going wrong except that if one's spoilt and has one's way over everything one doesn't know where one is. Do you know what I'm talking about? Does that make any sense to you?

Patient: My mum said that she could do with a good hiding.

Doctor: I don't know that a hiding would help. But I think perhaps knowing how far she can push you might. (child again starts crying) She's becoming a nag isn't she?

Patient: (laughing) She is. She's like it all day.

Doctor: Oh God you must be a saint, mustn't you, to live with it! (Mother says something to child.)

Doctor: What do you want me to do luv?

Patient: I don't know, I didn't know if you could give me something to make her eat. You know.

Doctor: She doesn't need to eat any more.

Patient: But today she hasn't eaten anything at all. Yesterday all she had was a piece of bread and peanut butter, and that's for two days.

Doctor: But look at her. She's beautiful.

Patient: Yeah, I know but...

Doctor: If you take her to a children's competition she'd win a beauty contest.

Patient: I know, but when she carries on like that how long should I carry on for? How long should I let it go on for? I mean before I do something about it.

Doctor: There are two things you can do: one is that there is very little you can do. Do you know when my wife was a child she was like that, and she used to hide food in the bookcases, under the beds, in the chairs, out in the garden? Children are far cleverer for one to be able to make them eat if they don't want to. So that's the first thing. The second thing is that I've never seen a child come to harm from not eating. I have seen children come to harm from eating too much.

Patient: Yeah.

Doctor: And what is true is that if you make a song and a dance about her eating she'll know how to have you on a string and you'll be like a yo-yo on a string and she'll play you up and down. She knows what I'm on about (child can be heard vaguely). (everyone laughs) Were you fat as a child?

Patient: Yes.

Doctor: Were you?

Patient: Yes. Oh yes.

Doctor: Because you're gorgeous now aren't you? You know it's the fat kids I'm worried about. I don't practically have to worry about the thin ones. She could live off her cheeks for a month couldn't she?

Patient: She's only got big rosy cheeks. But last week they were white. They're alright are they?

Doctor: Now look I don't want to examine her today. But I would be very happy, very happy, to examine her again if you brought her again, if you are bothered about her. At the moment she's a bit spoiled, she's a bit frightened of the examination. I got away with a reasonable examination of her tummy. She's discovered that it's no good fighting me, that I'm going to examine her anyway, and she's also discovered that it's not too bad, and not worth fighting over. So you bring her back in a few days if you want to and I'll have a look at her again. But I reckon she may have only a minor illness. I think she's got the feeling of the anniversary or something like that. People get much more upset about anniversaries than you'd believe. She may have a feeling that you're upset about the anniversary and she feels for you.

Patient: Well it gets on my nerves. I don't want to go about like this. I don't want her, when she's older (child interrupting). So, if I'm not satisfied with her I bring her back.

Doctor: If you're going through a bad patch.

Patient: Yeah. Alright then.

Doctor: I think you're going to have to have a spell of difficulty. Sometimes you will feel like hitting her and sometimes you will feel like shaking her and when you get like that come and talk to me.

Patient: Yes.

Doctor: People do, it's alright.

Patient: In the night, sometimes I feel at the end with her bottle. You know, when she keeps giving it to me and saying she wants more drink. You know. But perhaps she doesn't need a lot of sleep.

Doctor: That's absolutely true.

Patient: Yeah.

Doctor: Do you need a lot of sleep?

Patient: I do. But my mum doesn't you know.

Doctor: That's absolutely right. It's hard luck having a child that needs so little sleep. OK luv?

Patient: Bye bye.

Doctor: See you luv. Say something to your mum about the anniversary. Good. Bye bye luv.

Mrs Cumberland's consultation (which lasted nearly eleven minutes) is typical of the complex mixture of physical, behavioural and emotional problems encountered in general practice. The doctor seems to decide that the child is not 'ill' or at least has only a minor gastric complaint. Rather, he sees the problem as one of difficulty for mother and child in coping with each other. He does not prescribe any medication. His main advice is that the child should not be made to eat and that Mrs Cumberland should not concern herself with the child's eating behaviour too much. He supports this advice, which is the treatment in this case, in several ways. First, he says that it is children who eat too much, not those who eat too little, who have problems later. Second, he says that if Mrs Cumberland tries to make the child eat she will be manipulated by her like a 'yo-yo on a string'. The consultation took place in harassed circumstances with the child crying. None the less, in the course of it the doctor is caring, considerate and attempts to be empathic with his patient. He even goes out of his way to ask her opinion about what she wants him to do. However, the patient is not really able to make use of this offer (15) and it is unclear how far she really understands or accepts what the doctor has said. No specific check is made to see. Despite all the doctor's efforts to share his ideas what he and his patient do not succeed in sharing are her ideas and explanations, beyond the fact that she clearly thinks that a child who is not eating is a problem. How far the patient would subsequently understand or agree with the doctor is an open question (16). In a way the consultation has concentrated more on achieving a full diagnosis than on trying to communicate it. This will be evident in the next two consultations as well.

Mrs Jones

The second case concerns Mrs Jones, a fifty-six year-old married woman who worked as a part-time cleaner and lived in a tower block. She was relatively new to the doctor's practice, was in fact registered with one of his partners, and had changed to the practice when a short geographical move gave her an opportunity (as she told the interviewer later) to leave a practice with which she was not satisfied. As will be apparent from the transcript of the consultation that follows, but put in her own words as she described the consultation at her subsequent interview, Mrs Jones went to the doctor complaining of 'a lot of pain after eating and feeling really as though I don't belong to myself'. She reported at her interview that she had, in fact, been feeling this way for three weeks but did not like to trouble doctors unnecessarily ('obviously you don't. . . unless you really need to. . .'). It seems she needed three weeks of pain to convince herself that she really needed to go and she then made an appointment. However, having done so, she immediately felt better and nearly cancelled it. In fact she commented that she only kept the appointment because she felt it would be rude not to do so. The consultation began as follows:

Doctor: Yes?

Patient: I've been having a lot of pain on when I eat anything for this last couple of weeks and, er, I've been feeling generally really out of sorts and, er, for this last, well, nearly three weeks now, and, er. Eased up a bit the weekend but I felt dreadful all this week again and I popped in yesterday to see if I could see, you know, to see you yesterday but I just felt so ill I just feel as if I don't belong to myself. I know it's a funny thing to say.

Doctor: Yes.

Patient: But I've had this, er, pain on eating for you know on and off for years but they can't find anything wrong with me. I've been and had several. . .

Doctor: (interrupting) Who's they?

Patient: X-rays. Well the hospitals.

At this point the doctor, speaking gently and with concern, decided to inform the patient about what he has been reading in the notes he has audibly been leafing through:

Doctor: Well they, looking through your notes, they have in fact found something, um, in 1973, um, they did find that, er, on X-ray, that your duodenum cap was slightly deformed. Now what that means is it's a bit scarred so it does look as though you have had a duodenal ulcer at some time.

Patient: Yes.

Doctor: Now what that means is that from time to time you may well get pain of this kind.

Patient: (interrupting in an excited tone) Yeah. It seems to flare up about twice a year and it's really bad. I mean I cope with it, I get indigestion all the time, but it's just something they told me I've got to live with.

While the patient has been speaking the doctor has, audibly, been trying to stop her and to give her his views: twice he got as far as saying 'I think' only to find the patient has continued to speak. On his third try he succeeded, and elaborated to her a fairly detailed explanation, judged to give 'moderately elaborate' support for his view of significance but 'minimal' support for his preventive recommendations:

Doctor: I think the answer to this is: the BMA publish a series of booklets which was how to cure this and how to cure that, but with the duodenum...
Patient: Mmm.
Doctor: ...it was entitled *How to Live with your Duodenum.*
Patient: Yes.
Doctor: Do you see what I mean?
Patient: Yes.
Doctor: Now that's a little different and what happens is that if you're the kind of person that produces too much acid you can get the duodenal cap scarred, that's part of the stomach.
Patient: Yes.
Doctor: And once it gets scarred it stays that way and it does produce pain from time to time.
Patient: Mmm.
Doctor: And there are flare-ups. Now the important thing about it is that it never really goes bad it doesn't er...
Patient: No.
Doctor: You know, nothing terrible happens.
Patient: No. No, no.
Doctor: On the other hand it means that you must expect from time to time some kind of flare-up of your tummy pain.
Patient: Mmm.
Doctor: And all that we can do during that time is to give you something to control it.

At this point the patient appeared to be on the brink of saying something but was apparently interrupted as the doctor decided to examine her:

Patient: Well...
Doctor: Now let's have a look at you and see what's happening.

After a brief pause the patient starts again, leading to the first of several discussions of eating behaviour:

Patient: I usually take, I've always got Bisodol because I find, er the Bisodol powder,

I find that that, er, you know is the easiest thing to relieve it. But, er, in the night-time it starts here then it goes down there and then it goes right through to my back.

Doctor: (interrupting) Yes. If you eat something does that make any difference?

Patient: No. No I don't.

Doctor: Does it make it better or worse?

Patient: Oh no I don't think it makes any difference at all whether I eat anything. I've tried that, you see my father had a duodenal ulcer and I've seen him, you know, he used to have milk and biscuits.

Doctor: So you know all about it.

Patient: Yes. Um do you want me to slip anything off or.

There was then a pause of about a minute during which the patient was removing clothes, and the doctor undertaking the examination. During this interval Mrs Jones explained she has put herself on a diet of *Patent Groats* (marketed as a baby food). The doctor did not respond to this information. Instead he began to indicate the location of her duodenum to her and to demonstrate its tenderness. After being told to dress Mrs Jones then thanked the doctor for being so communicative:

Patient: And it feels as if somebody's jumped on me, you know so it feels all sore when I've had these pains, all tied up. But you're the only one that's ever taken the trouble to explain it this way. They just say oh it's something you have to live with and the last time I went to the hospital the doctor said well we couldn't find anything wrong you know. I felt that he was thinking: 'Oh, just another female that's got nothing else to do but sort of come up and get herself X-rayed', which is, you know, I don't trouble doctors unless it's really necessary.

During those parts of Mrs Jones' consultation that have been described, and throughout the remaining minutes devoted to discussion of treatment and eating habits (17), the doctor has been forthcoming with information and has undoubtedly sought to treat his patient as having a right to know. The patient has said she was grateful and made this clear at her subsequent interview. In this respect the consultation is a good example of the one third of consultations in which a doctor stated what was wrong clearly and also the one third of consultations in which doctors' reasoning was judged at least 'moderately elaborate'. At the same time it is also an example of the way in which the ideas the patient had were not given much prominence or attention. While the doctor clearly respected his patient and her intellectual capacities, at no point in the consultation did he try to elaborate the ideas he assumed Mrs Jones to have about the significance of an ulcer, its long-term implications, its most effective methods of treatment and so on. In particular, he obtained no idea of the explanatory hypotheses Mrs Jones possessed and on several occasions interrupted her when she might have been about to volunteer clues to her beliefs (18). Thus, while the doctor shared his ideas with the patient, he did not allow the patient to share her ideas with him or to try to meld them together. In this way, he appears to have conceived the consultation process as one in which doctors provide ideas to patients but not as one in which the patient is an expert with ideas of her own. Perhaps as part of this implicit conception he did not check to see if she understood her situation and what needed to be done: for example, it was unclear if she understood his distinction between curing and living with her difficulty, or appreciated the causal mechanism through which her eating habits would help her to do so (19).

Mr Nixon

The third consultation chosen illustrates much more graphically the problems most doctors encountered when patients hinted at their own theories. The patient, Mr Nixon, was a sixty year-old married man living in a detached house in a commuter suburb about twenty miles from London. He was a supervisor at an engineering plant. Mr Nixon had previously visited his doctor only infrequently and on this occasion had brought a rash on his leg. The consultation got off to a rather uncertain start but soon led to some very careful diagnostic inquiry work by the doctor:

Doctor: Come in please.
Patient: Hello.
Doctor: Take a seat. I won't be a moment. (pause) Mr Nixon is it?
Patient: Yes.
Doctor: Oh, I recognize you. Haven't seen you for a long time. (laughs)
Patient: How are you?
Doctor: Pretty well, thanks.
Patient: Are you? Good. Splendid.
Doctor: Eh, I shouldn't say how are you? Should I? (laughs) I should say what can I do for you?
Patient: Well, what I've come round about, doctor, on and off from time to time I seem to get like a leg aggravation. It, eh, it seems to be like a smarting type of feeling and eh, it aggravates like, itches.
Doctor: Itches, does it?
Patient: Yes. And it eh, it's like a smarting kind of thing. Not fiercely but mildly.
Doctor: Deep in the leg or on the surface?
Patient: No. No. No. On the skin. Surface of the skin. Yes.
Doctor: No aching in the leg at all?
Patient: Well, what I have found, well, if I have occasion to bend down, you know, (indistinct) eh, it's rather aching on getting up. I know age progresses and so forth but, eh, you know, over the best part of the weekend I wasn't bothered with it and then Sunday it sort of started again. I've had it on and off quite a while.

Doctor: On and off. I'm still not absolutely sure in my mind what you mean. It's not a skin irritation you're complaining of?

Patient: Yes, it's eh.

Doctor: Would you call it an itch?

Patient: It is. But the, it's also the sensation and feeling of it is, as I say a sort of slightly smarting as if the skin is a little sort of taut.

Doctor: Raw?

Patient: Yes, yes.

Doctor: Do you get this all the time or does it vary?

Patient: Pardon?

Doctor: Do you, is this a constant sensation or does it vary?

Patient: Eh, no. Some days I'm not bothered with it.

Doctor: No backache at all?

Patient: Oh no. No, no.

Doctor: You don't feel your leg is less strong than it used to be?

Patient: No, not really. I get, as I say, I sort of bend down and you feel a sort of achiness in getting up, sort of thing, but, eh...

Doctor: Do your legs ache when you walk?

Patient: No, no.

Doctor: No pain in the calf if you, um.

Patient: (very uncertain and speaking almost inaudibly) No. I didn't know, possibly you know, whether er, blood was a little bit rich or perhaps too much sugar on what I eat, or, you know. It's only a guess on my part, but this, it's not a lot.

Doctor: (interrupts) I see you're scratching now. Is this the sort of thing that makes you want to scratch, is it?

Patient: Yes it does. It's not a lot to be seen there. It's a little minute sort of blemish, but um.

Doctor: Just slip your shoes and socks off.

At this point the doctor began a very careful examination of Mr Nixon which lasted several minutes (20). Eventually a diagnosis was determined and this communicated to the patient:

Doctor: Ah ha. Bend your knees. Put your knee up. That's it. No. Everything is fine as far as muscles are concerned. I think it's a skin irritation, I'll give you a moisturizing cream.

Patient: Yes.

Despite this affirmative, the patient did not sound very happy. His discomfort was noticed by the doctor:

Doctor: All right?

Patient: Yes, as I say it's not for me to diagnose by any means, but, er, I wondered whether I might be having too much of rather sweet food. I'm rather a sweety er sort of person.

Doctor: Well, I don't honestly. Weight keeping steady by the way?

Patient: Yes. That's keeping pretty good.

Doctor: All right. You take a lot of sugar do you?

Patient: Well, I take my fair share.

Doctor: I don't think that has anything to do with that. I'll check your urine sometime. Drop a sample in. All right.

Like the previous consultation Mr Nixon's encounter with his doctor also illustrates an important feature of the way information was given in consultations. First, the doctor clearly tried very hard to understand his patient and to provide him with information about what was wrong – although this is one of the (minority) one third of consultations in which no reason-giving was actually rated as present. Second, the doctor was unable, apparently, to conceptualize his patient as having his own ideas and model of explanation. In consequence, the doctor seems to have found the few comments the patient did make difficult to comprehend and also confusing. He did not try to encourage the patient to elaborate his ideas – or could not find the words to help him do so – and on several occasions ignored what he was being told. However, in this consultation unlike the other two, there is much to indicate that the patient has been thinking and may be presenting a sub-jectively coherent complaint. For example, Mr Nixon mentioned early on that he knows that 'age progresses', he seemed determined to emphasize the sensa-tions he suffered very exactly (especially tautness), and twice he overtly hinted at some theory connected with sugar and sweet food. All these comments are ignored by the doctor until the last. At that point he responded not by seeking to understand but by action: the offer of a urine test 'some time'. In the absence of knowledge about Mr Nixon's theories or of attempts to check his understan-ding there was no way of knowing whether a urine test was a relevant considera-tion in his model of explanation. Indeed, the subsequent interview with him clearly revealed it was not (21).

Discovering patients' ideas

The consultations of Mrs Jones and Mr Nixon illustrate some important reasons why patients in the sample were not given explanations which related to their own ideas and models. Essentially, most of the doctors studied were not usually in a position to orientate their explanation to patients' theories simply because they had not tried to find out and elaborate the patients' beliefs. This point can be demonstrated more forcibly by a systematic exploration of doctors' efforts to discover or elaborate patients' ideas and of their response to the hints of such ideas offered by patients.

One way of examining doctors interest in patients' ideas was to seek evidence in each consultation of questions that indicated that doctors wanted to know the meaning patients placed on their symptoms, their explanatory framework or their ideas about appropriate treatment and prevention options. Questions such as 'What do you think it might be apart from a nervous headache ?' (2345) or 'Do you think any of them are serious?' (2139) or 'Did it make you think it might be due to anything other than arthritis?' (1851), or 'What can I do for you?' (Mrs Cumberland, 1910), for example, were considered instances of doctors inviting patients to tell them about their ideas and understanding. Such questions are to be distinguished from those which invited patients to give factual details about how they were feeling or what they were presenting (for instance, when Mr Nixon, above, was asked 'It's not a skin irritation you're complaining of?'). These questions may explore a patient's subjective view of his symptoms but do not address his ideas and theories about what is happening. Some other questions, like 'Looks like a wart, doesn't it?' (1962) or 'Do you want a prescription? ' (1444) are more ambiguous. The doctor might be asking a patient to develop ideas or he may simply be seeking an affirmative. Questions of this kind, therefore, were rated as 'ambiguous' invitations to patients to give their ideas (22).

Table 4.7 shows that there were very few occasions when the doctors in the sample were observed to make active efforts to ask patients to volunteer or to elaborate their ideas. Patients were invited to volunteer their ideas about significance in about

Table 4.7 *Discovering and elaborating patients' ideas in 405 consultations*

	information topics			
	diagnostic-significance (%)	*treatment-action* (%)	*preventive-action* (%)	*at least one of the three* (%)
inviting patients to volunteer ideas:				
some active effort	24 (6)	13 (3)	0	33 (8)
some ambiguous effort	42 (10)	70 (17)	16 (4)	102 (25)
no invitation	339 (84)	322 (80)	389 (96)	270 (67)
total	405 (100)	405 (100)	405 (100)	405 (100)
asking patients to elaborate ideas:				
some active effort	23 (6)	6 (1)	2	31 (8)
passive acceptance	52 (13)	30 (7)	9 (2)	77 (19)
no effort or interruption	330 (81)	309 (91)	394 (97)	297 (73)
total	405 (100)	405 (100)	405 (100)	405 (100)

Note: 54 (13%) consultations contained active invitations either to volunteer or to elaborate on at least one topic. 118 (29%) contained ambiguous or passive efforts on at least one topic and 233 (58%) contained no efforts.

one in seventeen consultations (6 per cent) and to present their ideas about treatment-action in one in thirty (3 per cent). No patient was asked for ideas about prevention and in less than one in twelve consultations were there any active efforts to inquire on any topic at all. Ambiguous attempts were more frequent but by no means common.

A second way in which doctors could show they wanted to know about the patients' ideas and theories would be by responding with interest to what patients themselves say. In some circumstances patients also explicitly stated their diagnosis of the problem or their specific expectations of treatment. In other situations, like Mrs Jones and Mr Nixon, discussed above, patients might hint at their ideas either in response to the doctor's invitation to do so, or in the course of presenting their troubles or answering questions about details of their condition. Mr Nixon introduced ideas about sugar, for example, and Mrs Jones mentioned that she had experience of stomach trouble from her father's illness. Whether patients were explicit or just hinted at their ideas doctors could try to get patients to elaborate on them by explicitly asking them to say more and perhaps by commenting (at what might be termed a meta-level of communication) that the more they understood the patients' ideas the easier it would be to explain to them what they think (23). *Table 4.7*, however, shows that such efforts to clarify or encourage patients to elaborate on points they have made are no more common than invitations for them to volunteer ideas. Only about one in twelve consultations contained an instance of this doctor behaviour. Moreover, in only one in five, did doctors appear even to tolerate patients' ideas passively – that is listening without either trying to encourage elaboration or to discourage continuation by interrupting.

Another way in which the doctors' response to patients' ideas was examined was by exploring consultations as a whole to ask how doctors controlled the verbal interaction with their patients and in particular how they reacted to any sign of patient theories. Pilot observation suggested that in some consultations doctors appeared to take very strong control and to ignore or inhibit the development of any ideas patients introduced. In others, patients expressed ideas which appeared to disagree with those of the doctors and in this situation three outcomes were observed: doctors might try to explore the ideas which were the source of disagreement; or evade disagreement either by 'backing off' and changing the subject or by altering their view without discovering what patients had in mind, or the doctor and patient continued to 'spar' until the end. Finally, there were consultations in which patients' ideas were tolerated or were not present at all, in which cases doctors' responses to them could not be determined.

Consultations in which doctors took control by interrupting or changing the subject so as to ignore or inhibit patient ideas will be termed 'inhibited' and those in which disagreement was evaded will be categorized as 'evaded' (24). Just over half the consultations studied were found to fall into either the inhibited or the evaded categories – the great majority being consultations in which doctors interrupted or changed the subject apparently to limit patients' expression of ideas.

The consultations of Mrs Jones and Mr Nixon were two examples. In both, the doctors interrupted and changed the subject in such a way potentially to discourage the patients from continuing to develop or volunteer ideas. Mrs Jones' doctor interrupted her several times when she was presenting ideas and before she had finished speaking (particularly when he asked 'Who's they?', and a little later when she was telling him about how she realized she had to live with her pain). In this way he may have created the impression that her theories were not important. In Mr Nixon's consultation the doctor took tight control at the beginning, losing very little time before proceeding to detailed history-taking. He subsequently ignored several hints about his patient's ideas – interrupting and changing the subject, for instance, when the patient first hinted at his sugar theory (25).

A fourth, rather different, way of looking at doctors' attitudes to patients theories was to consider the content of their explanations in terms of the extent to which they anticipated their patients' concerns and the decisions they would have to take after. In pilot interviews with patients after consultations, some appeared uncertain about whether they were experiencing side effects of treatment, about how they could fit a drug regimen into their daily lives, or about whether their illness was running its expected course. These uncertainties seemed to lead to 'unnecessary' return visits or phone calls to doctors, fears of the danger of drugs and failure to follow instructions – just as anticipated by authors such as West (1976) and Zola (1981) who have described in detail the interpretive work patients must often do to make sense of medical instructions and the damage to their confidence in their doctor that can be created if to make sense of them they have to conclude he was in error.

Three measures were developed to explore whether doctors inquired into the just mentioned aspects of patients' concerns and whether they responded with appropriate information. Using the measures it was found that very few consultations contained efforts to anticipate any of these areas of patient experience and decision-making. One in seven of the consultations contained even vague references to the future course of symptoms (26), about one in six contained any mention of drug effects (27) and one in about thirty contained any recognition that patients would have to adjust regimens to their life-style (28).

To summarize, the consultations that have been studied rarely contained active efforts on the part of doctors to invite patients to present their ideas and expectations and infrequently showed evidence of doctors picking up on hinted ideas or encouraging patients to elaborate. More than half were conducted in such a way as to actively discourage patients from thinking their doctor wanted to know their ideas. Moreover, examination of any attempts doctors made to anticipate decisions patients might need to make after leaving the surgery suggests that doctors did not usually conceive of their patients as 'active' thinkers or decision-makers. Finally, it is important to note that these conclusions cannot be explained as an artefact of the method of selecting which consultations to study in depth. When we examined the random sample of all the consultations we recorded, very much the same pattern to that we have reported emerged (29).

Who was given information?

Medical and social science literature has been hardly less silent about who is or should be given information than it has about exactly what giving information might mean. First, clinically-orientated writers have tended to assume that a prime determinant of who gets information would be the clinical characteristics of a patient's illness. Some illnesses might require a lot of information to be given, others might prevent it being given (Szasz and Hollender 1956). Second, social scientists have been interested in the effects on giving information to patients that flow from social stratification. Patients from lower social classes, minority ethnic groups, older patients or women have all been regarded as likely to receive less information than other patients (Cartwright and O'Brien 1976; Wallen, Waitzkin, and Stoeckle 1979; Pendleton and Bochner 1980). Third, doctors, mostly in conversation, tend to be concerned about the influence of time. Any discussion of giving information will often meet the objection that the six minutes thought to be the average duration of a general practice consultation is inadequate.

When the information given to patients in consultations was examined, however, the most striking finding was its relatively random distribution. Some relationships were discovered between what doctors said and aspects of a patient's illness (30). There was also some evidence of the influence of social factors and of the length of consultations. Which doctor a patient saw also influenced his chance of knowing more about what was happening. None the less, overall, it was very hard to detect a pattern or to understand why doctors gave information to some patients and not to others. Moreover, the same uncertainty pervaded attempts to explain why some consultations lasted longer than others.

The least influential variables were those associated with the individual characteristics of the doctors themselves. While individual doctors did vary markedly in what information they gave and how they gave it this did not appear to exert any statistical influence on the overall pattern. Knowing which doctor a patient went to gave an observer very little chance of predicting what information he would get (31). Only somewhat more useful was knowledge of whether doctors were in the Study or Comparison group. Doctors in the former (selected because of their teaching responsibilities and their reputation for being interested in communicating) were more likely to mention prevention to their patients, to state their diagnostic-significance hypotheses and to do so more clearly, to give reasons in support of their treatment advice, to make some attempt to check their patients' understanding, and to desist from inhibiting or evading their patients ideas (*Table 4.8*). Even so relationships were not all that strong. For example, while Study group doctors were less likely than their counterparts to inhibit or to evade their patients

Table 4.8 *Some statistically significant differences in the behaviour of study and comparison group doctors*

	study group (%)	comparison group (%)	gamma coefficient
proportion:			
mentioning prevention	35	26	0.22
stating diagnostic-significance clearly	46	32	0.29
giving moderately elaborate reasons for treatment-action	15	9	0.21
'inhibiting' or 'evading' a patient's ideas	52	38	0.29
some checking of a patient's ideas	11	3	0.54

ideas and were more likely to give 'moderately elaborate' reasons to support their advice, they still did not give 'moderately elaborate' reasons in more than four-fifths of their consultations and inhibited or evaded their patients' ideas in nearly half. They still did not check their patients' understanding at all in more than nine out of ten consultations. Knowledge of the group into which a doctor had been selected was not a strong predictor of their behaviour (32).

Various social factors were somewhat more predictive of the information patients were given (*Table 4.9*). The 22 Afro-Caribbean patients, for example, had a particularly low chance of being given reasons to support a doctor's view and were also unusually likely to be told these views in a way judged to be unclear. About half the proportion of Afro-Caribbean patients (18 per cent) compared to patients from all other ethnic backgrounds (32 per cent), were given 'moderately elaborate' reasons on at least one topic. Similarly, Afro-Caribbean patients (36 per cent) were half as likely to have views stated to them clearly on at least one topic.

Other social factors produced a rather less dramatic effect. For example, a third of the patients from service and intermediate backgrounds (middle class), compared to a quarter of those from working-class backgrounds, were given preventive advice (33). One in ten of the middle-class patients compared to one in seven of the working-class patients were given 'moderately elaborate' reasons in support of treatment advice. About two-thirds of the middle-class patients, compared to a half of working-class patients had doctors' views on at least one topic stated to them clearly. Factors such as educational background, marital and housing status, age and gender exerted little or no influence on the variables just mentioned and no social factors, with one exception, were related to the likelihood a patient's ideas would be checked, explored, inhibited or evaded. The exception was gender.

Table 4.9 *Some differences in information giving according to various social factors*

(a) *occupational background*

	service (%)	intermediate (%)	working (%)	gamma coefficient
proportion:				
mentioning prevention	37	32	25	0.19
stating diagnostic-significance	10	23	16	0.16
clearly stating a view on at least one topic	70	62	54	0.23
moderately elaborate reasons supporting treatment-action advice	10	10	15	0.07

(b) *gender*

	women (%)	men (%)	gamma coefficient
proportion:			
in which a patient's ideas evaded	15	6	0.41

(c) *ethnic group*

	Afro-Caribbean (%)	others (%)	gamma coefficient
proportion:			
giving moderately elaborate reasons on at least one topic	18	32	0.38
clearly stating a view on at least one topic	36	63	0.50

Women were twice as likely as men to find themselves in a consultation in which their ideas were evaded. Just under one in seven women (15 per cent), compared to over one in fifteen men (6 per cent), experienced this kind of consultation (34).

The influence the various social factors exerted on the information given in consultations was not large. While being working-class, Afro-Caribbean, or female did exert an influence, these phenomena explain only a small proportion of the variation in what information patients got or how they got it. Moreover, in the instance of occupational background influences were of an unexpected kind, at least to social scientists. Working-class patients actually had a greater chance of being given reasons than middle-class patients. From a clinical point of view there was also something rather unexpected and bizarre about the way Afro-Caribbean and working-class patients were treated. These patients, when they received information, were less likely to have it spelled out to them in a clear way. Yet it is exactly these patients who are most likely to require information to be given to them most clearly.

Rather more influential than variations produced by a patient's social background or which doctor he saw was the effect of the illness he had. The exact diagnostic category into which a patient's illness was classified (35) exerted little effect on the information he was given. However, those who attended with one of the 'special' conditions mentioned by a working party of the Royal College of General Practitioners as candidates for health education and preventive advice (36) and those with a condition we determined as 'diagnostically-significant' rather than self-limiting, did receive more information. *Table 4.10* shows that one and a half times as many

Table 4.10 *The influence of a patient's diagnosis on his chance of being given information*

	special diagnosis (%)	other diagnosis (%)	total
1 preventive advice			
given	32 (44)	92 (28)	124
not given	41 (56)	240 (72)	281
total	73 (100)	332 (100)	405
2 reasons given			
moderately elaborate	25 (34)	103 (31)	128
minimal	23 (32)	154 (46)	177
none	25 (34)	75 (23)	100
total	73 (100)	332 (100)	405

1 chi-square$=7.32$ 1 d/f $p<0.01$
gamma$=0.34$

2 chi-square$=6.52$ 2 d/f $p<0.05$
gamma$=0.08$

patients having a 'special' condition (26 per cent), compared to those who did not (15 per cent), were given advice about prevention. These patients were also a little more likely to be given reasons (*Table 4.10*).

Conditions we judged to be 'diagnostically-significant' were those where the problem the patient brought was in some sense 'bad news'. This judgement was based on medically 'serious' aspects of the prognosis for any given diagnosis but was not an assessment just of the threat to life. The judgement was mainly designed to distinguish conditions which would be a continuing source of discomfort or anxiety from those which would not. 'Diagnostically-significant' conditions, therefore, were those which might require surgery (for example, gall bladder trouble), which appeared to threaten life (for example, carcinomas or high blood pressure), or which were going to go on being a nuisance (for example, arthritic conditions, chronic 'thrush', chronic back trouble) (37). Not surprisingly, the rather *ad hoc* arrangement of conditions covered by the category 'diagnostically-significant' were only very weakly correlated with formal diagnostic categories (38). Patients receiving such a diagnosis, however, were treated rather differently in terms of the information they were given (*Table 4.11*). Compared to those given 'not significant diagnoses'

Table 4.11 *The significance of a patient's diagnosis on the information they were given*

	significance of diagnosis		total
	significant (%)	not significant (%)	
1 *reasons given*			
moderately elaborate	53 (44)	75 (26)	128
minimal	49	128	177
none	19	81	100
total	121	284	405

chi-square = 14.17 1 d/f p < 0.001
gamma = 0.33

2 *diagnostic significance stated*			
clear	32 (26)	88 (36)	120
not clear	76	112	188
not stated	13	48	61

chi-square = 10.66 2 d/f p < 0.01
gamma = 0.03

3 *treatment advice stated*			
clear	66 (55)	110 (39)	176
not clear	51	148	199
not stated	4	26	30

chi-square = 10.51 2 d/f p < 0.01
gamma = 0.32

they were about twice as likely to be given 'moderately elaborate' reasons in support of a topic, about one and a half times more likely to have a doctor's view about treatment stated to them clearly, but about one and a half times less likely to have doctors' significance views stated to them clearly. In other words, doctors seemed to provide more reasons for their views and to make treatment decisions clearer to such patients, but to be less clear about what the conditions actually implied. Possibly, doctors were more unwilling to spell out bad news than good. The significance of a patient's diagnosis, in the terms being discussed, did not influence whether doctors checked patients' ideas, explored them, or inhibited or evaded them.

The influences on the information patients received that have been mentioned so far were not large and do not go very far towards explaining what happened to make doctors give more information to some patients than to others or how they did so (39). We turn now to the influence of giving information on the duration of consultations and to the determinants of how long consultations were.

The duration of consultations

Consultations ranged in duration from just over 2 minutes to just over 32 minutes in total length. The shortest allowed 1.75 minutes for conversation and the longest just under 25 minutes. The typical (median) consultation was just over 8 minutes long allowing for a few seconds short of 7 minutes for conversation (40). The correlation between the amount of time spent talking and the total length of a consultation was high (41).

Table 4.12 indicates that mean consultation times were somewhat longer if patients were given advice about prevention, a clear statement of a doctor's view about diagnostic-significance or treatment, reasons in support of diagnosis or treatment, and if doctors tried to explore or check patients' ideas. Differences, however, were small and correlations very weak. Looking in more detail it was interesting to note that although longer consultations were more frequently associated with giving 'moderately elaborate' reasons, many very short consultations also contained them. In fact, in nearly one in five of the consultations in which doctors and patients talked to each other for less than four minutes the doctor gave 'moderately elaborate' reasons. The same proportion of consultations contained such information (nearly two-fifths) if they talked for 7 to 10 minutes or over 15 minutes. Nearly a half of the consultations lasting from 10 to 15 minutes contained it. Shorter consultations did not preclude giving 'moderately elaborate' reasons, therefore, no more than longer consultations guaranteed it.

In general, analysis of how long consultations took did not suggest that there was any particularly clear set of reasons why doctors should spend longer talking to some patients than to others. The diagnostic category into which a patient's problem fell did make some difference. Patients with eye and ear problems, respiratory conditions, menstrual disorders, and injuries were most likely to have consultations lasting less than four minutes. Patients with endocrine complaints, psychiatric difficulties, cardiovascular problems, digestive complaints, and menstrual disorders were more likely than others to have consultations lasting over nine minutes (42). Knowledge of a patient's diagnostic category of this kind improved the chances of predicting how long their consultation would last by about 20 per cent over chance. How 'diagnostically-significant' was a patient's condition had a similar influence. Patients with more significant conditions had somewhat longer consultations in total length. They also had somewhat longer conversations with their doctors (*Table 4.12*).

Table 4.12 *Various influences on the duration of a consultation*

	mean total time	mean speaking time	correlation with speaking time
Doctor behaviours:			
1 giving reasons (at least one topic)			0.12
moderately elaborate	8.7	7.8	
minimal	8.2	6.8	
none	7.2	6.1	
2 stating views (about diagnostic-significance)			0.03
clear	8.0	7.1	
not clear	8.0	6.8	
3 mentioning prevention			0.20
yes	9.2	8.1	
no	7.6	6.4	
4 exploring patients' ideas			0.15
active efforts	9.0	7.9	
some efforts	8.9	7.5	
no efforts	7.5	6.5	
5 Reacting to patients' ideas			0.04
inhibiting	8.5	7.4	
evading	8.5	7.1	
neither	7.7	6.5	
6 checking patient's ideas			0.11
high/moderate	8.9	7.4	
low	10.7	9.8	
none	8.0	6.8	

	mean total time	mean speaking time	correlation with speaking time

Diagnostic and background variables:

1 significance of diagnosis			0.16
significant	9.3	7.9	
not significant	7.6	6.6	
2 ICCHP diagnosis			0.21
infections (I)	6.4	5.4	
endocrine (III)	10.8	9.7	
psychiatric (V)	10.4	9.2	
eye and ear (VI)	6.0	5.2	
cardiovascular (VII)	10.0	7.4	
respiratory (VIII)	6.5	5.6	
digestive (IX)	11.8	10.3	
urinary	8.4	6.8	
menstrual	10.1	9.9	
skin (XII)	6.5	5.3	
muscular-skeletal			
(XIII)	8.4	7.4	
injuries (XVII)	6.6	5.7	
social	6.9	6.5	
normalize	7.8	6.6	
other	9.4	7.7	
3 type of visit			0.14
new problem, or			
change of			
diagnosis	7.5	6.3	
old problem	8.6	7.4	

Table 4.12 (*cont.*):

	mean total time	mean speaking time	correlation with speaking time
Social variables:			
1 patient's gender and adult status			0.02
woman with child	6.9	5.9	
woman alone	8.8	7.6	
man	7.6	6.6	
2 occupational background			0.04
service	8.2	7.4	
intermediate	8.2	6.7	
working	8.0	6.8	
3 ethnic background			0.11
Afro-Caribbean	7.0	5.2	
other	8.2	7.1	
4 educational background			0.02
high	8.5	7.6	
intermediate	7.9	6.9	
basic	8.1	6.8	
5 age			0.10
18-35	8.1	7.0	
36-55	7.8	6.6	
56+	8.5	7.2	
Doctor variables:			
1 individual doctor			0.17
A	9.1	7.9	
B	6.2	5.7	
C	7.7	7.0	
D	9.4	7.5	
E	6.9	6.5	
F	12.8	8.9	
G	10.4	8.5	
H	7.9	6.0	
I	6.0	5.3	
J	9.5	8.6	
K	6.8	5.9	
L	9.2	8.6	
M	7.0	6.5	
N	5.2	4.3	
O	9.5	8.2	
P	7.2	6.8	
2 group			0.04
study	7.9	6.8	
comparison	8.3	7.1	

If how long doctors spent talking to patients in the consultations selected for study (43) was not influenced very strongly by the nature of their illness it was hardly influenced at all by social factors. Patients from different occupational and educational backgrounds, those of different ages, and those of different ethnic groups had consultations of very similar mean duration. Women were somewhat more likely to have longer consultations (if they visited for themselves and not children) and those who were Afro-Caribbean were given shorter consultations.

If neither patients' illness nor their social background seemed to exert much influence on how long they would talk with their doctors, it might at least be expected that the past history of dealing with the problem would make a difference. *Table 4.12* shows, however, that even this influence was marginal. Patients bringing an illness to their doctor for the first time or those being given a new diagnosis for an old illness were likely to have shorter consultations, but only just.

Bearing in mind how difficult it has been to account for how long doctors and patients talked to each other (even though there is enormous variation to explain), the finding that individual doctors varied considerably in their mean consultation times (*Table 4.12*) may provide a clue to explain what was happening. One doctor spent, on average, just over four minutes with every patient. Another doctor spent nearly nine minutes on average. In the light of the findings that the social and clinical variables we have examined do not seem to account for how long doctors talk to patients it seems possible that the main influence on how long a consultation lasted was idiosyncratic. Each doctor may have felt he had a clear policy about talking to his patients but if so it was hard to detect (44). It was not at all clear that consultations in which more time was spent speaking achieved more than short ones. Certainly taking more time to talk did not lead to an increased likelihood of a mutual exchange of information. We will return to this matter in Chapter 8.

Summary

Most consultations contained efforts by a doctor both to state his views on one of the topics and to provide a rationale for them. However, doctors very rarely initiated any discussion of the social and psychological implications of a patient's condition, introduced preventive ideas in only one third of consultations and often stated their views and gave reasons in a less than clear way. The reasons doctors gave as part of their rationale for their views were also rather parsimonious and virtually no doctor gave his rationale in a way that was 'reactive' to ideas expressed by the patient. This last finding was mainly because doctors not only did not ask patients to volunteer their ideas but when patients did so, spontaneously or in response to a doctor's initial inquiry, did not pursue them by asking a patient to elaborate them. Indeed, not only did doctors not ask patients to elaborate their ideas, they also quite often evaded them or inhibited their expression. Although there were some social and diagnostic differences between the patients who were given more and less information in more or less clear ways these were usually small. It was difficult to form a clear idea of why doctors gave information to some patients and not others or why they spent much longer talking to some patients than others.

The patient's part

The importance of the part
patients can play

In this chapter and the next we turn our attention to the ways patients can contribute to a process of sharing ideas in consultations. Like doctors they can both give information about their views and they can attempt to encourage a mutual exchange of ideas by trying to help doctors express or elaborate their views.

We have mentioned in the first chapter that in many cases the successful outcome of a medical consultation cannot be evaluated without knowing about the patient's ideas and values. However, a doctor's reliance on the active participation of his patient extends beyond setting goals. At the level of everyday life several social scientists have emphasized how much initiative is required from patients just to co-operate with a doctor's instructions. Zola (1981), for example, illustrated the confusion he felt could occur after a consultation if a patient tried to take literally an instruction to 'take this drug four times a day'. Would 'it mean every six hours? Must he wake up in the middle of the night? What if he misses? Should he take two if he remembers later?'. Doctors cannot tell them everything so patients must expand on or interpret what is said. Trying to obtain clarification or to question a doctor in the consultation may be part of this process.

In fact, if the patient's part in a consultation is analysed formally, it is soon apparent that in certain respects the patient has a greater expertise than the doctor. We could say that only patients know about the nature of the subjective experiences of which doctors need to be aware to make a diagnosis and only patients can exercise the value judgements necessary to weigh up the costs and benefits of different types of intervention – for example, whether for them the benefit of an operation, a drug or a procedure outweighs the risks and side effects that they may subsequently experience. Moreover, it is patients who are usually relied on to make the first contact with the doctor and it is they who usually have the legal right to consent to treatment and physical examination. It is they who are usually in a position to follow or not to follow instructions. It is they who have to make sense of, appraise and evaluate what they have been told in a consultation at the time and subsequently.

Authors such as Stimson and Webb (1975) and Hayes-Bautista (1976), have illustrated the ways some patients try to influence doctors covertly when they are unsure about the propriety of doing so openly. In their study of general practice patients in South Wales, Stimson and Webb observed how doubts and disagreements were generally hinted at rather than made explicit, questions were put tentatively and carefully and information was withheld or manipulated so that patients could try to constrain the doctors to see the problem and the required treatment in the way the patient intended. In general, commented Stimson (1978), 'patient strategies tend to be covert and subtle' in order to avoid open conflict and, therefore, not always easily visible or directly recognizable to doctors.

It seems that doctors can remain quite unaware of the extent to which patients spend time making sense, evaluating, and on this basis, altering, the advice they are given. An example provided by West (1976) concerns the mother of a fourteen-year old girl who had been having epileptic seizures on and off since she was three years old and lately with increased frequency. West reports that initially her mother said she took no action 'because two other children had similar episodes and "grew out of them"'. However, following a seizure after she was hospitalized, epilepsy was diagnosed and appropriate medication prescribed. Soon afterward, however, her mother reported she took her off the tablets 'because there were no symptoms'. The girl took no more medicine for five years during which she was apparently symptom free. However, according to West, 'in order to keep up the appearance of being a "good" mother, she regularly went to her GP to obtain repeat prescriptions' (West 1976: 29).

If a patient's attempts to contribute to consultations are not encouraged or are frustrated, it seems there may be several negative consequences, although as in West's example, these may not always be obvious to the doctor involved. For example, patients who leave a consultation with ideas they have not shared with the doctor may reach medically erroneous and disadvantageous conclusions about what is happening to them. This may cause them to lose confidence and respect in their doctor and/or to ignore his advice and fail to comply with treatment. Another negative consequence of patients' keeping their thoughts to themselves has also been noted. It has been suggested that many patients are reluctant to run any risk that their doctor might think they might be unco-operative (Skipper 1965; Tagliacozzo and Mauksch, 1958) with the result that according to Lorber (1975) they keep silent when they do not understand and thus fail to co-operate by mistake.

Of the several ways patients can help the success of the communication process, asking questions and expressing doubts may be the most important. Patients who ask questions can save their doctors from the impossibly laborious task they would otherwise have if they had to guess what their patients would not understand and also to anticipate all the possible confusions there might be. It is very difficult to communicate without making assumptions about what people know (for example, Garfinkel 1964; Cicourel 1964) and if patients help in the process, therefore, it ought to be advantageous. Ley and Spelman (1967), who subsequently became more preoccupied with how a doctor could make his message 'clear' without a patient's encouragement, always recognized that if patients would ask questions or express doubts, this would be an effective way of warning doctors that explanations and instructions were not being understood. In this way questions and doubts expressed to doctors can enable the latter to make their instructions more comprehensible and more comprehensive – a view endorsed by physicians such as Hawkins (1967) and Fletcher (1973).

The extent to which patients participate and its consequences

Social science literature on the subject of how far patients attempt to facilitate a process of sharing ideas in consultations is rather contradictory. There is doubt about how frequently and how freely patients volunteer their ideas or try to clarify what their doctors say to them. There is also uncertainty about the effect of such behaviour on doctors and what happens in the consultation. Doctors, on the basis of their experience, tend to suggest that most patients show little sign of wanting to share ideas. They tend to be sceptical as to whether most patients have ideas or are interested in sharing information at all (1).

On the one hand, quantitative research has mostly tended to support the idea that only a minority of patients are very active. This conclusion is apparent from several studies in which patient participation has been investigated by counting their statements, questions, and other utterances by means of Interaction Process Analysis (Bales 1950). The method does not discriminate the content of the information patients present or the kinds of information to which their questions are addressed. It was developed for purposes other than studying doctor – patient consultations and has been applied without discussion or formulation of the various ways a patient can contribute in a consultation or the purpose there might be for doing so. With those limitations in mind the research does suggest that patients talk much less than doctors, usually ask fewer questions, and are less likely to express open disagreement (Korsch, Gozzi, and Francis 1968; Bain 1977; Roter 1977).

Two smaller quantitative studies which specifically developed methods to explore one aspect of a patient's behaviour, asking questions, provide more detailed information about patients' tendency to be active participants. Boreham and Gibson (1978), in Australia, separated the questions patients might ask according to the topic they addressed. They found that the proportion of consultations in which questions were asked on each of the separate topics was low. Although patients seeing the doctor for the second time in an illness episode asked more questions on several topics than those making their first visit, the topic which patients asked about most frequently (the name of the drug they were prescribed) was addressed by only a quarter of them. Topics such as the causes of the condition, detailed explanation of diagnosis or the effect of the drug were asked about by less than ten per cent of the patients. In her New York study Svarstad (1974) also found that the proportion of patients asking questions on specific topics was small. Less than a fifth (18 per cent) asked questions specifically requesting more detailed instructions about treatment and two-fifths actually asked no questions at all. One third of the patients asked three questions or more. Svarstad also found that nearly half the patients (44 per cent) hearing the doctor mention a term with which they were not familiar stayed silent (Svarstad 1974: 171).

The quantitative studies observing what doctors and patients actually say to each other suggest that many patients do not actively seek information by asking questions in consultations. One rather different study has explored another aspect of patient behaviour, how far they are prepared to express doubt and criticism. About half the sample of individuals studied in the USA by Haug and Lavin (1981) by means of questionnaires claimed that they had taken part at some time in their past in a consultation in which they had told a doctor his advice was too difficult, too costly, not necessary, or not consistent with their opinion. Summarizing quantitative studies, therefore, it seems that there is evidence that patients are prepared to ask questions and express doubts as well as evidence that they stay silent even when they admit they do not know what the doctor is saying. How far divergences result from methodological or 'real' differences is unclear.

The proposition that patients actively seek information and negotiate what they want with their doctors in consultations is based, mainly, on the series of small-scale developmental studies mentioned in Chapter 2. Part of the thesis of some of those authors was that there is endemic conflict and negotiation in medical consultations and, therefore, that giving and withholding information is part of a strategy of one person to control the other. Since these authors also usually consider that in formal terms the doctor is in a superior position of authority and knowledge, they have argued that it is inevitable that much patient activity is covert and, therefore, hard to recognize. If the argument is accepted it means that it would not be altogether surprising if doctors are less aware of patient's being active than research workers. It would also follow that sensitive approaches to measurement would be required to measure such behaviour quantitatively. One sociologist, Sharrock (1979), however, has argued an opposing view. He has suggested that when investigators have illustrated ways in which patients negotiate they have sometimes disproportionately emphasized patient efforts and so given a misleading picture of their activity in consultations. Sharrock takes West to task, for example, for emphasizing how a particular patient held his own against a doctor by asking a question, but for not recognizing how easily the doctor succeeded in ignoring it (Sharrock 1979: 134). Such difficulties of interpretation are accentuated when research workers select examples but do not indicate how frequently such cases occur in their data.

Hughes (1982) has made a rather different point about the interpretation of consultation data. Studying patients and doctors in a specialist (cardiology) out-patient clinic, he argued that a main communication problem they faced followed from patients' apparent difficulty in knowing how to develop their ideas. Often, he argued, the doctor gave them an open-ended opportunity to speak and they ran out of words. Long before the doctor had to interrupt the patients' flow of speech he had to prevent an uneasy silence. Hughes considered the problem as one of lack of communicative competence on the part of patients. Although he did not describe it explicitly Hughes identifies another problem for recognizing and measuring patient behaviour. As in the case of determining whether doctors gave information, the methodological problem is to distinguish lack of effort from not very skilled efforts.

The effect of patient behaviour

One effect if patients express their ideas, ask questions or air doubts might be to help their doctors to know what advice might best suit them or where their understanding is deficient (from a medical viewpoint). How far such advice or information is forthcoming if patients behave in this way, however, has rarely been the subject of study. The Interaction Process studies mentioned before, although detailed in their own way, were insufficiently sensitive to throw much light on this subject. The only two studies of which we are aware, therefore, are those by Svarstad (1974) and Boreham and Gibson (1978). In fact one of Boreham and Gibson's aims was to test the hypothesis that patients might be able to influence the 'informative process'. Because few patients asked questions and doctors quite often gave information they concluded that doctors rather than patients were the main influence on whether information was shared. Put that way Boreham and Gibson's conclusion was reasonable. However, if the data they present is examined carefully by arranging it in the form of *Table 5.1* it is apparent that patients had more of an influence than the authors seem to have realized. Asking a question was nearly always associated with receiving the relevant information. Patients who asked questions were between twice and twenty times as likely to receive information as those who did not.

Svarstad (1974) also examined the effect of different questions patients could ask on the content of the information they were given. She found that many of the instructions given by doctors to their patients were unclear and incomplete. Patients would often have to guess about such matters as how long drugs should be taken, how regularly, and in what dosage schedules. However, if patients had doubts or were unsure during the consultation they could, she hypothesized, try to obtain information by asking their doctors to clarify instructions. Svarstad found that those patients who sought such clarification by asking questions were much more likely to obtain adequate instruction than those who did not ask questions. In 22 out of 23 of the consultations in which a patient specifically asked a doctor to provide more detailed instructions the doctors gave them. Furthermore, patients who asked three questions of any kind were also more likely than those who asked fewer than three questions to receive detailed instructions (Svarstad 1974: 177ff.).

The fact that some doctors respond to patients' questions by trying to share information may surprise some of those authors who have been concerned with the social conflicts in consultations. The work of Svarstad and Boreham and Gibson,

Table 5.1 *The influence of a patient's questions on the provision of medical information in Australia*

	patient asked a question (%)	patient did not ask a question (%)
proportion of consultation in which doctor gave information of various types:		
diagnosis	3/3 (100)	36/77 (47)
minimal explanation	7/7 (100)	17/73 (23)
detailed explanation	6/6 (100)	4/73 (5)
progress of condition (improving, etc.)	5/5 (100)	18/75 (24)
causes of condition	5/6 (83)	9/74 (12)
symptoms	2/2 (100)	11/78 (14)

Source: Adapted from Boreham and Gibson (1978: 412).

however, confirms the general idea that asking questions in medical consultations is likely to be an effective way of obtaining information. They do not, however, provide detailed guidance as to what sort of questions might be effective in obtaining different types of information: for example, a statement of a doctor's diagnosis or his reasons for believing it. Equally, they say little about the consequence of other possible patient behaviours, such as withholding information, telling doctors ideas and explanatory hypotheses, or expressing doubts.

According to the general practitioner Holden (1977), 'most doctors today' expect, indeed desire, their patients to be ill; to respect medical authority; to show no sign of questioning their doctor's diagnosis or medical advice; to recognize that most doctors are busy and important; to use only the proper channels to gain access; to accept prescriptions and to be medically ignorant. If this is what doctors do indeed desire, then a patient's wish to play a more active part is likely to be evaded and even to cause conflict between them.

The conflict of expectations that can occur between doctors and patients was considered by Danziger (1978) when she observed doctors and pregnant mothers during antenatal consultations in the USA. She suggested that conflicting ideas, especially about each other's areas of competence or expertise, produced hostility in doctors and patients. Hostility and conflict could be expected, for instance, if a patient saw herself as a 'knowledgeable participant' while the doctor saw himself as the expert. It could also occur if doctors looked for 'knowledgeable participants' but found 'passive recipients' instead.

Danziger's study was exploratory. Quantitative research examining conflicting ideas about how to behave in consultations provides some further evidence. Roter (1977) studied what doctors and patients said to each other quantitatively by means of a social experiment. She found that patients who were given some prior encouragement to ask questions and generally to take a more active part in their consultations, did so more often than those not given such encouragement. However, the doctors were observed to get angry more often and to be less sympathetic to those patients taking a more active part. No evidence was available as to whether patients were given more information or if doctors adjusted their behaviour or advice. Moreover, Roter was uncertain how far their more angry and less sympathetic behaviour was part of a process of adjusting to new experience or the result of a more fundamental dislike by doctors of patients who asked questions.

To summarize the research evidence, it seems there is some indication that patients who ask questions can influence the information they receive and also some confirmation of the idea that patients who behave in this way may be restricted or otherwise responded to negatively by their doctors. The evidence is somewhat contradictory about how active patients are in general, although it is also possible that those patients willing to ask questions or express doubts are on the increase. So far no study has examined quantitatively the effect on the information patients are given of a range of different patient behaviours such as presenting information, asking questions and expressing doubts. Little is known also about how usual or unusual it is for patients to behave in these ways. Finally, there is little quantitative evidence about the extent to which patients do select and withhold information from their doctors. Moreover, no quantitative study has explored how patients account for their behaviour in a consultation. Why, for example, if they do not understand what the doctor is saying, do they remain quiet and passive?

Measuring patient behaviour

In the light of the problematic nature of the evidence about patients' behaviour in consultations, there were three main objectives for investigating it in our study. First, we wanted to estimate how many patients seemed to take an active part in encouraging their doctors to exchange ideas with them. Second, we wanted to know what effect this behaviour usually had: did doctors respond by giving information or did they try to evade the fact that patients had their own concerns? Third, we wanted to know how patients themselves explained their consulting behaviour.

To examine the extent to which patients presented ideas to their doctors or encouraged their doctors to give them information an analogous approach was applied to the patient's behaviour as that already applied to the doctor's. It did not seem to us that previous attempts to count the number of questions, count the number of statements betraying affect, or add up the length of time patients spent speaking in different phases of the consultation, were sufficiently sensitive or meaningful indicators of how active a part they tried to play. Skilfully phrased, relevant and articulate utterances might be just as effective as a lot of talk. What was needed was a way of determining how far every aspect of a patient's behaviour in a particular consultation contributed to the task of conveying to the doctor that the patient was trying to explain his problems, was trying to indicate his priorities, was trying to understand his doctor's advice, and was trying to encourage his doctor to elaborate. More dimensions of a patient's behaviour than asking questions or expressing affects needed to be considered and more precisely. This was achieved by conceiving of asking questions as just one means of trying to take an active part in the consultation and also by distinguishing different kinds of questions from the point of view of what they addressed.

Eventually, the five dimensions of patients' behaviour listed in *Table 5.2* were identified for study. Based on the ideas reviewed earlier in the chapter it seemed that patients might influence the flow of information in consultations by the way they selectively presented their problems, by choosing to volunteer aspects of their explanatory models, by asking questions to clarify a doctor's view or his instructions, by asking questions to find out the doctor's rationale and by expressing doubts.

Table 5.2 *Five dimensions of patient behaviour*

---

1 Setting the agenda: presenting details of the problem and elaborating the influence of the problem on concerns, feelings, plans.

2 Presenting and elaborating explanatory models or theories about which they would like the doctor to comment.

3 Seeking clarification of a doctor's views and instructions.

4 Asking for a doctor's reasons and rationales.

5 Expressing doubts.

Setting an agenda

The first means of influence was investigated by trying to determine how much information about their illness, its treatment and its implications, patients mentioned to their doctors and how much they kept to themselves. In most of the consultations observed in the pilot study the doctor normally invited the patient to indicate his reason for coming and so offered him the chance to set the agenda.

This is when a patient could talk about the problems he had been suffering from and his efforts to deal with them. He could talk about any physical symptoms, states of mind, or other problems that he had. He could mention the medicines he had taken, if any, and the extent to which he had or had not followed any advice he might have received from the doctor on a previous occasion. In doing so he could be more or less precise about such matters as the quality of symptoms, the time-scale in which he had experienced them and the context or situation in which they had arisen. If he wished, he could extend his description beyond the 'narrow' biological aspects of symptoms to mention his problem in other dimensions. He might, for instance, talk about the impact of symptoms on his life – for example, by telling his doctor that the symptoms make him feel ashamed, guilty, frightened, or likely to lose his job. According to those who emphasize the negotiation aspects of consultations a patient has the chance, both in presenting the details of his problem, what he has done about it and the impact of it, to emphasize or de-emphasize different aspects and he can choose which bits of information to put in and which to leave out.

To look at how patients set agendas, what they said in their consultation was compared with what they said at the subsequent interview. What they told the doctor about any symptoms, efforts at treatment or self-treatment, and social and psychological problems was compared with answers they gave to a short check list used during the research interview with them (2). An estimate of how regularly patients shape the agenda of their consultations by selecting and withholding relevant facts from those they could have mentioned was then prepared.

Overt and covert behaviour
The other means of influence – presenting explanatory models, asking questions and expressing doubts – have been examined by exploring the whole consultation for more and less obvious signs of each behaviour. Everything a patient said was considered, in turn, from the point of view of whether it could be understood as presenting aspects of an explanatory model, asking the various kinds of questions or expressing doubts. In the case of asking questions and expressing doubts what patients said was explored in relation to each of the topics of information used to examine doctors' behaviour: diagnostic-significance; treatment- and preventive-action.

The arguments that patients may have been coerced by normative or interactional constraints to adopt only 'covert' ways of trying to participate in their consultations (Lorber 1975; Stimson and Webb 1975; West 1976; Sharrock 1979) and also that they may sometimes lack the skill to indicate to the doctor what they want to tell him or to find out (Hughes 1982), presented a problem for assessing their behaviour. To try to understand the phenomena further it was decided both to try to recognize more obvious (overt) attempts by patients to participate and also less obvious ones (covert). For this purpose it was necessary to consider what each of the patient activities might involve, and when they could be considered 'overt' and when 'covert'.

The criteria used to determine how active a patient was in regard to presenting explanatory models, asking questions and expressing doubts, were based on the idea that patients who spoke in such a way as to make it quite clear to an observer that they had an idea, question or doubt were considered to have been 'active'.

Explanatory models

Attending a consultation provided a patient with the opportunity to inform a doctor about how he thought what was happening might be explained. Patients, for example, may consider that they have a 'not normal' infection, a vitamin deficiency, a problem caused by stress or tension, a social problem, a crippling or life-threatening disease, etc. They may also have particular reasons for believing in a particular theory which they could convey to the doctor. For example, they might have developed a clear view of why their symptoms are not following (what they consider) the usual pattern for a normal infectious illness or how their symptoms are exactly like those their grandmother had before she died.

Patients who volunteered any kind of explanatory hypothesis (for example, a diagnostic name) were considered to present their explanatory model at least 'covertly'. Those who also gave the doctor some opportunity for insight into their reasons for explaining matters in their particular way could be regarded as attempting a more 'overt' influence. The distinctions could be made reliably (3).

Asking questions

Once patients had been given the opportunity to present their problems doctors would usually start to try to understand them and then begin to arrive at a more or less tentative diagnosis. As this was happening the patient would have an opportunity to ask questions addressed to several different types of information. First, the patient could try to clarify what the doctor was thinking or he could attempt to ascertain the doctor's underlying rationale. To clarify the doctor's thinking on a topic he could ask him a question which might encourage him to state his views more clearly. A question might be addressed to his views on one of the three topics (diagnostic-significance, treatment- or preventive-action) or to clarify the details of how to follow instructions. To help the patient to evaluate the doctor's advice, the patient could ask the doctor to explain his rationale. The doctor could be asked why he thought the patient had a particular condition, why he did not consider a treatment or procedure appropriate, why he thought the patient was suffering from an ordinary problem rather than a more complex one, why he thought the patient should lose weight or give up alcohol.

Asking for clarification and asking for reasons were two sorts of patient activity which it seemed worthwhile to distinguish. While the former might not be understood as conveying a desire to participate in making choices, the latter is far less ambiguous in this respect. The two types of questions might also have different effects. They might stimulate different attempts to share information by a doctor and might have a different influence on the consultation process. Questions seeking a doctor's rationale might be expected to increase the chance of a doctor realizing his patient wants him to facilitate choice. This might lead him to try to share information more or it might make him annoyed and evasive. The reactions anticipated by Danziger and observed by Roter might be an outcome.

To decide how far patients had made it clear they wanted to know what the doctor's view was, about his instructions or about his rationale, all interrogative statements a patient made (judged by content and tone of voice) were examined. The rater was then asked to take on, as it were, the role of participant in the consultation and (following a set of rating guidelines) to use his intuitive communication skills to determine to what a question seemed to be addressed. Questions were considered to be clearly (and therefore 'overtly') addressed to discovering the doctor's rationale if the rater felt quite confident this was what a patient was asking. Most obviously, questions which stated or implied a 'why' query fitted into this category. Questions aimed at clarifying how an underlying causal mechanism or diagnostic process 'worked' might also be of this type. Questions, on the other hand, which seemed to ask 'what' were much more ambiguous in their meaning. They could be considered both as 'covert' examples of questions addressed to obtaining rationales or 'overt' examples of trying to obtain clarification – a feature of the rating procedure in all aspects of the study was that the same word or phrase could be considered to convey more than one kind of idea. Still more ambiguous questions like 'Tablets?' or 'Wednesday?', depending on the context, could be considered only 'covert' examples of trying to seek clarification. Distinctions of this kind, which are illustrated by examples in the next chapter, could be made reliably (4).

Expressing doubts

The possible consequences for consultation outcomes of ignoring patients' ideas have been discussed several times. Patients may leave with biomedically inaccurate ideas intact and unchallenged and also react by ignoring advice. Also they may have their doubts after the consultation, discuss them with a friend and at that point decide to ignore what a doctor has said. If doubts and disagreements do not surface in a consultation the doctor has no opportunity to change his advice or strategy so that it is more suited to the patient's beliefs. On the other hand, expressing doubts may be felt by doctor (and patient) to be a criticism and may be a cause of evasion and discomfort in a consultation. For all these reasons, a way of identifying whether patients did give more and less obvious signs of their doubts in their consultations required development.

Any doubts a patient might express and the extent to which a patient gave a doctor reasons for being doubtful were the focus of observation. Sometimes patients might express their doubts quite openly by means of a direct statement. Alternatively, they might express a doubt more indirectly. This might be done through a question (said in a particular way at a particular juncture) or by still less direct means indicating disquiet: such as by making abrupt changes of subject, constantly repeating ideas, frequently re-introducing new symptoms, or vaguely sounding dissatisfied. It was decided to judge patients adopting more indirect means as expressing their doubts covertly. Those who made more direct statements, leaving no uncertainty what their doubt was, were judged to behave overtly. Such distinctions could be made reliably (5,6).

Summary

Evidence about whether patients play an active information-seeking and sharing role and with what consequences in medical consultations is contradictory. Quantitative studies have not explored the full range of ways patients could influence the consultation process (by selecting what to bring to the doctor, by presenting him with their explanation of what is happening to them, by asking questions and by expressing doubts) and have mostly been restricted to counting statements or time units without attending to the ideas a patient is introducing. Developmental studies, on the other hand, have been queried because of the way data has been selected to present findings. An approach to measuring how far patients try to influence the sharing of information in consultations, and whether they do so more or less overtly, has been described.

CHAPTER 6

The way patients played their parts and its consequences

We have noted that neither the clinical characteristics of patients' illnesses nor their social characteristics had much effect on the probability that they would be given information, or even on how it was given if it was. It was, therefore, all the more interesting that the efforts a patient made to encourage doctors to share information could influence the information they were given, and in several ways. Patients who asked questions or expressed doubts were much more likely to receive information from their doctors than those who did not. Also, patients who offered an explanation for their illness were more likely to have their views explored than those who did not behave in these ways. We start, however, with the first research question concerning patients' behaviour: how active were they?

The extent to which patients were active

The device of comparing what patients mentioned to doctors in their consultations with what they mentioned at interview, revealed that most of the patients studied did select what to tell their doctors. This was evident because they kept a great deal of information to themselves (*Table 6.1*). First, about two-thirds of those patients who reported symptoms in answer to the brief health questionnaire they were given had not mentioned some of these in their consultation. Second, just under two-thirds of those taking some kind of medication had not mentioned this behaviour in their consultation. Third, over two-thirds of those reporting themselves to be depressed or anxious (either as a consequence or independently of their illness), or of those reporting that they smoked, were overweight or drank alcohol to a degree that seemed to cause them concern, also did not mention these facts in their consultation. Finally, just under two-thirds of those with social troubles (either as a consequence or independently of their illness) failed to mention to their doctor those aspects of their relevant experience which they had reported at interview (1). Such estimates of how much patients kept back from their doctors are consistent with more general findings that the symptoms taken to a doctor for help are a small proportion of all those experienced (Tuckett 1976: 161). The findings demonstrate the interpretive and evaluative work that occurs among patients when deciding what to tell their doctors and also the extent to which the doctors studied were reliant upon

Table 6.1 *Setting agendas: what patients said they had not told their doctors*

	content areas			
whether or not doctor knows	general health (%)	pill-taking (%)	reaction to symptoms/mental state/habits (%)	consequences of symptoms/ work/housing relationships (%)
something relevant and not mentioned although patient thinks doctor does not know:	65 (66)	62 (63)	69 (70)	61 (62)
something relevant and not mentioned although patient thinks doctor knows from before:	12 (12)	9 (9)	14 (14)	9 (9)
patient told the doctor everything relevant or had nothing relevant to pass on:	21 (22)	27 (28)	15 (16)	28 (29)
total	98 (100)	98 (100)	98 (100)	98 (100)

them to volunteer information (2). We did not, however, attempt to understand why patients withheld the information and what were the consequences of this.

Many patients also showed that they were trying to influence the consultation by providing some explanation for their symptoms, asking questions or expressing doubts (*Table 6.2*). Using the method of assessment described in the previous chapter, just over a quarter (26 per cent) of the patients were estimated to offer their doctors some kind of explanation for their symptoms. Nearly half (47 per cent) asked their doctor to clarify some aspect of his diagnostic hypothesis, treatment-action or preventive advice and about the same number (49 per cent) asked their doctor to supply a rationale for his view on at least one of the topics. Just over half the patients (56 per cent) expressed a doubt. In all just over four-fifths (85 per cent) offered an explanation, asked a question or expressed a doubt. Over a half (53 per cent) behaved in one of these ways overtly. Overall the results suggest a high level of patient participation (3).

Table 6.2 *Patient behaviour in 405 consultations*

	no sign *(%)*	*covert participation* *(%)*	*overt participation* *(%)*	*total*
indicating explanatory models	297 (73)	54 (13)	54 (13)	405
seeking clarification of a doctor's views	206 (51)	62 (15)	137 (34)	405
seeking clarification of instructions	214 (53)	177 (44)	14 (4)	405
asking for reasons and rationales	206 (51)	185 (46)	14 (4)	405
expressing doubts	180 (44)	116 (29)	109 (27)	405
at least one of the above	60 (15)	130 (32)	215 (53)	405

Just over one in ten (13 per cent) of the patients studied was reckoned to offer an explanation of their symptoms in a covert fashion. This means that a patient would have volunteered to the doctor a diagnostic hypothesis as an explanation of the symptoms. An example was Mrs Morrison (1027) who brought her daughter to the doctor saying 'She's so whacked out, this is what I wanted to check with you, could that be the penicillin?'. Although she did not elaborate why she thought penicillin could explain her daughter's symptoms and, therefore, provide a doctor with any clues as to why she explains matters in the way she does, it is apparent she has a hypothesis. A fragment of her explanatory thinking has been mentioned and this was enough to justify a 'covert' rating. Just over one in ten patients (13 per cent) went beyond presenting a diagnostic hypothesis to mention some of their reasoning in support (*Table 6.2*). They were considered to present aspects of their explanatory model 'overtly'. Mrs Cord's consultation (1074) was an example. She explained that she thought her child might have the same illness as she had, because of various aspects she had noticed about the way the illness started. Mrs Cord was considered to offer her explanation 'overtly' because she provided the doctor with some indication of the reasoning behind her hypothesis.

Turning to the questions patients asked, it will be noticed from *Table 6.2* that less than 1 in 25 patients (4 per cent) were considered to make it clear 'overtly' to their doctor that they wanted him to clarify instructions. A third (34 per cent) asked a doctor 'overtly' to clarify some aspect of what he had said and less than 1 in 25 (4 per cent) made it quite clear they wanted to know a doctor's rationale. Patients were considered to make it clear to a doctor that they wanted to know his rationale only if they asked questions which it took very little inference to recognize as attempts to obtain reasons. They asked, for instance, 'What happens if I don't have it done?' (2457) or, 'I see, and what effect will it have on me, the antibiotic?' (1412). Both these questions appear to address themselves to discovering the advantages and effects of treatment and so to providing the rationale for it.

By contrast, questions considered as 'covert' examples were those which required more inference to decide they might have such a goal. They would quite clearly be interrogatives (detected by a form of words or by tone of voice and context) but would be questions which left it open whether or not a patient wanted a doctor to clarify concepts or offer his rationale. They were questions like 'Do I have to have my eye bandaged or anything like that? ' (2457) or 'And no after-effects at all? ' (2457) or 'But won't it bring up the phlegm?' (1412). These questions are all examples of interrogatives (judging by the way they were said) which could be seeking information relevant to evaluation, but may not have been doing so. They were much more common than questions 'overtly' asking for reasons and occurred in nearly half the consultations studied (*Table 6.2*).

Whatever the difficulty of deciding if some questions were seeking a doctor's rationale, it was not too difficult to infer that many of them were at least seeking clarification of what the diagnosis was or what the treatment concerned. They were, therefore, rated as 'overt' questions seeking clarification. Nearly a third of the consultations contained at least one question of this kind (*Table 6.2*). Some other questions were not so clearly seeking clarification of a doctor's view on a topic. Patients might repeat what doctors said in an interrogative form by saying 'Rheumatism?' (1437), or 'Distalgesic?' (1051). Such questions were 'covert' examples of seeking clarification because, although it seemed likely patients were asking for more information, their question was not necessarily obvious as such and they did not make it very clear what they wanted to know. Questions of this kind could be found in about one in seven consultations (*Table 6.2*).

Turning to the issue of how often patients expressed their doubts, we estimated that over a quarter did so in a relatively obvious manner (*Table 6.2*). One circumstance in which an 'overt' doubt was rated was if the reasons patients had for doubting could be recognized quite easily. An example is Mrs Dennison's consultation (1745) about the problem of her child's bed-wetting. The following interchange was observed mid-way through the consultation:

Doctor: Well, you get him up at night?
Patient: No, I did try that but it didn't work. I think he wets in the early hours

in the morning. About 4 o'clock.
Doctor: Yes, but it's worth trying.
Patient: I have got him up in the night.
Doctor: Yes, but it is worth doing that.
Patient: But it hasn't made any difference, I mean I've tried all sorts. Not giving
   him drinks and so on.

In this example the patient's tone of voice and the content of what she said
made it easy to draw the inference that she was doubtful about the doctor's suggestion and that this was because she felt it had been tried and found wanting.

An 'overt' doubt was also rated if patients repeated a pattern of behaviour so
markedly that it was certain they were doubtful, even if the details of why they
were so was unclear. In one consultation Mrs Dawson (1911) was not prepared
to let her doctor conclude the interaction without trying to get some treatment:

Doctor: Right, I think you need more time, it's just a matter of a bit more time.
Patient: Could you give me something to try and pick me up?
Doctor: Oh, I don't think it will help, honestly.
Patient: You know I feel so down in the dumps.

In this exchange the patient did not explicitly doubt the doctor's decision that
she should wait before having further treatment. But the pattern of the discourse,
the tone of the patient's voice (quite easily identified in the recording), and the
context, all combined to suggest she was certainly doubtful, even if we must guess
to know why (4).

'Covert' doubts were recognized in just under a third of the consultations (*Table
6.2*). They would be rated if, during their consultations, patients seemed to indicate
they might be in doubt or have a disagreement but it was not possible to be sure
that this was so. The following extract from Mrs Verra's consultation (2282) is
an example:

Doctor: Yes there's no problem about that.
Patient: Mmm.

In this instance, what the patient said and how she said it seemed to indicate there
was some doubt in her mind but it is hard to know what was the difficulty.

To summarize the findings so far, most patients withheld information from their
doctors and nearly four-fifths either presented an explanation of their symptoms,
asked questions or expressed doubts. Far fewer, however, offered explanations, asked
questions or expressed doubts in an obvious (overt) way. Indeed as few as 4 per
cent asked doctors to give their reasons in an articulate and clear way. Rather,
they showed evidence of wanting concepts and instructions to be clarified, of wanting
to know doctors' reasons, and of having their own explanations for their symptoms, but not unambiguously. They employed hints, vague questions, and generally

more covert forms of behaviour. Such findings, therefore, are consistent with those that would be expected by authors who have emphasized that patients' behaviour is extensive but, because of a belief that they are not meant to be active, largely covert. The observed behaviour was consistent with the idea that patients thought that their doctors would disapprove if they displayed their wish to participate more openly. On the other hand, the findings might also be explained, at least in part, by the fact that patients were not particularly skilled in phrasing their contributions and in knowing quite what they wanted or how to get it across. Before taking this debate further the influence of patients' behaviour will be examined.

The influence of patient behaviour

A second objective of observing patients' efforts to tell their doctors what they thought, or to try to get their doctors to elaborate to them, was to examine the effects when they did. First, it was clear that the way patients behaved could exert an influence. Patients who offered explanations, asked questions and expressed doubts were treated significantly differently to those who did not. By acting in these ways patients appeared to influence their doctors to be more interested in their lay ideas and beliefs about what was wrong, to state more clearly what was wrong or what should be done and to give them 'moderately elaborate' reasoning in support of judgements.

Patients who themselves indicated they had an explanatory hypothesis were more likely to take part in consultations in which doctors appeared to show interest in their ideas. On average only about 1 in 16 consultations contained 'active' efforts by a doctor to get patients to elaborate their views about diagnostic-significance. However, when patients spontaneously presented their ideas and gave their reasons for believing them doctors responded to them in about 1 in 11 consultations (*Table 6.3*). Moreover, even patients who volunteered ideas about diagnostic-significance without explaining their reasons were more likely than those who did not do so at all to have their ideas explored (5).

Patients who asked doctors to give them information about their treatment recommendations (6) were more likely to obtain such clarification. Nearly a third of the patients 'overtly' asking for clarification (64 per cent), compared to two-fifths of those asking 'covertly' or not asking at all, had the details of *what* doctors advised stated to them in a clear way (*Table 6.4*) (7).

Third, patients who asked doctors to provide reasons to support their ideas greatly increased their chance of obtaining from them 'moderately elaborate' reasons in support of their ideas. *Table 6.5* shows that patients who asked for reasons quite directly, although rare, were twice as likely as those not asking for reasons to obtain 'moderately elaborate' reason giving. They were also a great deal more likely to be given 'moderately elaborate' reasoning than those who asked indirectly (8). The effect of asking questions was particularly dramatic if patients also had a 'diagnostically-significant' condition (pp 69–70). *Table 6.6* shows that the proportion

Table 6.3 *The influence of presenting explanatory models on whether doctors asked patients to elaborate their ideas*

	patients who indicated explanatory models			
	overtly (with reasons) (%)	covertly (without reasons) (%)	not (%)	total (%)
extent to which doctors asked for elaboration				
some active efforts	5 (9)	2 (4)	16 (5)	23 (6)
some ambiguous efforts	10 (19)	13 (24)	29 (10)	52 (13)
no effort or interruption	39 (72)	39 (72)	252 (85)	330 (81)
total	54 (100)	54 (100)	297 (100)	405 (100)

chi-square = 12.04 4 d/f p < 0.05
tau^c = 0.07 p < 0.001
gamma = 0.31

Table 6.4 *Asking for clarification of treatment advice and being given a clear statement about it*

	asking for clarification of treatment-action			
	overt (%)	covert (%)	not (%)	total (%)
statement of treatment-action advice				
clear	37 (64)	15 (40)	124 (40)	176 (44)
not clear	21 (35)	21 (55)	158 (51)	199 (49)
not present	1 (2)	2 (5)	27 (9)	30 (7)
total	58 (100)	38 (100)	309 (100)	405 (100)

chi-square 13.02 4 d/f p < 0.05
tau^c = 0.10 p < 0.001
gamma = 0.30

of patients given 'moderately elaborate' reasons on one topic rose from one-fifth (if they did not have a significant condition and did not ask questions) to three-quarters if patients both asked a question overtly and had a significant condition. Several case examples illustrate the process through which such questioning seemed to lead to the receipt of information.

Table 6.5 *The effect of asking for reasons and expressing doubts on whether a patient was given reasons*

	asking for reasons			expressing doubts		
	overtly (%)	covertly (%)	not at all (%)	overtly (%)	covertly (%)	not at all (%)
reasoning						
moderately						
elaborate	8 (57)	67 (36)	53 (26)	40 (37)	43 (37)	45 (25)
minimal	5 (36)	83 (45)	89 (43)	43 (39)	55 (47)	79 (44)
none	1 (7)	35 (19)	64 (31)	26 (24)	18 (16)	56 (31)
total	14 (100)	185 (100)	206 (100)	109 (100)	116 (100)	180 (100)

chi-square = 14.29 4 d/f $p < 0.01$ chi-square = 12.28 4 d/f $p < 0.05$
$tau^c = 0.15$ $p < 0.001$ $tau^c = 0.11$ $p < 0.05$
gamma = 0.28   gamma = 0.18

Mrs Lane's consultation (2457) was an example of a consultation in which the patient's behaviour appeared crucial to the information she received. Mrs Lane was a sixty-four year-old dress-making cutter who lived in a pleasant council flat. She went to her doctor (whom she had been with for many years) following an out-patient appointment at an opthalmic hospital which had caused her considerable anxiety. Essentially, her consultation appeared to have the sole purpose of establishing her doctor's view about the specialist's opinion. The specialist had diagnosed a partially detached retina and had recommended laser surgery. As she put it at her interview this advice had 'frightened the life out of me. I just sat there and thought I was part of Star Wars for a minute. I was so taken aback I really couldn't. . . I wanted to question the doctor. . . but. . . I just asked how long it would take and that's all. . . then coming home I thought I could speak to (my general practitioner). . . I'm always able to speak to him.' At her consultation Mrs Lane came directly to the point telling her doctor what had been advised briefly and then saying what she wanted from him: 'Really I've come to ask you what you think about it.'

Her doctor examined her without asking further questions and after several minutes concluded:

Doctor: I would say definitely have it done.
Patient: Have it out?
Doctor: No question about it.
Patient: Only I. . .
Doctor: (interrupting) The laser. . .

Table 6.6 *The combined effect of the significance of a patient's diagnosis and whether he asked a doctor for reasons on his chances of being given reasons*

	no question; diagnosis not significant (%)	covert question; or diagnosis not significant (%)	overt question; or significant diagnosis (%)	covert question and significant diagnosis (%)	overt question and significant diagnosis (%)
proportion of consultations in which the reasons given (on one topic) were:					
moderately elaborate	31 (20)	42 (33)	24 (40)	25 (42)	6 (75)
minimal	70 (46)	55 (44)	22 (37)	28 (48)	2 (25)
none	51 (34)	29 (23)	14 (23)	6 (10)	0
total	152	126	60	59	8

chi-square = 28.17 8 d/f p < 0.001
tau^c = 0.21 p < 0.001
gamma = 0.30

Patient: (also interrupting) When he said laser beam it got me a bit. . .
Doctor: (interrupting) Well I'll explain to you. . .

In the course of the doctor's explanation of the intended surgery Mrs Lane made encouraging sounds indicating he should continue. She then began to probe for further details – 'No effects? He said I will only be there two hours? They said it will take about five minutes? But there's no anaesthetic at all? Is it because it's so fast? And no after effects at all – it doesn't sort of effect the eye lid or anything like that?' All of these the doctor answered economically. Mrs Lane then asked a direct question, considered by raters to be seeking his rationale overtly: 'What happens if I don't have it done?' It was in answer to this question that the doctor gave her a detailed justification for the treatment: 'You could progressively lose your vision in that eye. . .I don't think you have any choice in the matter. . .it really is a very effective treatment. . .in fact I have never known it fail. . .it's very effective and painless. There's no question, you've just got to have it done.'

Mrs Lawn's consultation (1087) is another example of a consultation apparently illustrating the finding that questions seeking reasons are causally influential in obtaining reason-giving explanation. Mrs Lawn was a thirty-two year-old self-employed women running a small business with her husband. They owned their own home. She visited her doctor because pains in her body were disturbing her sleep. Her doctor explained that her condition was a consequence of her pregnancy (Carpal Tunnel syndrome) and that she might be helped by a more potent diuretic. To this the patient responded 'Why am I getting it in one wrist (only)?' The question, which was also considered an expression of doubt, seemed to have prompted the doctor to explain the nature of her condition and to indicate the mechanism by which such pain was caused – in other words to justify the diagnosis in some detail. Other examples of such apparently successful direct requests for reasons were similar. For example, one patient asked 'Why does thrush come back?' (1337). In reply, her doctor explained the causal mechanism and gave preventive advice. Another patient queried the reasons for the treatment she was offered: 'What effect will it have on me? It'll stop the cough? What will it do?' (1466). She was given an explanation of why antibiotic treatment is advantageous for treating a chest infection. Finally, a third patient asked a doctor to explain why her daughter was miserable with her sore throat symptoms: 'Normally, when they get it they grizzle with it, don't they?' (1547). She was given reasons to support the possibility that the diagnosis might not be an ordinary sore throat but glandular fever.

A patient wanting to know why his or her doctor takes a view, therefore, appears to be wise to ask for the reasons quite openly. However, such questioning was also associated with a less desirable outcome. Patients who asked doctors to give reasons were more likely than others to experience a consultation characterized by evasive attitudes and behaviour on the part of doctors who chose not to explore the source of any disagreement. In such consultations tension was noticeable as the doctor and the patient were observed to talk at cross purposes, to change the topic of conversation dramatically and without exploration or acknowledgement, or to spar with each other in a confused and contradictory way (9). We found that 29 per cent of those overtly asking the doctor to give reasons experienced a consultation marked by evasion compared to 16 per cent if they asked covertly, and 7 per cent if they did not ask at all (*Table 6.7*).

Ms Anchor (1287) took part in a consultation which illustrates this less desirable outcome of seeking reasons. Like the other consultations in which questioning and 'evasion' were associated, the case also shows how sometimes patients' attempts to be treated as 'knowledgeable' could be wholly unsuccessful. Ms Anchor was an eighteen year-old sales assistant complaining of swollen ankles, spots and feeling miserable, some of which, she hinted, could be linked to the contraceptive pills she had recently started to take. Her doctor did not think her hypothesis likely (he did not offer reasons or ask her to elaborate her explanatory hypothesis) and implied to her that none of her complaints seemed to merit treatment. Ms Anchor re-introduced her spots for the third time at a stage when the doctor had twice denied her pill hypothesis. At this point the doctor advised they were caused by her diet – specifically fried foods – and subsequently invited her to choose between spots and chips. At this point the patient asked her question:

Table 6.7 *The effect of patients' behaviour on their chances of their ideas being evaded*

	asking for reasons			expressing doubts		
	overtly (%)	covertly (%)	not at all (%)	overtly (%)	covertly (%)	not at all (%)
consultation atmosphere						
no evasion	10 (71)	156 (84)	191 (93)	78 (72)	100 (86)	179 (94)
evasion	4 (29)	29 (16)	15 (7)	31 (28)	16 (14)	10 (6)
total	14	185	206	109	116	180

chi-square = 8.86 2 d/f p < 0.05   chi-square = 10.45 2 d/f p < 0.01
tau^c = 0.10 p < 0.001 tau^c = 0.25 p < 0.001
gamma = 0.43   gamma = 0.70

Patient: Well, why haven't I ever had them (the spots) before? Could my ankle (be swollen) because I am carrying too much weight?'
Doctor: Partly.
Patient: Could it? How much should I weigh for my height?
Doctor: How tall are you?

Her question was not answered and they talked at cross purposes for the rest of the consultation – the patient continuing to make suggestions and the doctor continuing to ignore them. The consultation ended with the doctor emphasizing how he did not need to see the patient for six months (and only then, it seemed, because it would be time to prescribe more contraceptive pills) and the patient interrupting to ask if he really meant that by saying, 'Say if I'm not well?'.

Ms Anchor's questions were not answered and appear to have been part of a consultation in which patient and doctor had different preoccupations and achieved little meeting of minds. The patient's attempts to introduce ideas were ignored or even not welcome. The interaction has some of the characteristics of true farce.

Ms Anchor's experience was shared by under one-third of those patients who, like her, made it clear they wanted to know the doctor's reasons. By contrast, the other patients who made it clear they wanted to know a doctor's reasons (the other two-thirds), like Mrs Lane and Mrs Lawn, were rewarded by being given 'moderately elaborate' explanations. Only one of these patients also found themselves in a consultation characterized by 'evasion'. Thus, while asking for reasons apparently carried a risk of an evasive and uncomfortable consultation, it carried a still higher probability of obtaining a positive response in the form of 'moderately elaborate' reasoning.

Patients who expressed doubts about what they were being told had a similar experience to those who asked for reasons. In the first place expressing doubts, albeit less frequently than asking for reasons, increased the likelihood a patient would be given 'moderately elaborate' justification. Just over a third of those who expressed doubts (whether in overt or covert ways) received some 'moderately elaborate' reason-giving compared to a quarter among those who did not (*Table 6.5*). However, to express doubt (still more so than to ask a question) was also to increase the chance of experiencing a consultation in which communication was observed to be at cross purposes or evasive. Twenty-eight per cent of those expressing an overt doubt, 14 per cent of those expressing a doubt covertly but only 1 per cent of those not doing so at all, had 'evasive' consultations (*Table 6.7*). Doubting, therefore, still more than asking for reasons, most often took place in consultations in which patients' ideas and opinions did not seem to be considered or perhaps appreciated.

To summarize, patients could influence both the quality of the information they received and the extent to which doctors responded to their ideas. Patients who behaved more directly as experts, that is those who engaged in overt forms of behaviour, were generally more likely than other patients to receive the kind of information needed to help their decision-making. When this outcome did not occur (i.e. when their efforts proved unsuccessful) the expressing of ideas, asking of questions, or airing of doubts seem to have contributed to creating consultations in which disagreement or talking at cross purposes were apparent. While on most occasions doctors seem to have responded seriously to questions, at other times, and particularly if doubts were expressed, they seem to have been unable or unwilling to respond to patients as 'knowledgeable' participants. In these consultations clues provided by patients (in the form of explanatory hypotheses, questions or doubts) were not used to try to achieve mutual understanding (10).

Patients' experience of their consultations

We have argued that the preponderance of 'covert' rather than 'overt' attempts to participate in consultations (if this is how patients' efforts to present explanatory models, ask questions and express doubts can be understood) has been explained in the past in two ways. It could indicate that patients lacked the skills to participate more clearly and to be articulate or it could be the product of the cultural stereotype of the 'good' patient as one who is supposed to be passive and not to have ideas, questions or doubts.

To explore what patients themselves thought about their behaviour and the reasons for it a random sample of ninety-eight patients was selected from among those interviewed (11). They were asked, whenever during interviews they appeared to exhibit gaps in their knowledge or had misgivings about what doctors had said, to tell interviewers their reasons for not expressing such doubts or not asking questions and so to try to fill gaps in their knowledge (12). The accounts patients gave of their behaviour by means of this device must be treated with caution. They represent, after all, situated accounts which patients may have constructed to display their competence as interview respondents. After the consultation they may try to tilt the unfavourable balance of power they have experienced in a consultation and to appear more rational and sensible than perhaps they are (Webb and Stimson 1976). None the less they are also accounts which can be read as demonstrations of their ideas about what is adequate behaviour for a doctor and a patient (see for example, Voysey 1975; Locker 1981; Baruch 1981). In any case, three-quarters (76 per cent) of the patients interviewed in this way mentioned specific doubts or questions which they had had during the interview but had not mentioned to the doctor. The answers they gave to explain why they had not asked questions or expressed doubts were then recorded verbatim and grouped together into several categories.

The most common answers patients volunteered suggested that they explained their behaviour in one or more of the following ways: they thought it was not up to them to ask questions, express doubts or behave as if their view was important; they said they had purposely left queries and doubts till next time when they could be more certain of what they thought was reasonable; they said that they doubted if their doctor could tell them any more at the moment; they said they felt hurried or unable to think about what they were being told or unable to formulate their views in the heat of the moment; they reported they were afraid of being thought less well of by their doctors; they reported that they were afraid of a negative reaction from the doctor (*Table 6.8*). Only a fifth (19 per cent) of those not asking questions gave as a reason that they were not interested in the answer. Only one in ten (9 per cent) of those not expressing a doubt gave fear of the truth as a reason for not doing so (*Table 6.8*).

Patients who said that they felt it was not up to them to express doubts or ask questions and those who said they were 'not interested' in asking questions are those whose answers best typify the attitude that there is a competence gap between doctors and patients. They expect to take advice 'on trust' and don't envisage trying to evaluate what they are told.

About a fifth (19 per cent) of the patients gave one reason suggesting that 'knowing' about medical matters was not for them: they were not interested. One patient, Mrs Warren (1376), expressed surprise at the idea anyone would be interested. 'I don't know I don't suppose I ever thought about it. I never really thought about asking him how they [the tablets] work and what is wrong or anything like that. As long as they can be corrected I don't mind. I'm not really interested really – as long as he can do something for me.'

One-third of the patients (36 per cent) reporting they had a question which they had not asked said they did not feel it was up to them to initiate matters in this way. Mrs Furnace (1934) was an example. She told the interviewer that

Table 6.8 *The reasons patients gave for not asking questions and not expressing doubts*

Number and percentage of patients giving each reason for:

	not asking for reasons[1] (%)	not expressing doubt[2] (%)
felt hurried	16 (27)	2 (6)
frightened of a bad reaction from doctor	8 (14)	6 (19)
frightened doctor will think less well of patient	13 (22)	11 (34)
forgot/will tell or ask next time	21 (36)	8 (25)
feels it is not up to patient to ask/mention	21 (36)	14 (44)
doubts if doctor knows answer (yet)	13 (22)	
not interested	11 (19)	
frightened to know the truth		3 (9)

1 59 of the 98 patients (60%) volunteered questions they had but which they had not expressed. These patients gave a total of 104 reasons for staying silent.

2 32 of the 98 patients (33%) volunteered they had a doubt which they had not expressed in the consultation. These patients gave a total of 44 reasons for staying silent.

she would have liked to know what her doctor was doing when he examined her. But, when asked why she had not asked him, she said 'I don't ask questions because even if doctors explained to me I wouldn't have a very good understanding – I think anyone who hasn't had a medical training [doesn't]. And I do feel the doctor mentions things. . .[when it's appropriate].' Another patient, Mr Biggs (2300), had doubts about the lump his doctor had found. When asked why he hadn't mentioned his doubts, however, he said: 'If he said it's only a cyst, that's it.' He was among the two-fifths of patients who gave at least one answer to suggest they kept doubts to themselves out of deference.

Other patients also did not seem to feel asking questions was appropriate. But their reasons suggested that they keep quiet from fear. Indeed, as many as half (47 per cent) the patients who failed to express doubts they had and about a third (32 per cent) of those who did not ask questions gave at least one reason falling into this category. They said they kept quiet because either they were frightened that their doctor would somehow demean them or they feared he would be annoyed and react 'badly'. Mrs Farriman (1466), for instance, told the interviewer she was very interested to know how her drugs worked but never 'bothered asking' because, 'his answer would be: "What do you know about it? It's nothing to do with you"'. Mrs Warner (2216) wondered if her daughter had pneumonia but did not ask because of a fear she would be considered 'neurotic'. She said: 'I don't have medical knowledge. That's why we go to the doctor. I don't like going because you get a lot of pressure that you are being neurotic and...are wasting their precious time.' Another patient, Mrs Forrest (1714), was worried whether she had a tumour but had not asked because, 'He does know his job but I think he doesn't like to be told. He likes to be the one to diagnose what's wrong, not for me to tell him what's wrong'. Finally, a fourth patient, Mrs Fawcett (1312), was unable to ask her doctor about problems with her voice: 'I don't know, probably he'll think I'm trying to question his judgement or something, you know.' Some of these patients went on to volunteer examples of the way they or their friends had been treated in the past.

Another reason for not asking questions given by a quarter (27 per cent) of the patients was that they felt hurried. Mrs Farriman (1466) (who also thought her doctor would tell her it was not her business to ask questions) was one such patient. She told the interviewer that she would have liked to know more about the lump on the back of her neck and what the doctor thought it was. She said: 'I think I made a mistake in not saying, "can you tell me what it is, will you look at the back of my neck and tell me what it is?" I should have said so. But I feel sorry for them because they're always so busy.' Many patients clearly did not find it easy to formulate their thoughts and questions in the 'heat' of the consultation moment and were not practiced in doing so. This was particularly obvious in interviews when the experience of reviewing what had happened and being asked questions about their doctor's understanding clearly became a learning process for many of them. They suddenly saw what they might have said and how. Mrs Jones, whose consultation was discussed at length in Chapter 4, was a respondent who was able to talk at some length about her consultation behaviour and illustrates this phenomena. Despite her pleasure and relief at finding a doctor who had told her the facts the detailed questioning of the interview still revealed a number of important gaps and uncertainties in her knowledge. In reply to a query about this she said:

'I think that when you go to the doctor, well I do,...You go and you think, especially if you don't feel well, and you don't know how to explain to the doctor what's wrong. You sit in the waiting-room with all those things going round in your mind: where shall I start, what can I say to him first, how can I explain how I feel?...You can't explain...I get all panicky inside...Obviously if you don't give him a definite statement...how does he know?'

Why had Mrs Jones stayed silent about the fact that she still didn't really know what was wrong? Her answer indicated that she had not been able to think through what she was told in the consultation and that she had not been able to formulate her uncertainty:

> 'Well, if I'd have spoken to you yesterday and then I'd have gone to the doctor then I'd have said. . .I would have said I didn't understand. . .I'd have said "so, you tell me this: I've got a scar, but what's that? Why does it flare up? Is it the food I eat?" I just couldn't think at the time.'

Difficulties in formulating thoughts, such as experienced by Mrs Jones, might be explained in terms of lack of practice and lack of communication skill. It was also apparent that emotions such as relief or anxiety put patients out of their stride: 'I should have asked but I didn't. When he said everything is OK I was so relieved I forgot', said Mrs French (1248), an example of the one-third (36 per cent) of patients who said they had not asked a question because they forgot. Because patients forgot it does not mean the question was not important. In fact the question Mrs French had forgotten subsequently returned to her mind to make her doubt her doctor's judgement. Similarly, the questions Mrs Jones never formulated left gaps in her knowledge which undermined the effectiveness of her doctor's advice.

Patients' opportunities to collect their thoughts and formulate their questions were undoubtedly made worse by the feeling of being hurried or by the lack of any guidance or encouragement to ask questions. Feeling hurried was a salient feature of most patients' experience. It was astounding that no matter how ill a patient was he invariably referred to doubts about taking a doctor's time based on the theory that other much more needy patients were outside. Still less happily, as we have seen, some patients also feared their doctor's response to activity on their part. Few, if any, thought their doctors actually wanted them to question or to express doubts.

The fact that patients often gave reasons suggesting that they felt their understanding was not relevant, it was not up to them to ask, or doctors would not welcome questions and doubts, together with the fact, as we saw earlier, that doctors did not encourage patients to indicate their ideas, suggests that the norms governing consultation behaviour are not currently conducive to overt patient activity. The cultural stereotype of the patient that doctors think of as 'good' remains one who is passive. In this respect our findings are similar to those of Duff and Hollingshead (1968) and Svarstad (1974) in the US. Patients did not feel free to question or doubt and were rarely encouraged to do so.

How patients feel, however, may be strongly dependent on their sensitive observation of their doctors' behaviour. Certainly Svarstad found that the way doctors behaved could influence patients. She found that doctors who tried to solicit patients' ideas but avoided behaviour calculated to turn patients off (such as watching the clock, mumbling incomprehensibly, interrupting patients, ignoring what they said, or even walking out of the room before patients had stopped speaking) were likely to take part in consultations in which patients asked more questions than if they behaved in a less approachable way. Patients who asked more questions were more likely to obtain better information and more likely to take their drugs properly (Svarstad 1974: 204 ff.).

The influences on patients' behaviour

We mentioned in Chapter 4 that few systematic relationships could be found to explain how much information patients were given or how long their consultations took. The attempts patients made to influence the information they got were only somewhat more explicable. Whether patients had brought the episode of illness to their doctor before, their occupational background, and their gender were the most important influences. The significance of the diagnosis a patient was given also exerted a limited effect.

Table 6.9 shows that whether patients asked questions or expressed doubts and how obvious they were about it, depended on what they had talked about with the doctor before and whether he had changed his mind since then. Patients who were visiting for an illness they had experienced before (provided the doctor did not change the diagnosis) were more likely to ask the doctor to justify his treatment (but not his diagnosis) and to clarify his views on at least one topic. They were also more likely to express doubt about treatment (but not about his diagnosis). Differences were quite large. In fact they were twice as likely to ask questions (whether obviously or less obviously) and about 50 per cent more likely to express doubts.

Table 6.10 shows how patients from higher occupational backgrounds were more likely than those from lower ones to be active. Compared to those from 'intermediate class' and 'working class' occupations three times as many patients (6 per cent) from 'service class' occupations asked a doctor to give his reasons overtly. Nearly half (46 per cent) of the patients from 'service class' backgrounds, compared to less than a third of those from 'intermediate class' or 'working class' backgrounds, made overt attempts to ask the doctor to clarify what he said (*Table 6.10*). In the case of presenting explanatory models the differences among patients from different occupational backgrounds, although less marked, were still obvious. Whereas four-fifths of those from 'working class' occupations gave no hint of an explanatory hypothesis, this was true of only two-thirds of those in the two higher occupational categories. Those from 'working class' occupations were also least likely to mention a hypothesis overtly.

Interestingly, although patients with higher educational attainment (13) were more likely to ask questions connected with treatment issues they showed no greater tendency than others to ask questions on other topics. One-third of higher educated patients asked a question indicating an interest in a doctor's reasons compared to a quarter of those with intermediate education and a fifth among those with basic education.

Table 6.9 *The effect of the history of an illness on patients'*
consulting behaviour

	history of the illness		
	new illness or old illness with a new diagnosis (%)	old illness (%)	total (%)
asking for reasons for treatment-action			
overt	2 (1)	5 (2)	7 (2)
covert	22 (13)	67 (28)	89 (22)
none	145 (86)	164 (70)	307 (76)
total	169 (42)	236 (58)	405 (100)

chi-square=14.52 2 d/f p<0.001
gamma=0.44

requesting clarification of a doctor's view			
overt	14 (8)	44 (19)	58 (14)
covert	10 (6)	28 (12)	38 (9)
none	145 (86)	164 (70)	309 (76)
total	169 (42)	236 (58)	405 (100)

chi-square=14.53 2 d/f p<0.001
gamma=0.43

expressing doubts			
overt	17 (10)	40 (17)	57 (14)
covert	18 (11)	41 (17)	59 (15)
none	134 (79)	155 (66)	289 (71)
total	169 (42)	236 (58)	405 (100)

chi-square=8.93 2 d/f p<0.05
gamma=0.31

The third influence on whether patients asked questions was the diagnostic-significance of their illness. Although the precise diagnostic categories into which patient's problems fell did not appear to influence how they behaved, the extent to which their condition appeared to convey bad news did show an effect. Patients with diagnostically significant conditions in this sense were more likely than those who were not, to ask a doctor to give reasons (14).

Table 6.10 *The influence of patients' occupational background on their consulting behaviour*

	social class			
	service (%)	intermediate (%)	working (%)	total (%)
1 presenting				
explanatory models				
overt	17 (13)	24 (18)	11 (9)	52 (13)
covert	24 (18)	18 (14)	11 (9)	53 (14)
none	93 (70)	91 (68)	105 (83)	127 (32)
total	52 (13)	53 (14)	289 (73)	394 (100)

chi-square = 10.75 4 d/f p < 0.05
tau^c = 0.08 p < 0.01
gamma = 0.19

	service	intermediate	working	total
2 seeking instructions				
overt or covert	74 (55)	56 (42)	59 (47)	189 (48)
none	60 (45)	77 (58)	68 (54)	205 (52)
total	134 (34)	133 (34)	127 (32)	394 (100)

differences not statistically significant at the 5% level

	service	intermediate	working	total
3 seeking clarification				
(all topics)				
overt	61 (46)	39 (29)	34 (27)	134 (34)
covert	16 (12)	27 (20)	16 (13)	133 (34)
none	57 (43)	67 (50)	77 (61)	201 (51)
total	134 (34)	133 (34)	127 (32)	394 (100)

chi-square = 16.06 4 d/f p < 0.01
tau^c = 0.14 p < 0.0005
gamma = 0.23

	service	intermediate	working	total
4 asking for reasons				
(all topics)				
overt	8 (57)	3 (21)	3 (21)	14 (4)
covert	69 (39)	63 (35)	47 (26)	179 (45)
none	57 (28)	67 (33)	77 (38)	201 (51)
total	134 (34)	133 (34)	127 (32)	394 (100)

chi-square = 10.72 4 d/f p < 0.05
tau^c = 0.13 p < 0.001
gamma = 0.24

In contrast to the pattern of question asking and presenting ideas about what was wrong, occupational and educational background and diagnostic-significance had no statistically significant effect on whether patients expressed doubts to their doctors. The most important determinant of this behaviour, however, was gender. Women and men did not differ in their propensity to ask questions or to offer explanations. But, although women were only somewhat more likely than men to express doubt at all, they were nearly twice (31 per cent) as likely as men (18 per cent) to express their doubts overtly (15).

Many factors did not make a difference to any of the patient behaviours. There was no evidence, for example, that the patient behaviours being discussed were in any way influenced by which doctor they saw. Knowledge of which doctor patients saw gave no guidance to predict how they would behave (16). Neither was there any difference between the patients of Study as compared to Comparison group doctors. It also seemed unimportant whether patients and doctors had ever met each other or not, and other aspects of a patient's social background (such as their ethnic group, age or housing status) were not associated with any of the patient behaviours in which we have been interested. Neither owner-occupiers compared to council or private tenants, nor patients of different ages, nor patients from particular ethnic groups differed in their consulting behaviour.

The influences on patients' behaviour can be summarized to say that the main determinants of asking questions were a patient's occupational background, whether his illness was a new one to him and whether it represented bad news. The main determinants of whether patients expressed doubt were their gender and whether their illness was one they had experienced before. Occupational background also exerted some influence on whether patients presented aspects of their explanatory models.

The fact that occupational background should influence behaviour comes as no surprise to the social scientist. Communication skills would be expected to vary by social class and those patients from professional and service backgrounds would be expected to behave more freely in consultations and to be able to articulate their ideas more to doctors as their higher status equals (Tuckett 1976: 145). What might be surprising is the magnitude of the effect and the relative lack of relationships between educational achievement and patient activity: educational attainment was related to only one patient behaviour and social class variables accounted for no more than a fifth of the variation in any one.

The fact that patients coming for an old illness and those with more significant diagnoses were more likely to behave more actively requires more interpretation. Asking questions later rather than earlier in an illness episode is perhaps consistent with the 'wait and see' attitude some patients gave for not asking questions or expressing doubts. These patients indicated that, although they wanted more information, they felt it was best to wait until the doctor's advice had had time to take effect. To explain the influence of the significance of the diagnosis a patient was given, two hypotheses come to mind. One is that doctors were somehow more open to patient activity when a condition was more threatening and potentially bad news. Another is that in these circumstances patients cared more about knowing what was happening or were more likely to be disappointed and so dissatisfied. Against the idea that doctors somehow became more open to patient questions is the finding, if patients had a more rather than a less significant diagnosis, that doctors were less likely to state clearly what was wrong, no more likely to give more attention to patient's views and just as likely to inhibit or evade patients' ideas. In favour of the proposition that patients tended to behave more actively the more 'serious' they thought their diagnoses to be was the fact that many of them indicated that they were very reluctant to be thought of as wasting a doctor's time with a trivial illness. Perhaps, if they thought their illness was more significant and not trivial, they felt both that they wanted to know and had more of a right to do so.

Perhaps the striking fact about patients' and doctors' behaviour, is how little of it could be explained by the social, diagnostic, or historical variables we have explored. It is possible that the wrong variables have been examined. On the other hand, perhaps the relatively random occurrence of patient activity reflects what has been said earlier about the causes and consequences of being active in a 'covert' way. First, it seems that norms about not bothering a doctor or not trying to appear knowledgeable in a consultation may have taken root equally among individuals of different social status and education. From the social conflict perspective on medical consultations it might be said that members of all occupational groups are equally intimidated. At the same time, perhaps, if the extent of 'covert' behaviour is treated as an indicator of poor communication skills rather than the product of intimidation it may be that members of all occupational groups are equally unable to formulate ideas, questions and doubts in an obvious and articulate way. Like doctors, patients may have expertise to share but may also often lack the communicative competence to do so most effectively.

Summary

Using the approach developed in the previous chapter it was found that most patients showed signs of attempting to influence the sharing of information in their consultations. As many as half of the consultations contained obvious signs of this behaviour on the part of patients. Nearly every consultation contained less obvious signs of it. We also found that patients who presented their explanation of what was wrong with them and their reasons for believing it, those who asked a doctor for his rationale quite overtly and those who asked other questions or aired doubts, were more likely to have their ideas attended to by the doctors or to be given more information more clearly. At the same time it was also apparent that patients who behaved more actively in the ways just mentioned were more likely than others to experience a consultation in which their ideas were evaded and tension was evident. Such experiences in the past, it seemed, together with feelings of deference and difficulties in formulating thoughts in the heat of the moment, were among the main reasons patients did not ask more questions more openly or air doubts more clearly. Social, diagnostic or historical variables had little influence on the chances a patient would behave more actively and it seems likely that patients, largely regardless of what was wrong with them or their social background, shared a feeling that they should not openly try to share information or at least had equal difficulty trying to do so.

PART 4

Understanding and evaluating medical ideas

CHAPTER 7

The problem of patients' understanding

We have noted in earlier chapters that research workers and their clinical colleagues have been uncertain as to exactly what constitutes 'informing' a patient or why they might want to do so. The same problem permeates thinking about patients' understanding and the conditions under which it can be said to be 'correct' or 'successful'.

We will suggest that to reach reasonably clear and relevant conclusions about how accurately patients understand what their doctors tell them one requires four research implements: a method of determining which are the matters that a doctor mentions which patients might be supposed to know about subsequently; a method to determine what important points a doctor makes concerning these matters; a method of finding out patients' accounts of what they have learned; and a clear set of criteria to determine whether they have learned them. For reasons which we will shortly discuss the three dimensions of patient learning which we chose as criteria were the 'correctness' of their recall of what was said, the 'correctness' of the sense they made of it and the degree of commitment they had to what their doctors had to say.

There have been at least six published attempts to observe how many statements patients 'correctly' remember following a consultation (Joyce *et al.* 1969; Ley *et al.* 1973, 1976; Bertakis 1977; Anderson 1979; Pendleton 1982b), three previous attempts to examine the 'correctness' of patients' comprehension of what they remember (Svarstad 1974; Bain 1977; Larsen and Smith 1981) and one previous attempt to assess whether patients evaluate what they are told in a manner which demonstrates that the doctor has been successful in conveying his rationale (Svarstad 1974). However, with the exception of the last mentioned, these studies have usually not included a theoretical consideration of what was being assessed. They have also arrived at results which are difficult to interpret. It is, therefore, unclear whether there are established circumstances in which patients are likely to remember the most important points of what they are told, how far (if they do remember them) they are likely to make 'correct' sense of the information and how far (if they make 'correct' sense of it) they are likely to evaluate what they are told favourably. In these circumstances it is very difficult to support the different claims made about patients' capabilities for sharing medical information, to understand much about the process of communication or to advocate effective methods for improving it. To develop and test new measures which might help in this task was a major objective of the study.

The essential characteristic of every study of how successfully doctors inform patients is that what a doctor has told a patient in a particular consultation has been compared by research workers with an account of the consultation gathered from the patient later (1). To make such comparisons it is necessary to decide what a patient is supposed to know and then to decide in what way he is supposed to know it: for example, whether he is able 'correctly' to repeat what his doctor has said, to make the 'correct' sense of this information, or whether to agree with the doctor's rationale.

Some cognitive outcomes

All but two of the studies just mentioned chose to equate a successful cognitive outcome of a consultation with the situation in which patients' accounts of their consultations reproduced the information statements their doctors made. In other words they focused solely on patients' capacity to recall medical information. While what patients remember may provide a rough and ready estimate of how far doctors achieve a shared understanding with their patients (whether their aim is to persuade patients, to facilitate their choices, or to help structure their experiences of illness and to reassure them) it is clearly inadequate for testing the main issue with which we are concerned: how far it is possible for doctors to share with their patients their understanding of such matters as the diagnostic-significance of their illness or the purpose and value of possible treatment- or preventive-action.

One dimension of patients' understanding which would be worthwhile studying is indicated by the theme of meaning which is so central to many sociological and social anthropological discussions of the processes before, during and after, medical consultations. Patients, like everyone, can be seen as social actors subjectively giving meaning to what is happening around them and to the sensations and ideas to which they are exposed (for example, Schutz 1953; McCall and Simmonds 1966; Garfinkel 1967; McHugh 1968). From this perspective they may be supposed routinely to make sense of and to evaluate what their doctors do and say and to do so in terms of whatever models of understanding they bring to the situation. Such models of understanding are likely to be based on their understanding of the ideas and experiences to which they are exposed in their own cultural settings and also on any information they receive in medical settings. Patients' ideas may also be influenced by their past experiences of medical care or by other people's reports of it. The important thing from this perspective is that patients are expected to try to make some sense of what their doctors say to them and to do so with the knowledge at their disposal.

The 'explanatory model' concept (Kleinman 1975, 1980) is one way of conceptualizing the influence of patients' ideas on their understanding of what their doctors say. Kleinman argues that in any given situation individuals operationalize the many diverse and inconsistent health beliefs to which they are exposed, into a subjectively consistent explanation of such matters as the cause of their illness, its pathology, expected course and prognosis, and the treatment that they believe will be or should be administered.

The utility of the explanatory model concept for exploring the divergences between doctors' and patients' understanding of a medical condition and its treatment has been explored by Blumhagen (1980). He examined the explanatory models held by patients who had been treated in a clinic for hypertension for several months. By attending for a period of time it was assumed that these patients had been given an opportunity to integrate their personal beliefs with the knowledge they gained in their visits to a clinic. Blumhagen described how, none the less, the patients he studied shared two major sets of ideas about the cause of their illness, each of which significantly diverged from biomedical views and which had important consequences for their reaction to treatment advice. He argued that although lay and medical views of hypertension may appear similar in various ways they are in fact radically different both in their detail and in their implications. However, Blumhagen did not link the patients' ideas to what their doctors actually told them nor observe what happened in consultations.

The subtleties of the differences in understanding that can occur between doctors and their patients have also been discussed by Harwood (1981) who formulated five sources of potential difficulty. First, patient and doctor may use the same term but attach to it different meanings. For instance, doctors usually differentiate what they call the side-effects of a drug from effects caused by what they term an individual's allergies to it. Patients may use either term interchangeably. Second, doctor and patient may use the same term in the same way but mean something quite different, because they conceive of its causes differently. The patients described by Blumhagen, for instance, agreed with their doctors that high blood pressure is termed hypertension but differed from them in their views of its cause. Patients tended to emphasize the role of social and psychological stress – 'too much tension' – and in consequence tended to misconstrue or underplay the role of medication in treating their disorder (2). Third, doctor and patient may share the meaning of terms and causes but have different ideas about the significance of a condition. For instance, patients may regard a peptic ulcer as a step on the road to cancer, or a fracture as a precursor of crippling arthritis, while doctors would usually not do so. To the patient a diagnosis of a peptic ulcer or fracture may be effectively synonymous with cancer or crippling arthritis. Somewhat differently, the way terms can vary in their emotional meanings, whether it is a diagnosis, treatment or other procedure, is a fourth kind of conceptual difference. A social stigma, for example, may attach to some conditions or procedures, and may suggest attributions of blame or guilt. For instance, a patient whose headache is diagnosed as psychological rather than physical might take such a diagnosis to mean he is weak-minded and somehow to blame. Finally, there are also 'simple' linguistic differences. A word or term can mean something quite different in the patient's culture to what it means in the doctor's – for example, the term pain-killer may be used by doctors to describe to patients the ameliorative effect of analgesics but be understood by patients in the different sense that an antibiotic, for instance, is popularly and correctly known as a germ-killer. In these circumstances analgesics may be mistakenly considered curative.

The importance of the processes of assigning meaning, such as those just described, was the reason we decided that one dimension of patients' understanding that should be assessed as well as 'recall' was how far patients could make 'correct' biomedical sense of what their doctors told them. How far patients understood the main points of what their doctors said in correct biomedical terms would provide a first estimate of the magnitude of the problem of achieving some degree of shared understanding. Moreover, given knowledge of the correctness of a patient's understanding it would then be possible to explore differences between patients who were and were not correct and try to draw conclusions about the processes in consultations which produce correct biomedical understanding.

To establish how correctly patients understand what their doctors say it is necessary to compare what doctors said and meant with patients' accounts of what they said and meant. In the past this has been attempted in only two studies (Svarstad 1974; Larsen and Smith 1981). In Svarstad's study patients' understanding of the instructions for taking medicine were explored. In Larsen and Smith's study patients were asked to give only brief answers to six simple questions. Patients' understanding across a wider range of issues and in sufficient depth to explore the meanings they attach to terms has, therefore, not been probed. We decided, therefore, to try to develop measures of how far patients made correct sense of what they were told across each of the three topics used before: diagnostic-significance, treatment- and preventive-action.

Evaluating what a doctor says

An interesting feature of the interpretive differences discussed by Harwood is that they indicate rather graphically how patients' usage and understanding of terms are likely to take place in the wider context of their explanatory models (as, of course, are doctors'). The meaning of a diagnosis or treatment term tends to depend on and to be consistent with other aspects of the explanatory model which may be elaborated (see, for example, Blaxter 1983). One possible outcome of this process is that patients may feel their doctors have made contradictory or incorrect decisions. Helman (1978) has illustrated this phenomenon in a discussion of the effect of the explanatory models he identified surrounding fevers and cold symptoms in British culture. He emphasized how patients evaluated a diagnosis both by considering whether it fitted the medical facts, as they saw them, and also by assessing whether it responded to questions to which they needed answers, such as about who is to blame.

The explanatory model hypothesis, like the ideas of those such as Stimson and Webb (1975), who have emphasized the bargaining and negotiation aspect of patients' approach to medical consultations and the extent to which consultations are only a small part of patients' everyday struggles with illness and its treatment, emphasizes the potential of exploring a third dimension of understanding: patients' evaluations of what their doctors tell them. Only Svarstad, among previous investigators, has explored both the 'sense' patients made of the medication instructions they were given and the extent to which patients evaluated instructions as 'sensible' and 'important' in their case. She approached the latter judgement by asking patients at their interviews a variety of detailed questions about their understanding of the purpose and value of medication. Using their answers she determined whether patients considered their medication to be important for them and to be likely to do much good. She summarized answers to these questions in an index of their overall attitude. A high score was given if patients thought drugs helpful or effective, thought they were important, could mention major benefits, and did not fear side effects. Intermediate and low scores were assigned when patients could not mention the beneficial effect of a drug, thought drugs were unlikely to be helpful, were not important, or would have undesirable side-effects (Svarstad 1974: 260 ff.). Svarstad did not, however, systematically explore patients' understanding beyond the issue of medication or the influence upon it of their explanatory thinking. Nor did she consider the extent to which patients' overall models of understanding might continue to conflict with those of their doctors.

We decided to explore how patients evaluated their doctors' ideas by focusing on two aspects of what we termed their 'commitment': how far patients felt they agreed with their doctors' key ideas and how far they considered their doctor's ideas to be inferior to or in conflict with alternative ideas deriving from their explanatory models. By classifying patients according to their level of commitment we hoped to be able to explore the processes which influenced it.

The problem of importance

Whether the task is to explore what patients remember, what they understand correctly or what they agree with, it is first necessary to establish a basis with which to compare the accounts they give subsequently. The attempts to do this in the studies mentioned at the beginning of the chapter have generally adopted an approach which is similar to that of those quantitative studies which have tried to measure the information doctors give to patients: everything a doctor says has been considered to contribute to one of several broad topics (number of problems, diagnosis, treatment, advice) and then the number of discrete statements made by a doctor on each topic has been summed without paying further attention to content (Joyce *et al.* 1969; Ley *et al.* 1973, 1976; Bertakis 1977; Anderson 1979; Inui *et al.* 1982). Results based on this method report the proportion of statements patients were able to remember but are difficult to interpret. Forgetting some statements may be potentially consistent with remembering all the 'key' or important points made by a doctor. The problem with these methods is that they imply that a patient should remember and understand each statement indiscriminately. As a result, when some inevitably do not understand or remember each statement it is impossible to know exactly what it is they have not been able to remember or understand and so how far any 'errors' or 'failures' of recall are important.

Svarstad (1974), Bain (1977) and Larsen and Smith (1981), adopted an alternative approach to those mentioned in the last paragraph. They determined precisely which specific items of information given by doctors were worth studying and restricted their investigations to them. Svarstad compared what was said in consultation with patients' reports of the names of drugs they were given, what was said in the consultation about the length of time for which the drugs should be taken, what they knew of the dosage schedule for each drug and what they knew of the time-scale for which they could be expected to take them. Less specifically than Svarstad, Bain compared patients' answers to various more general questions with various things a doctor could have said: what was wrong with them, whether they had been given a prescription and, if so, the number of drugs they had been prescribed, the names of the drugs, the frequency with which they should be used, for how long they should be used and whether they had been given any additional advice or instructions about what was wrong with them. Larsen and Smith adopted a similar approach to Bain. It is interesting that the authors of all these rather more discriminating approaches to patient understanding all report rather higher levels of patient recall or understanding than studies based on the first approach (3). They also make it much easier to judge the significance of what patients did and did not recall or understand.

The potentially greater clarity of the approaches just mentioned is illustrated by a third type of study. Pendleton (1982b) made a direct comparison between patients' recall of all information statements and their recall of just those considered by the doctor to be 'important'. He found that patients remembered what they were told in a discriminating way: they could recall a considerably higher proportion of 'important' statements than of statements not so classified. His findings suggest, therefore, that attention should be paid to deciding what it is important for patients to remember and to finding a method of determining when they do so. Conclusions about what patients remember would then be more easily interpretable.

As we have mentioned, studies by Joyce *et al.* (1969), Ley *et al.* (1973), Bertakis (1977) and Anderson (1979) made no attempt to differentiate the importance of different information statements. They would not have been able to do so without altering their methods – by conceptualizing and defining in an open manner which statements they considered important and how they would recognize these from tape-recordings of consultations.

When the problem of deciding which information is important has been recognized, two approaches to defining it might be attempted. In his study Pendleton (1982b) approached the problem by asking doctors to make the judgement. After their consultations they were asked to write down (under the broad headings of treatment and diagnosis) the important points they thought they had made. Svarstad (1974), on the other hand, determined what was important for patients to know by asking what points they needed to be aware of if they were going to stand a good chance of being motivated to take their medication correctly. After defining the important points, what doctors said on each was noted from a tape-recording of the consultation. The two methods have both advantages and drawbacks. While Pendleton's approach of asking doctors to make judgements has intuitive validity as a basis for comparison – the doctors being studied were clearly very appropriate people to determine which aspects of what they had said they particularly wanted patients to remember and understand – it is open to the criticism that what doctors think they said and what an observer thinks they have said may be different. In fact, Svarstad found that there were many occasions when what doctors reported they had said, what they had said and even what was on medicine bottles, diverged substantially. On the other hand, Svarstad's approach of deciding what was important herself is as strong or weak as the rationale she provides for making the decisions she has made.

The difficulties increase considerably when what a doctor means, and not just what points he has made, is to be assessed. Yet such a baseline of information is needed if a patients' understanding rather than just their recall is to be measured. In his study Pendleton did not attempt this further step. Had he done so and continued to use his approach, he would have had to interview the doctors or to give them very precise and demanding instructions in order to establish what they meant by each of their important points. In her study, Svarstad did make the attempt. She decided what doctors meant on important points by listening to what they said and making the judgement herself. In the case of such matters as drug frequency, name and dosage this may not be difficult. If, however, the task had been to determine what he had said the patient was suffering from or why he thought so, it might have been more problematic. An investigator's judgement of what a doctor said would not necessarily be correct or superior to that of the patient and would involve an understanding of biomedical knowledge and judgements. Problems would be especially acute if what doctors said was not clear. Complications of this kind may explain why most research has concentrated only on what patients remember.

Since we have argued the need to discover whether patients remember and whether they understand correctly what their doctors say (and to estimate the limits of the process of sharing information), it was clearly necessary to determine what doctors said on important points and what they meant by what they said. Only then could we compare patients' accounts of what they meant and estimate how often they remembered and understood correctly the essence of what a doctor said. To judge what doctors said we decided to use the 'key points' already adopted to study the information doctors gave (pp. 35ff.) and to make a 'third-party' assessment of the doctor's view on each topic (diagnostic-significance, treatment- and preventive-action). Ideally, the doctors taking part in the consultations or other medical advisers would have assisted in this task. However, since to make several hundred judgements in this way would have been too time-consuming given the resources available, the validity of the assessments were estimated from a medical point of view by means of two checks on a sample of the ratings.

To be in a good position to begin to evaluate a doctor's ideas and advice we have argued that patients need to remember and understand the key points doctors made and also their reasoning behind it. It would have been desirable, therefore, to obtain a baseline view both of what the doctor decided and his reasons for doing so. Patients' understanding of doctors' views and of their reasons could then have been separately explored. Systematic exploration of what doctors' reasons were was not attempted in the present study. Deciding what a doctor's reasons were and deciding if patients had got them right was attempted in a small number of cases. To do it systematically for all consultations would have required considerable biological and medical knowledge and would have magnified the inferential task and its complexities beyond the resources available. The issues examined, therefore, were patients' recall, understanding and commitment to the views the doctor stated.

Third-party judgement

To decide the view a doctor reached on each topic everything he said and did in a consultation was considered. Working from a tape-recording of the consultation, a verbatim transcript and an extract from the doctor's usual records (in which diagnostic names, drug names, diagnostic tests, and names of doctors to whom patients were referred would be present), the 'key points' of the view the doctor took on each topic were decided. Topics were not regarded as mutually exclusive (diagnostic information may well contain information relevant to treatment or prevention, and vice versa) and so anything the doctor said or did could be considered to provide information on any or all of the topics.

As the discussion of how far doctors stated their views has already indicated (pp. 46ff.) it was not usually a difficult matter to identify what had been conveyed on the 'key points' and therefore to know what the doctor had decided on each topic. The technical terms (diagnoses or drug names) the doctor used could be checked and clarified from medical sources and, in context, they were usually sufficient to indicate the significance of the condition or the purpose of treatment-

and preventive-action. A diagnostic term usually conveyed the diagnostic-significance of a problem and a drug name usually indicated whether the treatment was meant to be curative, ameliorative or preventive as well as its likely effectiveness in the patient's circumstances. For example, when a doctor prescribed an antibiotic after telling a mother her child had an ear infection, it was assumed, in the absence of contrary indications, that its purpose was to remove the bacterial agents. Similarly, it was plausible to infer that a patient with a chronic respiratory infection, who was advised to give up smoking, was being given advice with a preventive purpose. In both cases the advice was considered to be potentially effective in the sense that it would be usual to assume that failure to follow it would be likely to have a harmful effect.

Difficulties arose in making third-party judgements when the the decisions doctors made in consultations were not stated or if, even so, they were still unclear. About a fifth of the consultations contained problems of this sort. The investigator, like the patient, had to draw inferences about a doctor's views on very limited information. In some cases it was, none the less, not too difficult. For example, in one consultation the patient (Mr Fraser (1916)) was not told the diagnostic term which his doctor applied to his illness. Instead, the doctor gave the patient two less tangible items of information. From these it was possible to draw inferences relevant to the diagnostic-significance of his condition. First, the doctor said that, although he was not sure, he thought he knew what was the trouble. Second, he said, that although the trouble was 'too technical to explain', it could be likened to a kind of 'tennis elbow' of the knee. He elaborated on this analogy. In this way he appeared to be saying that the patient had a potentially bothering and chronic complaint but need not consider himself dramatically ill: a view strengthened by the fact the doctor did not propose any further investigation. The rater inferred that the doctor certainly had a hypothesis, it was one he considered probable and that it meant the patient's symptoms were not life-threatening but would probably go on being a nuisance. This view would be the one the patient would be expected to remember, and against which the sense he made and his commitment would be assessed.

In some other cases judgements were much more difficult to make and much more tenuous. An example is the consultation of Mrs Cross (2189). She was a middle-aged women complaining of blood in her stools which she had noticed after a family crisis. The doctor diagnosed the bleeding as a recurrence of her well-established chronic intestinal disease (Crohn's Disease (4)), and advised her not to worry, to try to relax, to have a rest, and to continue her valium (taken for a chronic anxiety state). The advice was given in the context of great efforts to reassure her, to calm her down and apparently to prevent dramatization of the situation. In this context he suggested that she might need a certificate to miss work for a few days, whereupon the patient said that she was thinking of giving up work. The doctor responded only indirectly and ambiguously: 'I think it will all settle.' Not perturbed by this, the patient then introduced the fact she had two part-time jobs – two mornings at one and one afternoon a week at another. He exclaimed 'You are a busy lady!' but then moved on to ask whether she was a member of an insurance scheme and what kind of certificate she would need. He ended the consultation as follows: 'So I think all we can really do is to give you a certificate for a week and see you in a week.'

Difficulties about deciding exactly what the doctor advised Mrs Cross arise from the question of what inferences were to be drawn about his attitude to her work. It was not difficult to be certain that his overall attitude was one of reassurance and a wish that she calm down and not over-dramatize the situation. To what extent, however, did he sanction or legitimate the idea that it was medically advisable for her to give up work? Should his refusal to be drawn on this be taken to indicate indifference, deliberate ambiguity or vagueness? After much debate it was decided that he had not sanctioned early retirement and probably did not care very much what she did. Retirement plans were certainly not an important part of his strategy and inconsistent with playing down the crisis. If the patient thought he had advised her to give up work and this was an important part of his strategy she would be wrong.

The third-party judgements described were made by the senior investigator, who has no formal medical qualification, after discussion with other members of the team. They were made well after the interviews had been conducted and after the interviewer and at least one other member of the research team had independently made an assessment of the 'key points'. Formal criteria and anchoring examples to make ratings were laid down at the beginning of the project with the idea that several members of the team could make the 'third-party assessment and that these judgements could be tested for reliability in the usual way. However, in the course of the study it became apparent that the criteria (as they were then developed) were not always sufficient to allow satisfactory agreement between the judges. The clinical problems encountered among the general practice patients that were studied were simply too many to draw up decisive rules at the beginning of the project. In particular, specialist knowledge and advice were sometimes required to make a judgement. Rather than risk confusion about the criteria being applied it was decided to standardize ratings through the judgements of one rater. He checked every third-party judgement, discussing points of disagreement with the initial judges and sometimes with a physician-adviser. He then made the final decision about the 'key points'. In future work, and with the benefit of the present experience, it would undoubtedly be more satisfactory to make 'third-party' judgements in a more formal way: two pairs of raters, each with one member with formal medical expertise, could be asked to make third-party judgements independently and their ratings could be compared. The method could also be extended to assessing the explanations and reasons doctors give for their decisions.

To make some estimate of the the validity of the third-party procedure, some of the judgements were explored in two ways. First, 60 consultations were discussed with the doctors who participated in them some weeks after they took place. Second, a sample of 24 randomly selected consultations was discussed with a panel of five general practitioners.

In the first check, 15 of the 16 doctors (the sixteenth had an extended illness at this stage) who had participated in the study were sent the verbatim transcripts of four randomly selected consultations they had conducted and asked to examine them and any case notes they themselves had. The four cases were then discussed in an interview lasting over an hour. In this interview the doctor was introduced to the notions of the 'topics' and 'key points' and was asked to state what he thought he had conveyed to the patient about them. His view was then compared with the third-party judgement of the key points. The doctor was also asked whether the transcript could in his opinion mislead anyone not familiar with the past history of the patient. Comparing what the doctors said with the third-party judgement, it was found that almost all the assessments were acceptable. Third-party judgements of the diagnostic-significance of the problems were confirmed by the doctor's account in 56 out of 60 (93 per cent) occasions; those of the action to be taken in 59 out of 60 (98 per cent) and those of the preventive measures to be taken in 58 out of 60 (97 per cent).

A high level of agreement between medical and third-party judgements also emerged in the second check. The group for this purpose was chosen by a senior general practitioner with a university teaching appointment and included physicians with reputations for divergent points of view. After an introduction and clarifying discussion of the notions of topics and 'key points', these doctors were presented with a verbatim transcript of each consultation and information about the age and sex of the patients. They were asked to decide what the doctor said relevant to the 'key' points for each topic. After a discussion of each consultation they had no difficulty in summarizing an agreed view and the interpretations they arrived at agreed with the third-party judgement used in the investigation in each case. They usually found, given their medical training, that the symptoms which the patients presented or the doctors discovered suggested only a narrow range of diagnostic possibilities (and thus the diagnostic-significance). Diagnostic and treatment terms used by the doctors in the consultations usually both narrowed the possibilities and indicated the broad purpose and value of any action or prevention. There was, of course, sometimes uncertainty among the group about the details of what was being diagnosed but this was always limited to choices between two or more equally 'significant' diagnoses.

The two ways used to explore the validity of the third-party judgements suggested that it is a viable method for providing a meaningful and reliable basis against which to compare patients' recall and understanding of the key points. One reason for this, undoubtedly, was that the task involved was not particularly ambitious. To make more detailed ratings of what the doctors had decided, for example to decide on exact differential diagnoses or exactly how doctors had reasoned, might have been much more difficult. In any case, it was the 'third-party' judgements made in the way we have described that have served as the standard against which patient's accounts have been compared.

Summary

In deciding on which aspects of patients' understanding to focus and on how to do so, an attempt has been made to explore some dimensions of understanding suggested by current sociological and cultural concerns and to combine several methodological aspects of previous work. First, we decided to explore three dimensions of understanding: recall, making sense and commitment. Second, we determined to assess patients understanding of the 'key points' on the three topics already introduced in Chapter 3: diagnostic-significance; treatment- and preventive- action. Third, we decided to use a 'third-party' approach to decide what a doctor had conveyed in the tape-recorded consultation and, therefore, what patients should know if communication was successful. The ways patients' understanding were assessed and the understanding they had will be described in the next two chapters (5).

CHAPTER 8

Remembering and making sense of medical ideas

We have suggested that one way of estimating how much patients can correctly remember is to compare their account of what doctors said about the key points of information with a third-party judgement of what they were told. After interviewing patients and making the appropriate judgements we found that very few of them were not able to remember all the key points their doctors made. Only one in ten of them could not remember the key points of their doctor's view on all the topics on which he expressed one. As few as 7 per cent forgot a key point on diagnostic-significance, and still less (3 per cent and 6 per cent respectively) a key point on treatment-action or prevention (*Table 8.1*). These findings are in striking contrast to the impression given in earlier studies that patients forget a third to a half of what they are told.

Table 8.1 *Remembering the key points made in 328 consultations*

	information topics			
	diagnostic-significance (%)	*treatment-action* (%)	*preventive-action* (%)	*any one of the three* (%)
number of consultations where topic was introduced[1]	297	328	100	328
number of consultations after which the patient was able to remember the key points correctly	277 (93)	317 (95)	95 (95)	294 (90)

1 i.e. the number of consultations (out of the 328 studied) in which the doctor said anything on each topic. Patients' understanding was not assessed if the doctor appeared not to take a view on a topic.

The extent to which the patients were aware of their doctors' views was already apparent in the interviews conducted with them. After the interviewers had explained to the patients that they had no knowledge of what had happened in their consultation and had made it clear that they would like patients to talk in as much detail as possible, most respondents easily provided an almost verbatim account of the encounter. By discussing in turn each symptom (or logically connected set of symptoms), the interviewers then established the diagnostic-significance the patient believed the doctor to attach to it and any treatment- and preventive-action the doctor had advised. Respondents were asked to state what it was doctors did or said that made them think as they did. They were also asked to confirm that nothing else was said or talked about and were reminded of possibilities by means of various standard check lists (1). This standardized non-schedule interview procedure allowed interviewers to probe and cross-question respondents as they saw fit (2). Because interviewers were previously unaware of what had happened in the consultations questioning could take place without fear of contaminating patients' memories.

A patient had remembered the 'key points' correctly on each topic if he could report (or at least paraphrase) the things a doctor had said which had been judged to convey the key points of his view on that topic. Mrs Lawn (1087), for example, was judged to recall the key points her doctor made about diagnostic-significance because she remembered him saying that her painful wrist was definitely caused by Carpal tunnel syndrome. (She would also have been rated correct if, instead of being able to mention the exact diagnostic term used by the doctor, she had recalled that the doctor had said the pain was a side-effect of her pregnancy.) As we have noted more than nine out of ten of the patients studied were able to recall all the 'key points'. Mr Fraser (1916) was an example of the small minority of patients unable to recall a key point. His consultation, in which his doctor said that the mysterious pains in his legs were like a kind of tennis elbow, was discussed in the previous chapter. When he was interviewed Mr Fraser talked at length about the doctor's comments about his trouble being 'too technical' to explain and also about the doctor's comment about being unsure. He was very dissatisfied with what the doctor had said and, despite the normal probing, he could attribute no other relevant remarks to him. He thought the doctor did not know what was wrong and appeared to have no memory of the 'tennis elbow' comments or at least to have forgotten them as insignificant. The method of rating a patient's recall in this way was proved to be highly reliable (3).

Making sense

When deciding if the patients had recalled the key points it was necessary to ignore, as far as was practicable, the sense patients attached to what they remembered or their attitude to it. This was because we wanted to estimate whether patients had heard or 'taken in' what was said, in a manner as far as possible independent of the sense they made of it (4). To establish how far patients were able to make 'correct' sense of the key points their doctors made to them, the judgements we made about what doctors said had to be compared with the sense patients made of it at the interview. Among those patients who managed to remember what doctors said, we found that most of them 'correctly' made sense of what they were told (*Table 8.2*). That is to say, four-fifths (80 per cent) attributed a correct meaning to what was said to them about the diagnostic-significance of their problem, nine-tenths (92 per cent) a correct meaning to advice about treatment-action and three-quarters (75 per cent) a correct meaning to advice about preventive action. Nearly three-quarters of the patients (73 per cent) remembering what was said made correct sense of what they were told on all the topics about which a doctor took a view (*Table 8.2*).

Table 8.2 *Making correct and incorrect sense of the key points made in 328 consultations*

	information topics			
	diagnostic-significance (%)	treatment-action (%)	preventive-action (%)	any one of the three (%)
number of consultations after which the patient could remember 'key points' 'correctly'	277	317	95	294
number of consultations after which the patient made correct sense[1]	221 (80)	292 (92)	71 (75)	214 (73)

1 The denominators for recall (*Table 8.1*) and making sense are different because whether patients made sense was rated only if recall was correct.

To find out the sense patients attached to what was said, interviewers explored the significance each patient believed his doctor attached to his symptoms by asking about what the doctor called the conditions, whether the patient thought the diagnosis likely, and what (in the patient's case) the prognosis was likely to be. Any terms that patients used were carefully questioned to establish exactly what they thought the doctor meant in everyday language and behaviour. The interviewers also established exactly what actions each patient thought the doctor had advised, how effective and important they were supposed to be, and whether their purpose was ameliorative, curative, investigative or preventive. The interviewers continued until they felt they had a clear picture of the views about diagnostic-significance, treatment- and preventive-action that each patient attributed to the doctor.

After the interview, the interviewers had then to compare the sense the patient made of the 'key points' with the third-party judgement of those points. Patients were rated as making 'correct' sense of key points if their understanding was identical to that reached by third-party judgement or if any 'errors' they made would be unlikely to impair their idea of the significance of what was wrong with them or the purpose and importance of any treatment- or prevention-action. They were rated 'not correct' if they did not know the significance of their condition or the purpose of treatment- and preventive-action or if they over- or under-estimated the significance of a diagnosis or the importance of treatment and prevention (5). Mr Izard (1653) was a patient who was rated as not making the correct sense of what his doctor told him about the diagnostic-significance of his condition for the former reason. He suffered from double vision diagnosed by his doctor as due to his 'blood pressure'. At interview Mr Izard recalled quite precisely what the doctor had done to measure his blood pressure and that his doctor had said that his double vision was due to it being too high. However, this information apparently gave him no idea of the significance of his condition. When asked what the diagnosis meant he said that he had 'no idea'. All he knew was that 'as soon as any doctor finds out a patient has high blood pressure they immediately try to get it down. Whether it could do anything more [than give double-vision] I don't know. It may do'. Because Mr Izard was unable to say whether his condition had any future consequences and what it implied he was considered to be unable to make 'correct' sense of the significance of the diagnostic hypothesis his doctor had mentioned to him. Distinctions of this kind between patients able to make 'correct' sense and those not able to do so could be made in a reliable way (6).

Some correlates of a patient's understanding

Distinguishing patients who could and could not remember and 'correctly' make sense of the key points their doctors made allowed us to explore the possible influences there might be on the process of remembering and understanding medical ideas. Interestingly, many of the variables which were examined were unrelated to whether respondents remembered or made sense of what was said in the consultation: for example, the patient's age, gender, occupational background, or ethnic group; whether the patient was an adult or a child brought by an adult; whether he had met the doctor before; or whether the problem was a new or old illness. Nor did which doctor a patient saw or whether he was in the Study or Comparison group make a difference. The formal diagnostic category into which a patient's illness fell also had no detectable effect.

Two aspects of the strategies doctors might adopt to help their patients remember and understand what they say were mentioned in an earlier chapter: doctors have been advised to be as clear as possible and to encourage a mutual exchange of views. On the basis of work by psychologists, such as Ley and his colleagues (Ley 1979), we could expect that at least some of the variation in patients' understanding would be accounted for by variations in how clearly information was conveyed in a consultation. After consultations in which doctors stated their views clearly to their patients, compared to consultations in which they did not, patients should be more likely to remember and make correct sense of what they were told. This hypothesis was not, however, supported by the data (*Table 8.3*). There was no evidence that doctors who clearly stated their views about diagnostic-significance, compared to

Table 8.3 *The relationship between how clearly a doctor stated the key points of information and whether patients remembered and made correct sense of the key points*

| | how doctors stated their view on: | | | | | |
| | diagnostic-significance | | | treatment-action | | |
	clearly (%)	not clearly (%)	not at all (%)	clearly (%)	not clearly (%)	not at all (%)
recall and sense:						
correct	78	106	37	131	141	20
incorrect	20 (20)	46 (30)	10 (21)	12 (8)	19 (12)	5 (20)

diagnostic-significance:
chi-square=3.58 2 d/f n.s
tau^c =0.06 n.s.

treatment-action
chi-square=3.19 2 d/f n.s
tau^c =0.03 n.s

those who were unclear or didn't state a view at all, were more likely to succeed in helping their patients to make correct sense. In the case of what doctors said about treatment-action, although there was a tendency for views that were not stated at all to be forgotten or made sense of incorrectly this difference was not statistically significant.

While we were not able to confirm the hypothesis that doctors who stated their views more clearly enabled their patients to remember and understand more correctly, it was quite impossible for us even to attempt any direct assessment of the theory that doctors who undertook a mutual exchange of views were more successful in this respect. A patient's understanding was so rarely checked and clarified by a doctor that no test of the hypothesis was possible (7). Some indirect evidence supporting the idea that a mutual exchange might have been beneficial was, however, apparent. Consultations in which doctors inhibited or evaded their patients' ideas were quite a lot more likely than those in which they did not to result in failures of recall and understanding (*Table 8.4*). Four out of ten patients whose ideas were inhibited or evaded (40 per cent), compared to three out of ten whose consultations showed no evidence of this behaviour (29 per cent), subsequently did not correctly recall or make sense of their doctor's views on at least one topic.

Three other variables also influenced how correct was a patient's recall and understanding: whether his condition was diagnostically significant (bad news); the duration for which doctors and patients spoke in a consultation and a patient's educational background (*Table 8.5*). More than half (55 per cent) of those patients

Table 8.4 *The influence of inhibiting and evading patients' ideas on his subsequent recall and understanding of key points*

	patients' ideas		
	inhibited (%)	not inhibited (%)	total
recall and sense:			
correct on			
all topics	108 (60)	106 (71)	214
incorrect on			
any one topic	71 (40)	43 (29)	114
total	179	149	328

chi-square = 4.18 1 d/f p < 0.05
gamma = 0.24

with a 'significant' diagnosis did not make sense of or remember correctly one of the doctor's key points compared with about a quarter (26 per cent, among those who were able to do so. A quarter (25 per cent) of those who spoke to their doctor for less than five minutes, compared to a third (32 per cent) who spent five to seven minutes talking and nearly a half (45 per cent) who spent more than seven minutes in conversation, either did not remember or correctly make sense of at least one key point. More than two-fifths (43 per cent) of those with a basic educational background, just over a quarter (28 per cent) of those with an intermediate education and just under a quarter (22 per cent) of those with a high educational background, did not make correct sense or did not recall one of the key points made in their consultations.

The four variables which have been mentioned and which did influence patient understanding were combined in a simple index which was then used to predict the likelihood that patients would not remember or would not correctly make sense of what they were told. Patients were assigned points on the index as follows:

+2   if a patient's diagnosis 'significant'
+2   if conversation time of consultation > 7 minutes
+1   If conversation time < 7 but > 5 minutes
+2   if a patient's educational background basic
+1   if a patient's educational background intermediate
+2   if a patient's ideas were inhibited or evaded in his consultation.

Table 8.6 shows that the higher patients scored on this index the less likely they were to remember or understand correctly what a doctor said. In fact, three out of five (58 per cent) of those patients who scored highly on the index did not remember or make sense correctly of at least one of the key points their doctor made. Conversely, only one in ten of the patients (11 per cent) with a high educational

Table 8.5 *The influence of the significance of patients' diagnoses, their educational background, and the length of time doctor and patient spent speaking on whether a patient remembered and made correct sense of the key points*

	diagnostic-significance		education			duration of speaking		
	signif-icant (%)	not sig-nificant (%)	high (%)	inter-mediate (%)	low (%)	>5m (%)	5-7 (%)	7< (%)
recall and sense:								
correct on all topics	43(45)	171(74)	50(78)	65(72)	90(57)	80(76)	63(68)	71(55)
incorrect on any one topic	53(55)	61(26)	14(22)	25(28)	75(43)	26(25)	30(32)	58(45)
total	98	232	64	90	174	106	93	129

diagnostic-significance: gamma=0.55
educational background: gamma=0.35
duration speaking: gamma=0.31

Table 8.6 *Predicting whether a patient will remember and make sense of the key points*

	index score				
	0 (%)	1-3 (%)	4-5 (%)	6+ (%)	total (%)
recall and sense:					
correct on all topics	24	87	66	37	214
incorrect on any one topic	3 (11)	24 (22)	38 (36)	49 (58)	114 (35)
total	27	111	104	86	328

chi-square=33.97 3 d/f p<0.001
tau^c=0.34
gamma=0.50

background, who had a consultation in which conversation went on for less than five minutes and in which there was no evidence that their ideas were inhibited or evaded, and a condition diagnosed as of no diagnostic significance, could not remember or correctly make sense of key points.

Some causes of remembering and understanding

Doubt about the validity of the finding that there was no relationship between the clarity with which doctors stated their views and patients' understanding prompted us to examine a small number of cases in detail to check whether there was anything about the way ratings had been made that could be responsible for the results. The check gave no cause for concern. Even when doubtful or marginal ratings were modified in a direction to suit the 'clarity' hypothesis, no statistical relationship emerged. Instead, detailed case studies drew our attention to a paradox which seemed to explain the absence of a relationship. Some patients were given what seemed a perfectly clear and well-organized statement but misunderstood it. Other patients were given what seemed wholly inadequate information but made sense of it correctly. In both cases what seemed to matter most was not the clarity of the information the doctor gave but the detailed ideas the patient brought to bear to interpret it. The impression we gained was that patients appeared to elaborate the explanations given to them by doctors with the result that they could make sense of what the doctor said correctly when they were told very little or could make sense of it quite incorrectly when they were told a lot.

To explore further these impressions about the role of the ideas patients brought to consultations, it was decided to compare in more depth the consultation and interview material of those patients who remembered and correctly made sense of what they were told and those who did not. The interview data, although not ideal for the purpose, was a rich resource for exploring a patient's thinking. Patients had been asked to give an account in their own words of their reasons for going to the doctor and of their detailed ideas about possible diagnoses and treatments (8).

Comparing interview and consultation material in depth amounted to a large scale case study which, if it was to be done systematically for all 328 cases, was likely to be very time-consuming. Instead, therefore, we selected a subsample of 60 cases by choosing, at random, 40 cases on which to examine how patients remembered and made sense of diagnostic-significance and another 20 cases to consider how they remembered and made sense of treatment-action (9). Patients were chosen so that half of them had remembered and 'correctly' made sense of the key points and half had not.

The case study comparisons proved worthwhile. They suggested not only why the four factors included in the index were so important but also why the clarity with which doctors stated their views was relatively unimportant. Broadly, patients did not remember or correctly make sense of what their doctors told them because the information given to them presented particular difficulties of understanding (in contrast to that given to other patients) when it was compared with the ideas they themselves had. The views doctors took in these cases, considered in the light of the explanation the patient had himself developed prior to the consultation, were more likely to be unfamiliar, unwelcome, unexpected or intrinsically confusing than the views doctors conveyed to those who did remember and correctly make sense of what they were told. In these circumstances the limitations the doctors (and to some extent patients) usually placed on achieving a mutual understanding (because they did not explore patients' ideas or emotional reactions and did not check their understanding) were crucial. First, the relatively unorganized and contradictory approach doctors often adopted to conversing with their patients, meant that patients had considerable scope for misinterpretation. Drawing on their prior theories patients could arrive at a completely different version of what doctors had meant without either of them realizing it had happened. Second, also in the context of not exchanging ideas with their doctors, patients brought lay theories to the consultation which caused them to misinterpret ideas which were unexpected or unfamiliar. Of course, those who remembered and correctly made sense of what doctors said also had to do so without ideas being exchanged and without there being a check on what they understood. But the difference between these patients and those who forgot or did not correctly make sense was that they had less opportunity to misunderstand what the doctor said because it was already familiar to them, was expected, or happened to be consistent with the prior explanations they had already developed.

The statistical finding that patients with diagnostically-significant conditions and those with only a basic educational background were less likely to remember and correctly make sense, is consistent with the idea that some information may have been more intrinsically difficult and unfamiliar than other information. The finding that longer consultations were more likely to lead to misunderstanding is consistent with the idea that they provided more scope for contradiction and ambiguity. The finding that consultations in which patients ideas were inhibited or evaded caused more misunderstanding is consistent with the idea that they indicate both that a patient had ideas and that there was a failure to allow an exchange of them with the doctor. To support these contentions we will now describe the characteristics of the information which was more likely to be misinterpreted and the two processes that increased the likelihood it would be so.

The characteristics of the information patients misunderstood

The hypothesis that the process of forgetting and misunderstanding began with what doctors had to convey was quite clear in the sub sample of sixty patients. Patients who remembered and made sense of what their doctor said, compared to those who did not, more often received diagnoses which were already expected and more often were given treatments they had requested or which were routinely repeated. As indicated by the statistical findings, their conditions were less likely to be significant and were more likely to be straightforward and, therefore, familiar.

First, patients who remembered and made sense of what their doctors told them very often attended for an illness which had already been diagnosed in the previous consultation or in an earlier episode. The illness was, therefore, seen by these patients, from the start, as the same as they had had discussed before. They already knew they suffered from conditions like recurrent earache, hay fever, insomnia, sinus headaches, shingles, housemaid's knee or thrush and from their experience anticipated the doctor would confirm this as he proceeded to do.

Second, and similarly, the treatment received by these patients was often what they had requested or had been given on a previous occasion. Treatments such as inhalers, pain-killers, antacids, eye drops, nose drops, antihistamines, antibiotics and sleeping pills were prescribed. New treatments had often been anticipated by them (for example, antibiotics for a urinary tract infection) or by the recommendation made earlier by a hospital specialist (for instance, for minor surgery) and their doctor now concurred.

Third, among these patients, if their illness was new it was very often diagnosed as self-limiting (good news) or as a diagnosis they expected. These patients presented a disproportionate number of minor, clear-cut symptoms with diagnoses like conjunctivitis, tonsillitis, dermatitis and urinary tract infections all of which are reasonably familiar and non-problematic to the lay public. In these cases the doctor's role was often limited to confirming a diagnosis the patient had anticipated.

By contrast to those who remembered and made sense of what their doctors told them, those who did not were much less likely to be given a diagnosis which was the same as one that had been agreed before, much less likely to be given a well-established and expected treatment, much less likely to be given a self-limiting and clear cut diagnosis that they expected, and much more likely to be told their illness was diagnostically significant (bad news). In general, the characteristics of the information conveyed to these patients was frequently problematic in that the patient had not expected it, was not familiar with it, or had cause for an emotionally charged reaction to it.

First, although they might have presented their problem before, it appeared that these patients had not previously reached a basic understanding of it that was the same as the doctor's. They were more likely to be returning with such symptoms as those of nausea, back and shoulder pains that had not responded (in their view) to the treatment or advice given previously. Sometimes they or the doctor had changed their diagnostic ideas since their last meeting and sometimes it was clear that patients had understood the significance of their diagnosis quite differently from the doctor at the previous consultation.

Second, patients who did not remember or make sense correctly were more likely to have been given new treatments which they had not previously experienced or anticipated. Among these patients were some who had been asked for the first time to return to have their blood pressure monitored, or to see a social worker, or to take advice given in the form of psychosocial counselling which was novel to them.

Third, although these patients also presented problems which their doctor diagnosed as minor and self-limiting their problems tended to be more unusual (for example, loss of interest in sex), more open to explanation in several ways (for example, feeling feverish, a crying child), or subjects of popular misconception and controversy (for example, weight-gain due to being on the pill or menstrual problems). The information doctors gave to explain all these symptoms was inevitably less clear-cut, less obvious and less familiar than the information they gave to patients with the minor conditions found more often among those who could remember and correctly make sense.

Finally, these patients were more likely to be given diagnoses which were diagnostically 'bad news'. Sometimes these were conditions which are relatively unusual and so unfamiliar, such as an obstructed bowel. At other times they were conditions such as arthritis, migraine, high blood pressure, back problems and eczema which the lay public encounter frequently but it seems often have explanations for which are at variance with those of medical opinion.

To summarize, patients who remembered and made sense correctly very often received information that was expected, familiar and non-threatening. Those who did not remember or make sense correctly were much more likely to receive information that was unexpected, new, more complicated and more threatening. What happened in this situation was that the tendency noticed among all patients to understand what they were told in terms of the familiar and the expected led those given information the details of which were unfamiliar and unexpected to forget what they were told or to distort it in significant ways.

Ambiguous and contradictory cues

If information was unexpected, unfamiliar or potentially threatening the task of understanding was inevitably more difficult. It was especially so in consultations in which the doctor (from the point of view of the patient listening to him) provided information in an unstructured, ambiguous and potentially inconsistent way. In these circumstances patients very often selected out what they thought was familiar or sensible from the information doctors gave and used this to bolster and confirm the theories they themselves entertained. Sometimes, most especially when the important information was unfamiliar, unexpected and potentially threatening, this process resulted in patients missing the emphasis of what a doctor was telling them and so forgetting some parts of what he said or sticking to some incorrect way of understanding their problem or the purpose and importance of a treatment strategy. Because their ideas were not explored or their understanding checked, misinterpreting or forgetting of key points in this way would persist unmodified. The patient would have an illusion that his explanation and his doctor's were the same. One case example will illustrate how ambiguous or contradictory clues can be interpreted by a patient with unfortunate results for his understanding of the diagnostic-significance of his condition.

Mr Inman (1940) was diagnosed by his doctor to suffer from frozen shoulder syndrome. However, at his interview he reported only that his doctor was not certain whether his problem was a frozen shoulder or not and was unsure whether his doctor knew what was wrong at all. Mr Inman's doctor had begun his contribution to the consultation by interrupting his story about what had happened at the hospital. The doctor indicated he was doubtful about both the diagnosis of frozen shoulder and the physiotherapy treatment suggested by a hospital specialist. He then said: 'I'd like to examine your shoulder to see whether you have got a frozen shoulder.' He then added ' because if you have, if it is a frozen shoulder, it doesn't actually make much difference what you do. . . .' In the course of examining Mr Inman further the doctor made more remarks such as 'That's catching you, this isn't a typical frozen shoulder, but it's more like that than anything else.' Later on, however, the doctor had clearly made up his mind. 'I think that's what you've got' and 'Sometimes something else can mimic a frozen shoulder. . . but. . . there is nothing to suggest mimicking here.' Mr Inman questioned this last statement, reminding the doctor what the hospital had said. Mr Inman said 'No! He said that they had found arthritis quite a bit'. The doctor responded dismissively: 'Pooh!'

It is quite easy to see how many of the comments made by Mr Inman's doctor as part of a self-dialogue in which he came, at the end, to a pretty clear decision, might appear to be contradictory and indicative of uncertainty to the patient who is listening to him. The doctor's subtle shift in position *vis-à-vis* the frozen shoulder diagnosis provided the patient with much opportunity to introduce his own beliefs when actively trying to sort out and make sense of what the doctor said. In this connection what was important was Mr Inman's own prior misgiving (derived in part from the hospital) that his complaint might be a frozen shoulder or that it might also be something he considered more insidious like arthritis or tuberculosis. It was this uncertainty about what was wrong with him that he heard confirmed by his doctor and which caused him to feel his doctor did not know what was wrong. The consultation is particularly interesting, like many others in which doctors gave ambiguous and potentially contradictory clues, because it reveals some of the difficulties a practicing doctor might have with the instruction that he keep his advice simple, state the important matters first, or avoid jargon. Clearly Mr Inman's doctor could have summarized and clarified his views once he had reached them (and checked and elaborated on Mr Inman's ideas instead of ignoring and inhibiting them). But however clear he might have been at the stage of stating his view formally his communications would always be muddled in so far as a special feature of much medical work is that taking a history, making an examination and choosing between one or more possibilities without absolute certainty, are part of a social interaction. The patient will hear what a doctor says, observe what he does and be aware even of his silence. All these stimuli may enter into his efforts to try to understand what the doctor says and he may not easily discriminate between so-called 'information-gathering' and 'exposition' stages of the consultation (Fletcher 1973). The parts of the consultation devoted to formal explanation have to take place in this dynamic context and it is for this reason that a two-sided dialogue approach to communication, featuring an exchange of ideas, may be more appropriate rather than the largely one-sided 'expository' approach that was observed in most consultations.

Another way in which apparent inconsistencies within what doctors said could be misconstrued by patients arises from the patient's need to try to form a coherent model of explanation. In some consultations, for example, what a doctor advised about treatment was not obviously related to the diagnosis. Patients could then remove any dissonance they experienced by forgetting aspects of what was said or altering the sense of what they had been advised. One short example illustrates this process in its most simple form.

> Mr Inshape (1412) was told by his doctor that his blood pressure was satisfactory, his heart wasn't too bad and his chest, although it had lost elasticity because of bronchitis in the past, was not too bad. The doctor followed this by prescribing tablets to assist Mr Inshape's breathing (in fact a repeat prescription), a blood test to be done at the surgery immediately after and a chest X-ray to be done at the hospital.
>
> At interview, Mr Inshape reported being given the tablets to help his breathing and he mentioned the blood tests done by the nurse at the surgery. However, he did not recall and had not attended for the chest X-ray.

In this case the general impression the doctor gave that all was well (followed by tests which were not explained and for which the patient did not know the purpose) was potentially in contradiction with the need for a chest X-ray. Nothing was said about how the X-ray fitted into the overall strategy with the result it may have appeared inconsistent with the diagnosis. As far as could be judged from Mr Inshape's interview his understanding that he had been pronounced well led him to see no reason why any further action was necessary and and so to forget about the X-ray.

A second consultation is a more dramatic example of how patients could adapt what doctors said about the diagnostic significance of a condition so that it was consistent with the treatment and their own ideas.

> Mrs Bannen (1468) was making her second visit in ten days. She emphasized that she was no better than before: 'Doctor, I'm still feeling this sickness.' He tested her urine and afterward said, confidently, 'there's not much wrong with your kidneys actually at this moment'. At the same time, however, he asked her to remind him which kidney specialist she had been under ten years previously. Without further comment he then rang the hospital. In her presence, he was heard to ask about the patient's history and to ask whether she should be seen again. On replacing the phone the doctor told Mrs Bannen 'Well, they tell

me to send you up to see him, so I'll put a note at the back here. You go down there today'. The doctor gave no other information.

After her consultation Mrs Bannen tried to make sense of the consultation in terms of her belief that there was something pushing into her kidney and damaging it. To her this was not an infection but a chronic 'anatomical' problem which she imagined could be remedied only by a serious operation. Ten years previously, she told the interviewer, she had seen an X-ray of her kidney which she believed had shown something pressing into it. This idea did not emerge in the consultation but the hospital referral allowed her to attribute to the doctor the idea that he thought she had a physical object pushing into her kidney, to ignore his comment that all was well, and to believe that he thought she needed the urgent operation she had long thought would be necessary.

Distraction and divergence

Patients' own theories and ideas helped to make the information which they were given more or less difficult and allowed patients to interpret apparently ambiguous and contradictory statements in a way that was sometimes consistent with what their doctor believed and sometimes not so. Patients' prior beliefs interacted with what doctors said to make ideas familiar or unexpected and to determine how they interpreted ambiguity. The prior theories they brought to the consultation were also important in a third way. They could cause patients to be distracted from crucial elements of what doctors said and, when they diverged from those of the doctor in regard to crucial details, could cause patients to understand in an incorrect way the ideas he had mentioned apparently clearly. By the same token, when a patient's ideas and more detailed understanding were convergent with the doctor's views they served to create correct understanding. This process was encouraged by the fact that the detailed ideas patients had were not very often elaborated in consultations, and were quite frequently inhibited and evaded. As in the other examples, in this way patients' prior ideas influenced matters in an unseen and silent manner.

The way in which patients' ideas caused them to be preoccupied and distracted from the communication process is illustrated by two consultations: those of Mrs Illingworth (1401) and Mr Inland (2413).

Mrs Illingworth was a seventy-two year old whose brother, sister, mother and grandmother had all, she said at interview, died of cancer. She, herself, admitted during her interview that this was a source of constant fear. 'Well, there's always that dread – cancer,' she said. She presented her doctor with chest problems, and shoulder pain, both of which had been presented before.

After examining her shoulders and listening to her chest, the doctor told her that 'I think your chest is a lot better. I think we'd better get your shoulders X- rayed before we do anything to that. . . I think you have shown us that it is still that the caps, the landing of the joint that's bothering you and this is a condition that sometimes goes on for a long time but clears up in the end.' And it is not like rheumatism that sort of spreads elsewhere. It just stays in the shoulder but it is quite difficult to get rid of sometimes.'

At her interview Mrs Illingworth was not able to say what the doctor thought was wrong with her, nor was she able to say whether the doctor thought her trouble was serious and diagnostically-significant or not. She remembered, she said, that the doctor said it was arthritis but added that 'I'm no further' in understanding what was wrong (also implying he was no further as well). She indicated clearly that she had lost a lot of weight and had cancer on her mind. When asked directly she could not rule out the possibility that this was what her doctor thought was wrong.

Mrs Illingworth received a detailed explanation, albeit one which was based on the doctor's ideas of what she might be thinking and was stated in difficult language. None the less she appeared to have missed his confident conclusion that the chest condition was a lot better and the shoulder condition was temporary. The main influence on the fact that she missed that information and felt that her doctor was uncertain about what was wrong with her was undoubtedly her preoccupation with the possibility that she had cancer and was losing weight and experiencing symptoms because of it. The way the doctor spoke and the fact the X-ray might be considered inconsistent with a clear diagnosis increased the scope for her interpretation. She may also have suspected that she was not being told the truth.

Mr Inland (2413) went to his doctor with a badly swollen ankle. After a brief examination, the doctor said he had pulled the ligaments of it. Before he finished telling the patient this Mr Inland interrupted the doctor to say: 'It's very painful, actually.' In what then seemed to be a rather uncomfortable conversation the doctor did not explore the meaning of this comment but reiterated his view to an obviously doubtful patient. During this part of their conversation the doctor also mentioned that the ligament strain was likely to be chronic.

At interview, Mr Inland said that the doctor had said that he had a ligament strain but did not remember that the doctor had added that it would be chronic. Mr Inland thought that the doctor meant by ligament strain that the complaint was ordinary and not serious. He himself doubted this, as he implied in the consultation, and had gone the same day to the local hospital where he thought he could get a more reliable diagnosis. At the hospital he had received an X-ray and had been given an opinion which, he believed, was different from the one he received from his doctor and so confirmed his doubts about his doctor's clinical competence.

The fact that Mr Inland mistakenly believed he and his doctor had a different view of the significance of his condition seems to have been caused by the fact he and his doctor understood a strained ligament in a different way. Mr Inland was so preoccupied with the idea that something more was wrong than an ordinary ligament strain and so frustrated that the doctor would not or could not listen to him that he became distracted. In this way he believed the doctor had made a diagnosis that nothing much was the matter and felt it necessary to go to the hospital for an opinion. Given his preoccupation and the effect it had he did not hear what the doctor said about his problem being chronic nor try to discover more about what the doctor meant. The case appears to be an example of why, when doctors inhibited or evaded their patients' ideas and did nothing to explore obvious disagreement, it was more likely that patients would not remember or make sense correctly of what they said.

By contrast with the last two cases, there were some consultations among those of patients who remembered and correctly made sense of what their doctors said when the patient's ideas, although not explored in detail, were directly considered. An example was the consultation of Mrs Cecil (2340).

> Mrs Cecil thought her headaches might be caused by sinus trouble and told her doctor. He responded to this by considering it when he examined her. He then said that he thought a sinus origin was unlikely because her cheeks would be more tender than they were if sinus was the cause. Instead he preferred the hypothesis that her headaches were probably due to tension, although he mentioned that they might possibly be caused by migraine, or be a side effect of the contraceptive pill.
>
> It was noticeable from her account at interview, that Mrs Cecil felt her doctor had considered her ideas and was happy about his examination. She was able to make 'correct' sense of her doctor's hypothesis and correctly reported that he thought she had been run down, depressed and under a lot of tension, the outcome of which was headaches caused by tension. She reported to the interviewer that 'I suggested to him it was to do with my sinuses and he said, 'You've been under a lot of tension haven't you. It's probably migraine'.

Mrs Cecil, unlike the two previous cases, had her preoccupation sensitively taken into account. In the consultation it was quite clear that the doctor had considered the possibility of the symptoms being of sinus origin carefully. It seems likely that the main difference between the outcome of this consultation and the other two, in which patients also held views divergent to those doctors eventually reached, was that Mrs Cecil's ideas were not inhibited or evaded. These findings are particularly interesting in the light of the belief that the emotional aspects of illness preclude or limit reaching an understanding with patients (Parsons 1951: 442). In the two consultations which went wrong one was an example of a patient (Mrs Illingworth) who was made more anxious and unable to understand because her anxiety was not shared and discussed. The other (Mr Inland) was a patient whose emotions were also inhibited and evaded. On this evidence, at least, communication was being made more difficult because ideas were not being discussed and exchanged.

The second way in which patients' ideas influenced the chance that they would remember and correctly make sense of what doctors said was through the fact that sometimes the detailed understanding they had of what was wrong with them and what they needed led them to distort the meaning of what their doctors advised or said was wrong. Mr Ison (2276) is an example of a patient of this kind.

Mr Ison went to his doctor with a tight, needle-sharp, pain in his abdomen, tennis elbow, a complaint that he was full of wind, a worry that he might be impotent and a feeling of too much stuff in his throat. His doctor told him that the pain and probably the wind were caused by his discontinuing too early the tablets he had been given for a stomach ulcer and thought that the impotence might be a side effect. He advised him to stay on the tablets for another week, to be sure to eat regularly, to go off work for a week and to stop cigarette smoking. He was advised to return later to have an injection for the tennis elbow.

At his interview Mr Ison knew what he had been advised about the tablets, the tennis elbow injection, staying off work and giving up smoking. Despite a specific question about eating, however, he was unaware that he should eat regularly or carefully.

Careful examination of what Mr Ison told the interviewer reveals that his detailed ideas about what was wrong and his idea about how the treatment worked were responsible for his failure to appreciate that eating was in any way important. He believed that the tablets were designed to disperse the poison in his stomach and to dry up his ulcer. He described the ulcer like a 'boil in the stomach'. According to him it had a centre which was poisonous, caused by gathering up all the poisons in his stomach. To treat the problem, he imagined, the tablets would disperse the poisons and help to dry up the boil. This detailed understanding of what was wrong and how the treatment worked was markedly variant to the medical view and included no conception of the role of stomach acids and of the introduction of food (and alcohol) into the stomach. It seems likely that because of this divergent understanding of the details of what was wrong with him, Mr Ison had no framework within which to grasp what the doctor had meant about the tablets interfering with the production of acid in his stomach or about eating regularly. This had led him to forget a crucial aspect of what the doctor said to him. The example illustrates the potential shortcoming of approaches to giving information which focus only on making clear what a doctor has decided or advised, and which do not emphasize the need for patients' detailed understanding of causal mechanisms and rationales to be considered.

The illusion of shared understanding

The characteristics of the information patients were given, the ambiguous and contradictory cues their doctors gave them, the inclination of doctors to inhibit and evade patient ideas, and the divergence of some patients' detailed understanding seem together to go a long way towards explaining which patients remembered and correctly made sense of what their doctors said and which did not. A tentative statistical analysis of the differences between these two groups of patients in the sub sample of sixty provided some confirmation for each aspect of the hypotheses we have sought to illustrate (10).

The central argument that emerges from these analyses is that the explanatory frameworks with which patients entered the consultation were the crucial factor in determining what patients remembered and understood. A high proportion of patients remembered and made sense correctly of different aspects of a doctor's views because in terms of the predictions their framework indicated for the diagnostic-significance of their condition or the purpose and importance of treatment and prevention, they shared explanatory models with their doctors. At those relatively superficial levels most patients had nothing to learn. Their visit to the doctor confirmed the ideas they had or provided them with the advice and treatment they anticipated. Although doctors and patients never explicitly exchanged their ideas (both parties restricted such a dialogue) this did not influence for the worse the understanding of the majority of patients.

Two features of the construction of medical knowledge in contemporary society were partly responsible for this convergence of explanatory models, at the level at which we have examined them so far. In the first place, as Chrisman (1977) has argued, in societies such as Britain and the USA, lay health knowledge and explanatory models are developed in relation to the scientific health care system and lean heavily upon it. Second, at the same time, since primary care doctors tend to deal with self-limiting problems symptomatically rather than in terms of the underlying disease process, their 'operational models' are in many ways closer to the lay models of their patients than to the official biomedical models of disease (Helman 1978). At the relatively superficial level we have so far examined, therefore, the patients' lay health knowledge and explanatory models provided an adequate resource for them to draw on in 'filling in' the doctors' comments and making sense of the consultation. In the great majority of cases, doctor and patient shared the same ideas and terms at the level we examined and this enabled the patients to remember and make sense correctly of the doctors' views.

On most occasions the doctors escaped the consequences of being relatively unorganized and implicit in the way they conveyed information, only because the patients' own initial views were functionally similar to their own and so enabled them to make sense of the doctors' comments in an appropriate way. When the patients' initial views differed from those of the doctors, however, brief or vague comments from the doctors and views which were left implicit, did not convey to the patients (or doctors) that they viewed things differently. Instead, it allowed the patients to assume, incorrectly, that the doctors were confirming their own views. The clarity with which information was conveyed (and its detail) therefore would be important, not for mechanistic reasons, but largely to make it clear that the doctor views the patient's problem in a different way from the patient. This recognition of a difference in views is the first step towards exploring those views, shattering any false illusions about shared understanding, and eventually negotiating a shared explanatory model. The same task may be more effectively established, however, by checking what a patient has understood.

In this way, we see the role of clarity in conveying information very differently from how it has been conceptualized by Ley (1979) in terms of a formula which advises doctors to state their views more clearly, more simply and more explicitly. Familiarity with many of the consultations we have described makes it easy to say why such an argument might be maintained. But being clear in this sense, even if feasible given the dynamic setting of a consultation in which doctors must make decisions as well as convey them, would be to miss the nub of the problem. Similarly, the implication that a little information properly conveyed is most likely to be understood by the patient also makes the wrong emphasis. A little information, if for example it is understood as leaving out an explanation of the reasons for diagnostic hypotheses or treatment recommendations, may be insufficient if the point at which a patient's understanding diverges from that of the doctor stems from his causal understanding, not his literal ability to repeat what he is told.

In some cases, such as in Mr Ison's above and also in many of the cases to be described in the next chapter, it is likely to be necessary to explore with the patient his detailed understanding of relevant medical ideas. Otherwise there will be a major risk that the patient will misunderstand the purpose and importance of treatment and prevention or the diagnostic significance of his condition, or that he will evaluate it unfavourably.

The level at which patients' recall and interpretation of what their doctors said was studied was in many ways quite superficial. It would, therefore, be interesting to know the kinds of influences that determine deeper levels of patients' understanding. One could examine, for example, how far patients could remember and make sense of the reasons their doctors gave for deciding on a particular diagnosis or treatment and their understanding of diagnostic processes and treatment and preventive mechanisms. As we noted in the previous chapter for practical reasons it was not possible to make a systematic and quantitative examination of patients' understanding in this regard. However, two brief analyses were undertaken to explore some aspects of a patient's understanding of medical ideas at deeper levels. Both analyses suggest that the likelihood that a patient's deeper understanding of his doctor's views would be correct is dependent on many of the same processes which determine the sense he makes of the key points. Because interviews had not been designed specifically for the rather more demanding task of establishing what patients understood at deeper levels, the conclusions in this respect are more tentative than those reached earlier.

The cases of sixteen patients who had been given 'moderately elaborate' explanations by their doctors were considered by looking at what they said in their interviews about their doctor's rationales for his views. Of the 16 patients whose consultation and interview data was examined 10 (63 per cent) recalled exactly what the doctor said while the other 6 did not. It was apparent that those who did not remember the explanations their doctors gave them failed to do so for reasons which were very similar to those that influenced whether patients remembered and made sense of key points. Three patients had strong divergent theories and were preoccupied with them. One was also very dissatisfied with her treatment. The prior theories these patients had, which were not explored in the consultations, had apparently caused them to be inattentive to the details of what their doctors had said. Another patient missed an explanation which was embedded in a long and ambiguous discussion by her doctor and the sixth, an elderly patient with only basic education, did not understand the terms and processes the doctor was employing.

A second opportunity to explore patients' deeper levels of understanding of health issues was provided by a small study undertaken with only some patients in our main sample. The study explored how twenty-four patients who smoked understood the nature of the harm caused to their health by smoking (11). The results are interesting in the present context because they illustrate several features of the way lay health knowledge which is convergent with medical ideas at one level can be quite divergent when considered at another. All twenty-four patients questioned were aware of the government health warning and knew that smoking was considered by experts to be harmful to health. This level of understanding is, perhaps, slightly more superficial than that assessed by determining whether patients correctly made sense of their doctors' advice.

Despite their superficial understanding that smoking was harmful to health these patients showed that they usually did not understand exactly how their own smoking was currently doing them extensive harm, particularly in comparison to the other causes of ill health they perceived in their daily lives. Summarized very crudely, inhaling tobacco smoke was considered by these patients to be only one rather minor factor among the causes of ill health in their environment. The more patients were given an opportunity to spell out their views and beliefs the more it became apparent that their understanding of the risk was markedly divergent from that indicated by current biomedical evidence (12).

Some patients told us that cigarette smoking merely aggravated chest conditions which they believed to be caused primarily by other factors. They would point to the fact that if they did not smoke they would put on weight – an eventuality which they considered to place their health at as grave a risk as if they continued to smoke. Patients would often warrant this belief with reference to biomedical ideas about the effects of obesity on the cardiovascular system. In the context of the additional consideration that increased weight was undesirable for reasons of their body image, many patients concluded that to stop smoking might be worse for their health than to continue with it.

Other patients pointed to people they knew who had smoked heavily for many years and who had lived into their eighties, or to people they knew who had never smoked a cigarette but had died from cancer at a young age. Most patients had available a personal story of this kind. Indeed, 5 out of the 24 patients made a point similar to that made by Mrs Taylor (2356): 'My mother had cancer and she never smoked in her life.'

Still other patients felt that smoking was only one of several environmental risks, some of which were unavoidable, such as breathing exhaust fumes. Mrs Thomas (2346) was one of four who mentioned the large number of other environmental risks. She said: 'There's so many bad things to worry about like pollution and stuff like that – if we are worried about it all the time we'd be a lot sicker than we are.' As another patient put it 'I'm not firmly convinced that smoking will enhance my death. There are so many other things over which I have no control that are hastening my death' (2318). The same patient and nine others considered that the risks of smoking were outnumbered by the benefits. One of those benefits was the effect mentioned by two patients on 'the nerves': 'If I didn't smoke I'd be mad because of the kids' (2269).

While the comments made by respondents who smoked are not, by any means, an exhaustive explanation of why they under-emphasized the risks of smoking (and do not, for instance, take account of the role of cognitive dissonance (13)), our purpose in mentioning them here is to illustrate the complex and thoughtful patterns of explanation in which the patients in our sample tended to locate their understanding about their health. Information given to them on the topic of smoking or that given to explain a doctor's diagnosis and advice would be 'pitched in' to a cauldron of ideas and assumptions. As we shall show in the next chapter, if these ideas are ignored in medical consultations, they can not only lead to some patients being unable to remember or make sense correctly of what they are told, but they can also lead to very negative evaluations of what doctors say.

Summary

Comparing patients' accounts of the key points their doctors made in their consultations with the assessment of what their doctors said described in the last chapter, most patients were found to remember and correctly make sense of most of the key points their doctors made. However, many consultations were successful in terms of the patient's subsequent understanding of the doctor's views mainly because at no stage were there differences between the views of the doctor and patient.

Most consultations largely confirmed the patients' views or at least fitted into their preconceptions and health knowledge. Such consultations are probably in the majority in primary care where often there is little new or unexpected for the patient to understand. Where there were differences between the views of the doctor and patient, or where the patient's lay health knowledge was medically inaccurate, consultations tended to be unsuccessful. In those consultations, the patient's views and beliefs were not explored nor related to the doctor's medical views.

CHAPTER 9

Evaluating medical ideas

Most patients who remembered and made sense correctly of the key points their doctors made were also able to evaluate their doctor's views and advice in a manner that was judged to be favourable: over four-fifths of these patients (85 per cent) were committed to his view of the diagnostic-significance of the problem; and a similar proportion (79 per cent and 82 per cent, respectively) to his treatment- and preventive-action advice. Indeed, over three-quarters of the patients (77 per cent) who remembered and made sense correctly of the key points that a doctor made were committed to his view on all of the topics (*Table 9.1*).

Table 9.1 *How patients evaluated what their doctors said on the three topics*

	information topics			
	diagnostic-significance (%)	treatment-action (%)	preventive-action (%)	any one of the three (%)
number of consultations after which patients had remembered or made sense correctly	221	292	71	214
number of consultations in which patients were also committed to the key points	189 (85)	233 (79)	58 (82)	164 (77)

Note: The denominators for recall (*Table 8.1*), and making sense (*Table 8.2*) and commitment are different because whether patients made sense was rated only if recall was correct and whether patients were committed only if they made correct sense.

How patients evaluated the key points of what their doctors said was determined by exploring with them, in the interviews, how far they accepted what their doctor had told them and whether they evaluated what he said favourably against potentially competing theories they themselves had mentioned. Since it made no sense to assess commitment to attributions that were incorrect, the rating was made only for those topics on which patients had made correct sense of the 'key points'.

Once the patient had attributed views to the doctor and the sense he made of them had been established, the interviewer explored his evaluations of what his doctor said on the 'key points': particularly his own theories and relevant aspects of his explanatory model. Respondents were invited to comment on the value of a standard set of possible treatments and diagnoses that might be relevant to their problem. They were asked, for example, what kind of things could be wrong with them and what would that mean? What were the worst possibilities the patient could envisage? What were the best? Would problems persist or be self-limiting? Were there alternative or preferable treatments? Throughout this part of the interview the patients were reminded that they might have heard about medical ideas over the years from television, radio, newspapers, magazines, encyclopedias, doctors and friends (1).

When the interviewer felt that a patient's views of the potential diagnostic-significance of his problem, or the range of possible actions and preventive measures had been established thoroughly, a new phase began. First, the patient was warned by the interviewer that no suggestion was being made that the doctor was wrong. The purpose of the questions to follow was only that the interviewer wanted to know what he, the patient, thought. The patient was then asked in various ways what he thought, once he had got home, about the views he attributed to his doctor. Was he inclined to agree? Did he have any doubts? Had anyone else mentioned doubts to him? The interviewers were sensitive to any hints of doubt or disagreement that might be apparent from the patient's manner or tone of voice. How far the patient believed the doctor had ruled out any conflicting ideas that had emerged so far and what reasons the patient had for believing that any conflicting views were less plausible than those of the doctor, were then explored (2).

A feature of the way patients responded to the interviews, already noticed in the previous chapter, was that most were able to talk at some length about the views they had considered before their consultations. Sometimes their views were definite, at other times vague. Sometimes they reported views which they thought were confirmed by their doctor, at other times views they thought were not confirmed. What was particularly interesting, however, was that an individual patient's responses were not the same across topics. On one topic he might report vague ideas, on another he might have definite views. On one topic he might report that his ideas were confirmed, on others that they were not confirmed (3).

Most patients had quite strong views on at least one of the topics, which they believed to have been confirmed by their doctors. On these topics they accepted what the doctors said, saw it as self-evidently correct and were somewhat bemused by interviewers' efforts to assess their attitudes to any conflicting ideas.

Many patients also doubted their doctors' ideas on one or more topics. When they felt like this they usually mentioned spontaneously their own strong views and volunteered their doubts about the doctor's views. Low confidence in the doctor's views and an attachment to a competing theory seemed to go together. Patients expressing such doubts usually had an underlying framework of ideas that they believed to be in conflict with those of the doctor. Because their views were strong and definite it was usually easy to interview such patients without fear that the interviewers were putting ideas into their minds.

Other patients, however, also held vague and 'flexible' views on one of the topics. They did not entertain these ideas with any confidence or strong belief and they seemed to be keeping options open. Patients who held such views on a topic tended to report agreement with doctors' views but also indicated that they remained 'open minded' about competing alternatives. They were neither explicitly doubtful about doctors' views nor attached to an alternative. Interviewing patients about topics on which their views were vague and flexible in this way was difficult and so raised the problem of interviewer effects. To guard against the danger that the interviews might 'put ideas into the patient's mind' an interview procedure advocated by Kinsey, Pomeroy, and Martin (1949) in a similarly difficult context, was adopted. First, possible alternatives were 'suggested' to the patients in a leading way. Once the patients responded positively, however, the possibility that they might be trying to please investigators by their replies was carefully probed. Only conflicting ideas or doubts which patients defended against the interviewers' questioning were considered relevant for rating.

Ratings of the patient's commitment were made on the basis of the material obtained from the patients in the interview. Two separate components were assessed: the extent to which a patient believed the doctor to be right; and, the extent to which a patient believed conflicting views to be wrong. These components were then combined so that patients 'not committed' on a particular topic could be distinguished from those regarded as 'strongly' or 'weakly' committed. Patients were assessed as 'not committed' only when they both reported some kind of doubt about the doctor's view and were not inclined to reject conflicting alternatives. Most of these patients were the ones described above as volunteering competing views.

An example of how ratings were made is the case of Mrs Nolan (2467). She was a mother who brought her young child to see the doctor thinking that he wheezed a great deal. In the consultation her doctor seemed unwilling to label the child and did not actually supply a term to describe his hypothesis. Instead, he said 'It's just a wheeze' and then emphasized that it would continue and be something to which they would have to become accustomed. He added that it was not serious and nothing to worry about. When interviewed Mrs Nolan was indignant about what had happened but was able to give an accurate verbatim account of what the doctor had advised. She was also judged to make sense of the treatment-action recommended (in fact, inaction) correctly. But Mrs Nolan also said that she had no confidence that her doctor was right and believed that a proper investigation of the child's trouble would be more appropriate than inaction:

she volunteered that hospital tests, like those given to her friend's child who was 'unexpectedly' found to have bronchitis, would have been better. She did not feel the child's wheeze was something to be 'put up with' and also disputed the doctor's idea of significance. 'It is not right', she said, 'that a young child sounds like an old man' and, therefore, she believed that the doctor could not have got the diagnosis right when he said the child would continue to wheeze for years. Mrs Nolan's views were so clear cut that there was no difficulty in determining that she lacked commitment to the doctor's treatment-action advice as well as to his ideas about diagnostic-significance. She expressed disagreement at her interview, took a negative attitude to her doctor's recommendation, and suggested alternative action. She is an example of the one-fifth of patients who made correct sense of the key points of a doctor's treatment-action ideas but were 'not committed' to them. Ratings of commitment made in this way were reliable (4,5).

Some correlates of a patient's commitment

Distinguishing between patients who were and were not committed to the key points their doctors made allowed us to explore the possible influences there might be on the process of evaluating medical ideas. As in the case of whether patients remembered and made correct sense of what their doctors said many of the variables we examined did not appear to influence how patients evaluated what their doctors said: for example, a patient's educational and occupational background; the diagnosis he was given (both the formal diagnostic category and its diagnostic-significance as 'good' or 'bad' news); which doctor he saw; whether the doctor was in the Study or Comparison group; the length of time patients and doctors spoke to each other; and whether it was a new or old illness; all made no difference to whether a patient was committed or not. It was especially interesting that three of the four variables which influenced whether patients remembered and made sense correctly (a patient's education, the diagnostic-significance of his condition and the length of time doctors and patients talked to each other) had no influence on a patient's commitment.

The way we assessed how patients evaluated what their doctors told them made the theories patients had about what was wrong with them and what should be done about it a central focus. One purpose was to explore the effects of a communication strategy based on trying to enable a mutual exchange of ideas. We had expected that doctors who explored patients ideas and related their statements and reasoning to them (reactive explanation) would be more likely than doctors who did not to have their ideas and advice evaluated favourably by their patients. It proved impossible to test this hypothesis directly. No doctor provided reasons on even a single topic which were specifically related to precise information he had obtained about a patient's ideas on that topic.

If it was not possible to test directly whether reactive explanation influenced the evaluation a patient made of what his doctor said and advised, some indirect evidence could be established about the influence of the ways doctors dealt with patients' ideas. When this was examined we found that consultations in which there was evidence that a doctor had inhibited or evaded a patient's ideas were less likely to result in a patient being committed than those in which there was no such evidence. Over one in three (37 per cent) of those consultations in which a doctor evaded a patient's ideas and one in four (24 per cent) of those in which he inhibited them, compared to one in eight if there was no evidence of evasion and inhibition, resulted in a patient being not committed to what the doctor advised about treatment (*Table 9.2*). A similar influence was perceptible in the case of patients' commitment to what doctors said about diagnostic-significance but it was not statistically significant.

Table 9.2 *The influence of inhibiting and evading patients' ideas on their commitment to what their doctor said about treatment*

	reaction to a patient's ideas			
	evading	inhibiting	neither inhibiting nor evading	total
	(%)	(%)	(%)	(%)
committed to the doctor's view treatment advice	22 (63)	95 (76)	115 (87)	232 (100)
not committed to the doctor's view treatment advice	13 (37)	30 (24)	17 (13)	60 (100)

chi-square 11.57 2 d/f p < 0.01
tau^c = 0.17 p < 0.001
gamma = 0.40

The other variables which influenced a patient's commitment were different depending on whether it was diagnostic-significance or treatment-action on which patients were giving an opinion (6). In the case of diagnostic-significance women, women bringing children, patients aged under 60 and patients from minority ethnic backgrounds, were least likely to be committed. A quarter of those women presenting a child under ten (26 per cent) compared to one in six (16 per cent) of the women patients if they were adults on their own and only one in fourteen of the men patients (7 per cent), were not committed to a doctor's diagnostic-significance hypothesis. One in five patients under age 35 (20 per cent) compared to one in seven aged 36 to 55 (14 per cent) and one in seventeen (6 per cent) patients aged over 56, were also not committed to the doctor's view on this topic. Finally, as many as a third (30 per cent) of patients from all minority ethnic groups in the sample (Afro-Caribbean, Asian, Irish or continental European) were not committed to a doctor's ideas about diagnostic-significance compared to one in eight (12 per cent) among the majority group in the population.

In the case of treatment-action patients from minority ethnic groups, women presenting babies under two years old and patients who had not seen the particular doctor before, were the least likely to be committed. As many as two-fifths (43 per cent) of the patients who were Afro-Caribbean, Asian or Irish, compared to one in five (19 per cent) among those from continental Europe or the majority ethnic group, were not committed to the treatment doctors advised. Almost a half (47 per cent) of those women who presented babies, compared to 1 in 5 (19 per cent) men or women presenting themselves or older children, were not committed to what doctors said on this topic. Finally, nearly a third (32 per cent) of patients seeing the doctor for the first time, compared to 1 in 5 (19 per cent) among those who had already met their doctor, evaluated treatment advice unfavourably.

Two indices were constructed to see how far the variables so far mentioned could predict the likelihood a patient would not be committed to what doctors said on each of the topics. *Tables 9.3* and *9.4* show that with these variables it was possible to predict commitment but not very precisely. In the case of commitment to a doctor's action advice increasing combinations of the four factors (not knowing their doctor, coming from an ethnic minority group, presenting a baby, or having ideas inhibited or evaded) were more likely to lead to a situation in which a patient evaluated advice unfavourably. Patients with none of these factors had a one in ten chance of lack of commitment whereas patients with two or more had a one

Table 9.3 *Predicting patients' commitment to their doctors' treatment advice*

	index score			
	0	*1-2*	*3+*	*total*
	(%)	*(%)*	*(%)*	
committed	93 (89)	97 (82)	42 (60)	232
not committed	11 (11)	21 (18)	28 (40)	60
total	104	118	70	292

chi-square=23.11 2 d/f p<0.001
tau^c=0.23 p<0.0001
gamma=0.50

scoring: patient's ideas inhibited (+1); patient's ideas evaded
    (+2); not met doctor before (+2); women with baby
    under 2 (+2); minority ethnic group (+2) (max. score=8
    min. score=0)

Table 9.4 *Predicting patients' commitment to their doctors' views on diagnostic-significance*

	index score			
	0/1 (%)	2-4 (%)	5+ (%)	total
committed	40 (93)	118 (87)	31 (72)	189
not committed	3 (7)	17 (13)	12 (28)	32
total	43	135	43	221

chi-square=8.60 2 d/f p<0.05
tau^c=0.13 p<0.01
gamma=0.45

scoring: age 18-35 (+2); age 36-55 (+1); women and child under 10 (+2); woman alone (+1); minority ethnic group (+2); patients' ideas inhibited (+1); patients' ideas evaded (+2) (min. score=0; max. score= 8)

in four chance (*Table 9.3*). The five factors implicated in predicting commitment to what doctors said about diagnostic-significance (being younger, being a woman, presenting a child, being from a minority ethnic group and having ideas inhibited or evaded) were less influential. None the less patients with none of these factors had a one in fourteen chance of being not committed to what their doctor said compared to a one in four chance with two or more factors (*Table 9.4*).

Sources of commitment and lack of commitment

To explore in more depth the processes underlying the way patients evaluated what their doctors said the interview material of a sub sample of 50 patients, selected at random, was examined. Ten patients, who were committed to the key points doctors made concerning diagnostic-significance, were compared with 10, who were not. Fifteen patients, who were committed to the key points doctors made concerning treatment-action, were compared with 15, who were not.

Detailed analysis of the consultations and interview material of those who were committed to their doctors' ideas revealed that these patients had started consultations with views which were congruent with those their doctor settled on. As in the case of those patients who had remembered or correctly made sense of what doctors said those patients who evaluated a doctor's views favourably had very often anticipated, or even suggested, the diagnostic hypothesis or treatment-action with which they emerged. Their consultations served to confirm their views or perhaps to confirm which of several opposing views they had was correct. In the main they did not, therefore, have to understand and to adapt to ideas with which they were not familiar. Nine of the 10 patients we selected who were committed to what the doctor had to say about diagnostic-significance, for example, had already entertained the diagnosis they were given before the doctor arrived at it. Similarly, among the 15 patients committed to the doctor's view of treatment-action, 7 had themselves actually asked for the treatment they received, 4 were given the established and expected 'routine' treatment for their problem and only one patient was actually dissuaded from an initial view contrary to that advised by his doctor.

By contrast with those who were committed to what their doctors said, those not committed to it had usually started out with views that they thought contradicted those of the doctor. Among the 10 patients not committed to what their doctors had to say about diagnostic-significance, 6 started their consultation with a conflicting view of the diagnosis. Among the 15 patients who were not committed to treatment-action as many as 11 patients appeared to have started their consultation with an alternate view about the best treatment. Either these patients had attached a significance to their symptoms which differed from that implied by the treatment the doctor suggested or they had disagreed with the doctor's diagnosis. In either case they considered the treatment to be linked to an inappropriate causal model of their problems and rejected it in preference to an alternative. To illustrate how this could happen we will examine five sources of lack of commitment in detail.

Different diagnostic hypotheses

In analysing the consultations and the patients' interviews, it seemed that the majority of those patients not committed to what their doctor had said about the diagnostic-significance of the problem had arrived at a hypothesis to explain the problem, before going to the doctor, which differed from that which the doctor arrived at in the consultation itself. These patients' belief in their own view of the problem, usually unchallenged or avoided in the consultation, then led them to doubt the decision the doctor had made and concomitantly to doubt the way he had arrived at that decision.

Mrs Nugent (1093), for example, went to the doctor with the idea she might have an ovarian cyst. However, according to her doctor, she suffered from cervical erosion, trichomonas, and a bacterial infection. At interview, Mrs Nugent disagreed with this diagnosis, saying she did not think she had a trichomonas infection but one of another origin. She supported this view in her own mind by saying that her doctor could not know what kind of infection she had because he restricted himself just to looking and did not take a swab. Moreover, she considered, he could not have ruled out her ovarian cyst hypothesis in any definitive way because he did not palpate her abdomen. Mrs Nugent, therefore, was a patient who had a theory about what was wrong with her and clear ideas about medical procedures to test the theory. These latter ideas, which were not mutually explored in the consultation, permitted her to sustain her theory despite the doctor's diagnostic procedures and contrary diagnostic conclusion.

Mrs Nonelly (1841) was also a patient with alternative ideas which remained unmodified by her consultation. She had volunteered to her doctor that she thought her daughter had whooping cough. However, the doctor said that her daughter's cough was not whooping cough but an ordinary cough. At interview Mrs Nonelly said she had (in her mind) disagreed strongly with the doctor about this. The teacher at her daughter's school had suggested whooping cough and she sees many more young children than the doctor and sees them over a longer time. Also, since she had seen the doctor, she mentioned, she had talked to a friend whose daughter had the same symptoms. Her friend's daughter had been diagnosed as having whooping cough. She summed up her beliefs in the interview by saying, 'If I went to another doctor he might well say it was whooping cough. It just depends on which doctor you see.... He seemed to have enough difficulty in diagnosing in the first place'. In these last comments Mrs Nonelly demonstrated attitudes towards a doctor's diagnostic procedures which are of considerable interest. First, she has questioned her doctor's ability and competence to diagnose on the basis of observing the way he went about it. Second, she has used comments derived from her friend's doctor and her child's school teacher to support her view. In doing so she indicated their superior qualifications for diagnosing in the particular case.

The extent to which diagnostic procedures influenced patients is a matter about which it is very interesting to speculate. It is widely believed by many general practitioners that various symbolic examinations (such as taking the patient's blood pressure if he has a headache) are potent forms of reassurance. However, among the patients we studied it was clear that such procedures were often ineffective as methods to change patients' ideas. Patients who disagreed with a diagnosis seemed to have no difficulty finding arguments to discredit the validity of the evidence on which it was based. Like Mrs Nonelly and Mrs Nugent, they drew on ideas about proper medical procedures first, to question and then readily to dismiss what their doctor said. In part this may have been possible because the doctors did not explain their procedures or ask patients about their ideas concerning diagnostic rules. Nor did they relate their reasons to them. It is also possible that the diagnostic procedures which doctors use, in general practice at any rate, are far from appearing as rigorous systematic attempts to rule out all possible alternative diagnoses on the basis of 'scientific' evidence. Although patients tended to concede that doctors had greater medical knowledge to draw on in arriving at their diagnoses, they could discount this by attributing to them a more restricted knowledge of the 'normal' state of the patient, the current manifestation of the symptoms and the broader context in which they were located – information which patients would often not provide and often not be asked to provide.

Subjectively inconsistent diagnoses

Michael Balint (1964) warned eloquently of the dangers to the patient's confidence in his doctor if a patient's symptoms were dismissed with the assertion that 'nothing is wrong'. As Balint put it 'finding "nothing wrong" is no answer to the patient's burning demand for a name for his illness...he feels that "nothing is wrong" means only that we have not found out and therefore cannot tell him'(1964: 25). A second reason why the doctors' diagnostic hypotheses in our sample did not make sense to patients and were negatively evaluated by them involves an extension of Balint's argument. One group of patients were not committed because the way they understood the doctor's views made the latter appear to contradict the 'facts' in the case. Just as Balint argued that 'nothing wrong' cannot make sense of subjective experiences which patients feel are wrong, so (albeit in a more subtle way) we suggest that some diagnostic explanations simply made no sense to patients because they could not link them to their experience. What the doctor said in these cases seemed to the patients quite contrary to the characteristics of the situation as they understood them. This kind of discrepancy gave rise to the rejection of the doctor's view as inadequate or inappropriate to account for the patient's complaint.

Mr Anstey (2286) was one of two patients in the sub sample of ten who were not committed to a doctor's diagnostic hypotheses who felt they had been given a diagnosis which did not appear to 'fit the facts'. He presented his doctor with pain in the abdomen. His doctor thought this was caused not by cardiovascular problems (which the doctor assumed might be his worry) but by 'a muscle strain'. At interview Mr Anstey was doubtful. He volunteered that he had himself had thought the pain was sciatica and, when asked what he thought about that now, could still not reject the ideas that it really was. In his view his symptoms were not consistent with muscle strain: he could not recall lifting or pulling anything heavy and, since he was unaware that a muscle can be strained even lying in bed, could not make sense of the explanation. He stuck, therefore, to an explanation which did make sense.

Divergence of explanatory models

Patients who felt they could not make sense of the diagnosis they were given or who had doubts about it often doubted the validity of the treatment recommended. They tended to see treatment-actions as part of a coherent 'model' and, therefore, specific not to the symptoms or complaint as it was experienced, but to a particular diagnosis. As suggested by authors such as Blumhagen (1980), it seems that patients presumed that a diagnosis implied a view about the pathology and disease processes underlying the symptoms. The value and mechanism of an action, therefore, was seen to depend on the way in which disease processes operated and the effectiveness of actions was linked to this specific interaction. When the doctor's view on significance was rejected as incorrect, therefore, it seemed to follow that his treatment-action recommendations would also be questioned as inappropriate for the underlying problem. Among all the patients studied nearly two-thirds of those who were not committed to diagnostic-significance, compared to just over one-tenth of those who were committed, were also not committed to action advice.

In the sub sample 7 of the 15 patients who were not committed to treatment-action had doubts about the doctor's diagnosis.

Mrs North (1367) was one such patient. She presented pain in her leg which her doctor believed was of a muscular origin. He recommended rest and aspirin. At interview, however, Mrs North rejected 'muscular pain' on grounds similar to those which caused Mr Anstey to reject a similar diagnosis for pain in a different site. Mrs North thought it did not feel like a muscular pain and was more like a nerve pain because of the way it 'shoots'. In the context of this contradictory diagnosis Mrs North had doubts about 'rest' and 'aspirin' as the right treatments. She thought that she had a nerve being pinched by a displaced leg joint and expected the appropriate remedy to involve 'whacking' it back into place. She could not reject this or a variety of other treatments associated with other 'causes' of the pain in favour of the treatment on which the doctor decided.

Mrs North's case illustrates the way in which the rejection of a doctor's recommendation was generally accompanied by a preferred alternative which the patient considered to be specifically suited to the preferred diagnosis – demonstrating the importance of the model underlying patients' deeper understanding of what they are told.

Mr Norwich (1121) was another patient whose understanding and evaluation indicate the interrelatedness of some patients' thinking. Mr Norwich presented a sore toe which his doctor told him was gout and prescribed pills accordingly. At interview Mr Norwich was doubtful about the doctor's hypothesis (although he did not totally reject it) and could not reject his original idea that the true cause was that he had stubbed his toe in bed. He reported that he had been prepared to consider the doctor's view as plausible at first and had started to take the tablets. However, by the time of his interview three days later the pain in his toe had almost gone. This eventuality did not fit with his common-sense view of gout and of how the tablets worked. It did fit, however, with his original idea that his troubles might be caused by a stubbed toe which would get better within a few days if he rested it. Mr Norwich's case illustrates the way patients' views are tentative and constantly revised in the face of new evidence. As Stimson and Webb (1975) emphasized patients will nearly always have ample opportunities to revise their theories after the consultation and then to reject the doctors' ideas in retrospect.

Patients who misunderstood their diagnosis or the pathological processes underlying it, were another group who felt treatment-actions were inappropriate and so another group of those not committed to treatment-action recommendations. In the minds of these patients the effectiveness of an action arose from its specific interaction with causal processes underlying the complaint itself. Actions which did not correlate with what was understood about causal processes, therefore, gave rise to a rejection of the action the doctor decided on, in favour of an alternative treatment which was believed to act more specifically on the disease processes as they were understood.

Mrs Nathan (1058) was such an example. She presented with a new 'irritation' on 'her private parts' as well as continuing rashes on her face and wrists. Her doctor diagnosed the new irritation as similar to her 'adolescent acne'. He advised her to continue with the cream he had already given her for her wrists, to continue with the tablets he had prescribed for her face, and to use a new cream for her 'private parts'. At interview Mrs Nathan rejected the idea she should continue to take tablets for her face and could not disagree with her own alternative idea that a change in her diet would be better. This evaluation appears to arise because Mrs Nathan associated the spots on her face with 'poison' in her blood. She therefore regarded an action which would 'purify' her blood (such as a diet) as the most appropriate therapy and considered that the tablets she was given, which she did not think had this function, might accentuate the problem. Her deeper understanding and causal model of her troubles was in this way substantially at odds with the doctor's advice.

Four of the 15 cases in the sub sample misunderstood some similar vital aspect of the process underlying what was wrong with them in the way exemplified by Mrs Nathan. These patients, however, were not necessarily those who could not remember and make correct sense of what doctors said in the relatively superficial way described in the last chapter. They often knew what he had diagnosed and advised correctly. What was problematical in their case was the deeper understanding they had of the hypothesized condition or the mechanism of an action and the extent to which this led them to question what they were advised to do. This finding underlines the point made in the previous chapter when we argued that concern with patients' deeper understanding may often be essential to providing them with information they will understand and accept.

Faith in the doctor

Some doctors place very considerable emphasis on the importance of a patient's 'faith in the doctor' and have been doubtful about the value of a 'rational' knowledge of disease processes and their treatment. They regard 'faith' as a potent source of influence on patients' propensity to accept recommendations and, therefore, emphasize the importance of various stylistic aspects of how information should be made to sound convincing. In this context Parsons (1978) has even suggested that faith in the doctor might be undermined by increased efforts on the part of doctors and patients to negotiate a 'rational' understanding of biomedical thinking. It was interesting to find, therefore, that among the patients studied what might be termed 'blind faith' in doctors could actually cause low commitment.

Two patients among the 15 not committed to doctors' treatment-action recommendations, and 2, among the 10 not committed to diagnostic-significance, appear to have been unable to accept their doctors' ideas mainly because of a discrepancy between their 'optimistic faith' in the power of medicine and the real limitations of medical intervention as perceived by their doctors. These patients refused to believe that medicine could do nothing for their problem and that their conditions were as hopeless as the doctors said they were. Their rejection of the doctor's view seems largely to have been an emotional one, in which they put forward no specific alternative of their own but insisted that medicine must be able to do 'something' for them. These patients not only rejected the doctor's view but at the same time questioned his 'credentials' for making such a decision. They wanted, instead, to take their problem to someone more qualified like a 'specialist' at the hospital (perhaps someone who was seen as having access to more potent medical knowledge and 'magic').

Mrs Nancy (1338) was one of these patients. Her doctor told her that a post-operative mark on her breast was not a sign of any pathological process although it might not go away. At interview she disagreed that the disfiguration (as she saw it) was inevitable. She told us that her whole reason for accepting the previous advice to have a small operation to her breast had been to remove another similar mark. To discredit her doctor and to justify further help-seeking, she said, 'He's a GP and is not meant to know that sort of thing'. Mrs Neal (1284) was another example. Her doctor said that the pain about which she complained was 'a little early arthritis' in the hips, more marked on the right. He advised her to keep taking the pills as she had been doing and to come back if it got worse, so that they could discuss the possibility of physiotherapy or a hip replacement operation. At interview Mrs Neal rejected this strategy as inadequate and could not disagree that an immediate specialist referral for more 'careful' treatment would be more appropriate. She believed, she said, that 'Doctors had been doing research for a long time' and, therefore, must have come up with a more permanent remedy or pain reliever than her doctor had given her. She could not believe that in 1979 (the year of her interview) doctors could do no more than give her the pain relievers which her doctor had given her.

It was particularly interesting that among the 10 patients committed to the doctor's view of the diagnostic-significance of their condition and the 15 committed to his view of the appropriate treatment-action 4 also seemed to rely on 'blind-faith', but in these instances it helped them to accept their doctors' ideas. These patients could give no reason for accepting the doctor's decision other than their faith in him and to some extent resisted attempts by interviewers to get them to provide a rationale or warrant for their belief. However, these patients appeared to differ from those who were not committed to the doctor's decision only insofar as the doctor had lived up to their expectation that he could 'help' them. This suggests that faith in medical practice is a rather double-edged tool with which to achieve favourable evaluations of what doctors say. It could provide grounds for acceptance of a doctor's decisions but just as likely could be counter-productive in creating unjustified expectations which work against the doctor when medicine can do little. On balance, it would seem, little benefit can be envisaged from a strategy encouraging 'faith in the doctor' as a way to promote commitment and to persuade patients to follow the doctor's advice.

Value disagreement

Two patients among the 15 not committed to treatment-action recommendations can be described as patients who rejected their doctor's advice for a fifth reason. They preferred a treatment which the doctor was not willing to give and disagreed with his assessment more on value grounds than because they did not follow or understand a doctor's reasons.

An example of a patient who disagreed in this way was Mrs Newington (1955). Her doctor prescribed 'nothing' for her cough. At interview she appeared to understand why the doctor thought 'nothing' was desirable but disagreed with this decision. Cough medicine, she believed, was better than nothing and did no harm. She intended to go out and buy some. Her case and another like it were the only ones (among the fifteen cases not committed to treatment-action) in which a patient's lack of commitment reflected a relatively straightforward and verbalized conflict between the 'values' of the doctor and those of the patient concerning the 'best' course of action for a given problem. What each thought was out in the open to be negotiated and bargained with. The two cases, therefore, appear to be the only ones in which persuasive strategies (on either side) would appear to be relevant: a somewhat interesting finding in view of the extensive attention given to persuasion and negotiation among health educators and social scientists (7).

The process of evaluation

The striking fact about patients' evaluation of their doctors' ideas was that by far the majority of patients were committed to their doctors' views. Three out of 4 patients who remembered and made sense correctly of what the doctor said on the key points evaluated what was said favourably and rejected any conflicting alternative ideas on all three topics. As we have mentioned, however, the main difference between those who were committed to what their doctors said and those who were not depended on the relationship between the doctor's views and those with which the patient had arrived at independently prior to consulting the doctor and after. When the two coincided, the patient was likely to be committed to the doctor's decision. When they diverged, however, the patient was likely to reject the doctor's ideas, rather than his own. The doctors in the consultations we studied rarely paid attention to patients' ideas and asked them to elaborate them. They were not informed about a patient's thinking and could not, therefore, direct their explanations precisely to it. We believe that the analysis of the consultation and interview material of those who were not committed to a doctor's ideas support the argument that to allow more patients to make a favourable evaluation of their ideas, just as to ensure they correctly make sense of them, doctors need to establish what ideas patients actually have.

Some other conclusions about the way doctors dealt with their patients in the consultations also suggest the need for change. Many of the efforts which doctors made apparently to influence what their patients thought were ineffective. For example, the diagnostic procedures utilized by the doctors (such as physical examinations) did not convince patients that their decisions were correct when those procedures resulted in a decision which the patient himself could not square with his understanding or had not previously been inclined towards. Similarly, the explanations and reassurance doctors gave, given that they did not involve a mutual exchange of views, had no demonstrable effect on those who did not already agree.

The main finding, then, is the fact that about three-quarters of the patients were committed to the doctor's ideas about diagnostic-significance but that this was not due to the persuasive power of the doctors nor to the magical power of the diagnostic techniques they employed. Rather, it appeared to be due to the fact that in most instances the doctor and patient made sense of signs and symptoms in similar ways before the consultation started. On the whole, doctors simply confirmed what patients already 'knew'. When they did not, that is, when any persuasive work needed to be done, the doctor was on the whole ineffective.

The findings about the process by which patients evaluated what doctors said may appear similar to those concerned with the process by which they made sense of what doctors said. Both processes do indeed emphasize the role of the patient's prior ideas and understanding. However, there is one important difference. In the case of the process of making sense patients were largely unaware when they arrived at incorrect conclusions. This was much less so in the case of evaluation. Patients who were not committed to the key points doctors made were usually aware this was so during the consultation. Had they been asked they could have identified and elaborated to a considerable extent both their lack of conviction and the reasoning behind it. The point is particularly poignant in the light of an additional finding that patients who expressed doubts and asked questions in a consultation were more likely than those who did not to be uncommitted to doctors views afterward. A third (34 per cent) of those who openly doubted something a doctor said in the consultation, compared to just over a quarter (28 per cent) of those who doubted covertly and only a sixth (17 per cent) of those who did not do so at all, were found to be not committed to a doctor's view on one of the key points. Just under a quarter (24 per cent) of those asking the doctor to give reasons for his diagnosis in some way, compared to less than a tenth (9 per cent) of those not asking such a question, were not committed to diagnostic-significance. Those asking the doctor to give reasons for treatment-action were also much more likely not to be committed to it although this result (unlike the others) was not statistically significant. The findings indicate, however, that patients in a way warned their doctors of the need to take their views and thinking more seriously: to treat them as experts in their own health care and to exchange ideas with them. These potential warnings went largely unheeded.

It seems likely that the variables included in the two indices (mentioned above), which also predicted the likelihood that patients would not be committed, all indicate the presence before a consultation of divergent lay views. Patients from minority ethnic groups, women (especially with young children), younger patients and patients having their first consultation with a doctor, were all less likely than others to be committed to one or more of the key points a doctor made.

It seems likely that patients from minority groups (those not of Anglo-Saxon origin) probably live in communities and family settings in which they draw on a body of health beliefs and knowledge which diverges at times from that which the (usually Anglo-Saxon) doctor draws on. They may access different sources of health knowledge to make sense of their symptom experience or to make sense of the doctor's decisions, as they understand them.

As we have mentioned women were also less likely to be committed, especially if they brought their children for attention. As an aspect of their family roles, women in our society have been given responsibility for the family's health. It is likely, then, that women both attend to the signs and symptoms of ill health more readily than men, and discuss them with other people, especially other women, more frequently. They are therefore particularly likely to arrive at the doctor's surgery with well thought-out views on the nature of their problem and its treatment. This may be most noticeable among women with young children, who feel their responsibility for their family's health most keenly. Over a number of years they are likely to have become 'experts' in the area of health and illness, with an extensive body of lay knowledge about the problems pertaining to children and a unique sensitivity based on experience to the meaning of signs and symptoms in their own children. Similarly, other mothers and professionals such as teachers or health visitors, with whom they discuss their children, also gain status as expert alternate consultants by virtue of their extensive knowledge and experience. Mothers of young children, then, are particularly likely both to have arrived at their own well-developed views on issues of diagnosis and treatment, and to have faith in the validity of those ideas. While these ideas are likely to coincide with those of the doctor on many occasions, it is when they diverge from the doctor's view that their confidence in their own and their lay consultants' particular expertise leads them to believe their own views and reject those of the doctor. This is particularly likely given the high status accorded to 'personal experience' as evidence for health beliefs (Davies *et al.* 1982).

The younger patients were the more likely they were not to be committed to a doctor's ideas about diagnostic-significance. Just as membership of minority ethnic groups and being a woman seems to have been associated with well thought-out and perhaps more divergent health beliefs, so it seems possible that younger patients might be expected to be more informed and to have considered their health beliefs more thoroughly. It is at least consistent with the belief mentioned in an earlier chapter that patients are becoming better informed and more participatory in their health care. It has been argued, for example, that younger patients may be more likely to be critical of their doctors (Haug and Lavin 1981).

Patients meeting a doctor for the first time (42 per cent) were twice as likely as those who already knew him (21 per cent) not to be committed to his ideas about diagnostic-significance or his suggestions for treatment-action or prevention. This influence seems generally consistent with the idea that it was situations which were unfamiliar and unexpected which caused problems of understanding and commitment. Patients attending a new doctor are more likely to encounter unfamiliar ways of working and thinking which would be likely to increase the difficulty of the communication task.

Finally, it is interesting to consider what was happening in those consultations in which doctors inhibited or evaded the signs that patients had ideas and chose not to explore them. It seems likely (as, for example, in the case of Mr Nixon (Chapter 4) whose doctor was mystified by the patient's leg aggravation and dietary preoccupations) that doctors did not see the importance of the patient's communications and, perhaps, became agitated, uncomfortable or even irritated by them. The perceptions that some doctors had about how to practise medicine clearly did not include a recognition of the patients' ideas as particularly relevant. From these doctors' perception, and in the context of what doctors usually thought of as a busy surgery, patients' apparently meaningless preoccupations must have seemed incoherent and irrelevant. However, while doctors largely ignore the ideas their patients have, those patients who start with divergent ideas are likely to remain wedded to them. If this is so, it is a further finding which supports one of the theories mentioned earlier. So long as doctors ignore the detailed ideas their patients have, the explanations they give, the physical examinations they offer to reassure and the tests they take, will make little difference to the commitment their patients have to their ideas. If patients themselves arrive at theories consistent with what the doctor says and does, they will be committed to it; if they do not, they will not.

Summary

The overwhelming majority of patients who succeeded in correctly remembering and making sense of what their doctors told them about the various key points were also committed to their doctor's views. Those patients who were not committed to what doctors said were most likely to come from minority ethnic backgrounds, to be women bringing their children to the doctor, to be younger patients, to be patients who were new to the doctor, or those whose ideas were inhibited or evaded during the consultation. Closer examination of a number of cases suggested that patients usually evaluated what a doctor said favourably because they already expected him to say it and themselves already agreed with it. In those cases in which patients started out with views divergent to those of the doctor the consultations did little to change them. The absence of a mutual exchange of views between doctors and patients, rather than any inherent conflict between their ideas, was mainly responsible for this latter outcome.

CHAPTER 10

Stereotypes and the process of sharing medical ideas

We have emphasized, in the last two chapters, the extent to which it was usual for the patients we studied to remember what doctors said, to make sense correctly of the key points the doctor made and to be committed to these points. Patients so often managed to make sense correctly and to be committed to what doctors said, we have argued, mainly because they shared at the outset of the consultation much the same views as their doctors. Although doctors and patients rarely tried to clarify each other's views and consciously relate them one to another, this did not matter in the great majority of cases because of the congruence of views and thinking with which they began. At the same time, difficulties in remembering, in making correct sense, and in being committed, all resulted from the fact that these outcomes derived, in the context of doctors and patients not managing to exchange and clarify their respective views together, from a divergence in the initial views with which they started. Thus, 'successful' outcomes occurred when communication was largely unnecessary; 'unsuccessful' outcomes occurred almost every time it was. The lack of efforts to treat patients' views and theories as important and worth elaborating, and to find some way of relating medical models to them when they were divergent was the main cause of these 'unsuccessful' cognitive outcomes.

Despite the large numbers of patients who could remember, make sense correctly, and who were committed to so much of what their doctors said, there is also a way in which the results obtained can be characterized as a considerable failure in communication. This may become more evident if we represent the findings in a different way (*Table 10.1*). Although, as we have just reported, patients made correct sense and were committed to the great majority of the key points their doctors made, there were nonetheless a very large number of consultations in which something went wrong. In fact just over one third (36 per cent) of the patients given information about diagnostic-significance either had incorrect recall, made incorrect sense, or were not committed to the key points doctors made. Also, well over a quarter (30 per cent) of the key points made to patients about treatment-action and well over one third (42 per cent) of those made about prevention were not successfully communicated. Altogether in as many as one in every two consultations (50 per cent) patients either could not recall all the key points doctors

Table 10.1 *Remembering, making sense and commitment among 328 patients*

	information topics			
	diagnostic-significance (%)	treatment-action (%)	preventive-action (%)	any one of the three (%)
number of consultations where topic was introduced	297	328	100	328
number of consultations where the patient either did not remember or make sense 'correctly' or was not 'committed' to key points	108 (36)	95 (30)	42 (42)	164 (50)

made on the three topics, or could not make correct sense of them, or were not committed to them (*Table 10.1*). Bearing in mind that the key points were defined in such a way as to include only those important points patients needed to know about, an astonishingly high proportion could not do so on all of them. The study suggests, therefore, that there are major problems in doctor – patient communication in general practice. In half the consultations the patients in one way or another were not able to take advantage of the key elements of the advice their doctors gave them. As we have argued, the reason for this, in large part, appears to have been the failure of the doctors we studied to elaborate or to relate to patients' own ideas and explanatory models, despite the fact that patients gave many hints they had them.

Some crucial aspects of the interactions between doctors and patients that we studied made it unlikely that an elaboration and sharing of views would take place. The consultations appeared to occur, in the main, in the context of a medical ethos which cast the doctor as professional and expert and the patient as passive and ignorant. Nearly forty years ago Sir Morris Cassidy (1938), Senior Physician at St Thomas' Hospital, illustrated this ethos most aptly. 'A lot of valuable time would be saved', he felt, 'if our patients could be taught that all we want to hear from them is an account of their symptoms as concise as possible and chronological!'. Moreover 'What we do not want to know are the very things which they are just bursting to tell us – e.g., What Dr X of Freiberg or Prof. Z of Lausanne thought about them' (Cassidy 1938: 177). In so far as this view is widespread it may explain why any indication of a view on the patient's part, or any questioning of the doctor's views, often tended to be inhibited or evaded or even a source of some tension in the consultation. Such tension in the past was indicated in patients' accounts of why they did not, in a direct fashion, ask the questions or express the doubts that they had. The same tension was, perhaps, evident in the way doctors sometimes appeared to be quite puzzled by what was happening when patients presented ideas. There seemed to be a strained emotional atmosphere in many consultations with both parties avoiding or backing-off from the issues. Shifting and vague consultations of this sort may have evaded the tension that might have been caused by a direct confrontation of anomalies and it may have allowed both doctor and patient to cherish the illusion they shared each other's views. For example, Mr Nixon (the patient with a leg 'aggravation'), told the interviewer that he thought that his doctor had ruled out all forms of heart disease. It had not even occurred to his doctor, however, that this was required. By keeping their ideas to themselves the participants allowed hidden differences to continue unrecognized and unchallenged and encouraged a Kafka-esque parody in which different rules were apparently being used to play the same game. While this may have been felt by both parties to be a way of reducing interpersonal tension, it also precluded the possibility that they could achieve a real understanding.

Conventional stereotypes

In so far as they reveal patients' ideas and theories to be a critical and constructive element in the consultation process, the findings we have reported contrast markedly with many of the views commonly expressed within the professions of medicine. As Sir Morris Cassidy's views suggest, patients' beliefs have very often been considered a nuisance or a barrier to communication and patients themselves have been thought to be largely without knowledge of medical ideas. This latter view was cogently expressed by Sir Henry Brackenbury (1935), another force in medical thinking in that formative period of its development just before and after the Second World War. Brackenbury wrote;

> 'It is not altogether easy for the doctor to realize the colossal ignorance of the laity of things which are to him ingrained or even axiomatic. . .it is really extraordinary how such laymen, even if what is commonly regarded as well educated, seem unable to form any sort of clear image of anatomical or pathological conditions, or any true conception of physiological or pathological processes. . .This is no trivial matter, for it is not only a serious obstacle to a doctor giving a rational explanation or description. . .but is the major cause of all the superstitions, quackery, charlatanism and nonsense. . .in reference to medical matters still so astonishingly prevalent among persons who, in other spheres of which they have more knowledge, are able to think logically and well.'
>
> (Brackenbury 1935: 90)

Such views are still expressed in conversation and in postgraduate seminars. In one form or another, they seem to have underlaid the thinking of many of the doctors in our sample – particularly in the practical situation of consultations in which they were confronted with, what seemed to them, irrelevant patient ideas. As

Brackenbury's and Cassidy's comments indicate, if one views patients' beliefs and knowledge in this stereotypical way, their contributions are likely to be experienced as no more than a nuisance, especially if one feels busy.

The equation of inaccurate biological conception with no knowledge at all, is one that many have made since Brackenbury. In many hospitals, for example, teaching rounds are still conducted in front of the patient's bed but taking little notice of his capacity for making some sense of everything that is said and done around him. Latin terms or complex terminology are often used apparently to obviate the danger of patients being made anxious or confused by what is said.

The idea that patients are ignorant and usually not capable of understanding medical ideas, together with research implying that they very often fail to remember what their doctors have said, has undoubtedly had a less than encouraging effect on attempts to supply patients with information. We have just quoted Brackenbury's pessimistic conclusion in 1935. The following statement made in 1982 by a 'progressive' and innovative general practitioner confirms that little has changed in this respect: 'If we give six statements only four will be remembered...we have been trying to economize on the number of statements that we give to patients on the grounds that...you're not going to fill in the science behind it if he is merely going to forget most of it' (1).

The ideas that patients are biologically ignorant and that they frequently forget what they are told can be considered part of a powerful stereotype. Among other effects, it is associated with an aura of medical superiority. This provides a clue to some of its origins. The stereotype of the patient as biologically incompetent belongs, in part, to the events in the historical struggle through which the practitioners of medicine came to claim credibility as a profession. An essential part of this process (clear even in the Hippocratic Corpus) was that the doctor claims a monopoly of relevant expertise (Freidson 1970a).

What is new about the stereotype of patients as less than biologically competent is that, in the last twenty years, it has been revitalized by the assumed findings of those few quantitative studies which have been widely cited to support propositions derived from it. 'Many studies have shown', it is stated in one 'progressive' text, specifically intended to improve what the authors saw as inadequate communication in contemporary medical practice, 'that after routine consultations the average patient remembers only half of what he has been told. This is not really surprising: some patients are too anxious to listen attentively. It is easy for doctors to forget that although what they say is commonplace to them, it is quite strange to patients who may know nothing about anatomy, physiology, pathology, or therapeutics' (Walton *et al.* 1980: 22).

We do not claim that doctors and patients have an identical expertise or that they are equally competent in the sphere of biomedical knowledge – this is, after all, the doctors' 'raison d'être'. However, it will be apparent that the findings that we have reported so far suggest that patients might best be treated by doctors as biomedical experts, albeit possessed of different, rather than inferior or superior sources of knowledge. If our results (and the practical implications that stem from them) are considered valid, it may be worthwhile for a moment to pause and consider the basis of the medical stereotype about patients and how it comes to be maintained. What is particularly interesting is how doctors, despite their daily contact with patients, should maintain their view of them as largely ignorant and also how social science research, consistent with the stereotype, can be so widely believed to have reached such different conclusions to those which we have reported. In fact, consideration of the way the modern stereotype of the patient has borrowed from social science research seem to enlighten some of the reasons why many doctors have not noted how expert their patients are and may not have been able to put this resource to good use.

Ley's studies

Judging by citations in several medical publications in Britain and the USA the view that scientific research has demonstrated that patients are forgetful and biologically ignorant derives from the series of arguments and British research studies conducted by Ley and his colleagues (for example, Ley and Spelman 1965; Ley and Spelman 1967; Ley *et al.* 1973, 1976; Ley 1979). These studies have been summarized for medical audiences as evidence for the proposition that patients forget much of what doctors tell them. They are also cited to support several other propositions: for instance, that instructions and advice are more likely to be forgotten than other information; that the more a patient is told, the greater the proportion he or she will forget; that moderately anxious patients recall more than either those who are highly anxious or not anxious at all; that age and intelligence make no difference to what is remembered; and that the more medical knowledge a patient has the more he or she will remember (Becker and Maiman 1980; Cassata 1978: 498; Horder *et al.* 1972: 142). Students and young doctors are advised, in consequence, to put the most important advice first in sequence, to encourage patients to write down what they say and to beware about being too ambitious in what they tell (for instance, Royal College of General Practitioners 1981: 16; Walton *et al.* 1980: 24-9). They have also been warned that 'Only when the number of statements is limited to two is recall good' (Horder *et al.* 1972: 142) and that patients 'recall the first statements the doctor makes better than the later ones, regardless of their importance' (Walton *et al.* 1980: 24).

The quotations just mentioned indicate that Ley's work is widely believed to support two propositions. First, the idea that patients are unlikely to remember very much information and, second, that the communication of information to them should be kept fairly simple, be clearly organized, and avoid medical jargon. These propositions are frequently used, as in some of the comments earlier, to warn doctors to restrict the communication process. Curiously, however, such restriction misses the spirit of the objectives, central hypothesis and conclusions of Ley's work. His thesis was that communication was poor because patients were dissatisfied about how little information they received. They received very little, however, not because information had been withheld but because they had not been able to comprehend what they were told and had forgotten it. Ley's solution was to encourage doctors to improve their communication by making it clearer and better organized so that patients would comprehend it, remember it, and feel satisfied they had been informed. All his writings and studies set out or tested dimensions of this view.

The fact that the ideas for which Ley is known in medical circles, far more than the model he set out and tested, happen to be consistent with the conventional stereotype of the patient will not have escaped the reader. Those aspects of Ley's ideas which are relatively consonant with the stereotype have achieved prominence, those which are more dissonant have not. Ley's central conclusion that doctors have only to make more effort and to use appropriate skills to be more successful has tended to get lost. Two aspects of Ley's work are, perhaps, partly responsible for this development: his conception of the problem involved in communicating medical information and his empirical methodology.

Ley's conception of the problem of communicating medical information started from the basic premiss that the problem was how one person who knew communicated with another who did not. Specifically, since many patients did not possess adequate medical knowledge (demonstrated by an early questionnaire study), they faced a situation analogous to that of any individual asked to learn nonsense. Many patients were believed to be in this situation because they had no set of associations or system of encoding information and, in consequence, were faced with the task of remembering 'each individual item' (Ley 1979: 253). This approach leads to two, in the light of our conclusions, unfortunate implications. First, as in the view of Brackenbury (1935) mentioned above, what patients do know if it is biologically inaccurate is regarded as no knowledge at all and, therefore, irrelevant. Second, as in the conventional stereotype in which the doctor is in control, attention is to be paid to the message the doctor wants to communicate and its characteristics rather than to a two-way dialogue and process of learning by mutual clarification. In short, and essentially, the doctor has a monopoly of any expertise there is.

A problem with Ley's recommendations, based on his theories and research findings, is that they are all too easily equated with the beliefs implicit in the medical stereotype. Sir Henry Brackenbury, for example, as a solution to the problem of patients' ignorance, emphasized the need for doctors to keep information short and simple and to make very clear to patients what they said. Ley's recommendations, although more precise, are little different. Nowhere in the main recommendations is the potential for individual patients subjectively and systematically to give meanings to what they hear recognized (2). Clarity is conceived as an 'objective' matter, not as one in the mind of the listener.

If Ley's theoretical formulation directs attention towards the importance of what the doctor rather than the patient is thinking, his empirical methodology also emphasized the problems of doctor – patient communication in an unhelpful and ultimately misleading way. Ley's studies might lead one to expect vague and incomplete accounts of consultations. Yet when we interviewed patients we found that they seemed to remember most key points and also that during the interview almost every patient was able to give a comprehensive and detailed account of the encounter. While Ley assessed patients' recall of every statement a doctor made we assessed his recall of only the key points. As we have seen the two approaches cast patients' capacities in an altogether different light (3).

Ley's intention was always to improve communication in consultations and to achieve the situation in which a patient would remember and understand more information so as to feel satisfied with this aspect of a medical encounter. His statements about how little information patients could remember were never conclusions to his work. Rather he used findings about how little patients remembered (and about how they did not take medication) to try to motivate doctors to change what he and Spelman referred to as communication which was 'poor and in need of improvement'. In the event these efforts have had two discernible effects on doctors. On the one hand they sometimes quote his ideas to support the ideal – or at least to imply it – that there is very little scope for more than very basic communication. On the other hand, insofar as Ley has been very successful in influencing medical educators, it has been in terms of the idea that they must make their messages 'objectively' clear. Both effects bolster the conventional stereotype about communication strategies and, on the basis of the arguments we have made, are deleterious to the sharing of medical information. This result, which is certainly not what Ley intended, we suggest, follows from the social and interpretive processes involved in communicating information. Just as patients pick and chose which aspects of what doctors say to interpret on the basis of the familiar and the expected, so doctors have dealt with the contributions of Ley and his colleagues.

Health beliefs and the health belief model

A second source for contemporary medical opinions about patients and their beliefs has been research work utilizing the Health Belief Model. This work, quoted extensively by some medical educators, can also be considered to have reinforced some aspects of the medical stereotype and to have diverted attention from the pressing issues relevant to how patients' beliefs could be utilized in consultations. Health Belief Model research has contributed to the idea that patients influenced by social groups with 'inaccurate' beliefs present a major threat to improved care and has provided the theoretical backbone of attempts to provide 'health education'. Indeed, according to a working party of British General Practitioners influenced by it, the main barriers to patients' participation in preventive health care 'appear to depend chiefly on their beliefs and knowledge about health and disease' (Royal College of General Practitioners 1981: 1). The same beliefs are also widely held to influence inappropriate visits to doctors and non-compliance with treatment.

The Health Belief Model began principally as an attempt to organize and make theoretical sense of the diverse relationships between social and cultural groups and patients' utilization of medical services or compliance with treatment. The idea was that culturally based ideas about personal susceptibility, the potential severity of a disease, or the potential value of action influence a person's motivation to act. Thus if an individual's ideas on these dimensions are biomedically inappropriate, they are likely to be a main cause of failure to consult at an appropriate time, failure to follow instructions, or failure to utilize preventive opportunities (Kasl and Cobb 1966; Rosenstock 1966; Becker 1974). Exponents of the model have argued that changing patients' ideas about severity, susceptibility and the costs and benefits of action, that is making them congruent with biomedical ideas, followed as an educational strategy.

Research on the relation of health beliefs to health and illness behaviour has tended to support the general postulates of the Health Belief Model, although a great deal of the research is retrospective and thus potentially confusing (4). Health Belief research has, however, been applied only rarely to the direct study of doctor – patient communication or to how to improve it. An exception was a study by Becker, Drachman and Kirscht (1972), who concluded a study of how beliefs influence visits to pediatric clinics by arguing that: 'Ultimately, it should be possible to construct a brief and useful index of questions, the answers to which would help the pediatrician to estimate the likelihood of each mother's complying with the prescribed regimen and to identify the problem dimension or dimensions in each case. . .By knowing which model factors are below. . .the pediatrician will know where to direct this appeal' (1972: 852-3). In other words, if doctors believe their patients to think their condition insufficiently severe, to think they are insufficiently susceptible, or mistakenly to consider that the costs of treatment outweigh the benefits, the doctor will want to devote time to trying to modify their ideas on these issues. Arguments such as these, influenced us when we were seeking to define what might be the 'key points' patients would need to understand.

Proponents of the Health Belief Model have, undoubtedly, helped to indicate which aspects of patients' belief systems need to be changed, if they are to be made consistent with biomedical thinking. Recent research has also considered why some beliefs may seem more or less psychologically attractive to patients – because they enhance or threaten feelings of control or guilt (Wallston and Wallston 1978; King 1982). The striking feature of Health Belief Model research, however, is the recommendations reached by its proponents as to how a doctor might use their insights. Rather than attend to the subjective or cultural implications of the belief systems to which patients owe allegiance and the consequences for the process by which patients make sense of information, proponents have concentrated on advising doctors how to manipulate patients to take action. They found that beliefs themselves did not correlate very closely with health behaviours and so, despite the name of the model, have concentrated less and less on beliefs and more and more on what were originally conceived as potentially chance cues to trigger behaviour (such as the illness of a friend, stimulation by a newspaper article or a mass media campaign) (Rosenstock 1966; Becker and Maiman 1975). In consequence, suggestions for change have been concerned with experimenting with the degree to which communications successfully arouse fear (or other emotions) and thus motivate patients to action. The doctor's role becomes that of someone who induces fear. This development of the theory leads away from the doctor's efforts in a consultation and may suggest that the model is not easy to apply to it except in the most general terms. Certainly, most subsequent research has concentrated on assessing the effects of films or other potentially mass media material on an individual's behaviour.

Two more subtle aspects of the Health Belief Model may help to understand why it has recently begun to influence medical education and why it seems to us this may be a retrograde step. First, health belief theorists have conceptualized beliefs as relatively stable properties of atomistic individuals, as illustrated by the fact that they have always been investigated using hypothetical questions. They have ignored the role of beliefs as part of the everyday cultural process by which individual members of a society give meaning to their experience. Second, health belief theorists have constructed a role theory. As such it focuses on the expectations and beliefs to which 'rationally' a patient must subscribe if he is to achieve the role-prescribed end. If he does possess the relevant beliefs and attitudes he can behave rationally according to the ends prescribed by the role. If not, he cannot and will therefore be deviant. Both the conceptualization of health beliefs as properties of atomistic individuals and the role theory in which they are set contain flawed and potentially misleading assumptions. First, the underlying principles of the Health Belief Model make it logically unable to explain health behaviour except by resorting to some factor other than the patient's beliefs (5). Second, its location within a role theory makes it logically incapable of explaining individual errors or communication difficulties, or of understanding the process by which such errors and difficulties can be diminished. As a role model it describes what doctor and patient must agree on, but neither describes, explains nor gives guidance about how they might come to do so (see, for instance, Svarstad 1974: 27; Flavell *et al.* 1968: 15).

As is in other utilitarian theories, the suppressed or implicit premiss of the Health Belief Model is that a social actor has only one possible norm of behaviour – he must behave 'rationally' and, moreover, he must behave rationally in a very restricted sense (6) (Tuckett 1970). By this premiss a theory that appeared to set out to consider the importance of ideas and phenomena as they appear from the point of view of the individual must become a theory which relegates his significance very considerably. In the process the subjective meaning of belief systems, their ritual and semiotic functions and their potential relation to action in the mind of an individual are neglected. Moreover, when it comes to making suggestions to improve communication, the contribution of the health belief model is to identify which patient beliefs are wrong but to provide no help in understanding how this eventuality has occurred. As in Ley's studies or in the views of Brackenbury, the assumption remains that individuals possess 'correct' knowledge or no knowledge at all. The detailed way in which health beliefs, regardless of their 'biomedical rationality', may form an explanatory system which influences how new information is understood and evaluated, is not considered. Finally, and perhaps still more important, the Health Belief Model, like the model of communication used by Ley, encourages the belief that communication can be conceived in terms of a 'message', to be handed down from an authority which knows what is 'best'. In this way attention is directed away from the idea of a process of sharing meanings towards an emphasis on a one-way, relatively simple, and potentially authoritarian process, in which education becomes concerned only with the 'message' and with efficient techniques of persuasion. Such an approach ignores such difficulties as those introduced by the proposition that only a patient can know what is best for him.

To summarize, while the Health Belief Model and the research it has inspired may have helped to place patients' beliefs on the medical agenda, they have done so in a way which confirms the stereotypical idea that they are a nuisance and an indicator of patients' ignorance. Moreover, the Health Belief Model provides little guidance about how to deal with a patient's beliefs in a consultation and has inspired little or no research which examines directly what doctors and patients say to each other and its possible outcomes.

The role of beliefs about patients' beliefs

We have suggested that medical educators seem to have selected which parts of research on which to base recommendations, and have made sense of it, on the basis of the (probably implicit) explanatory models of the consultation with which they began. They have been able to find confirmation of 'old' stereotypes, in some aspects of the work by Ley and the advocates of the Health Belief Model, partly because of ambiguities in that research which have not been the focus of attention or comment in medical circles and partly because of its implicit 'utilitarian positivist' and authoritarian assumptions. We have drawn attention, particularly, to the ambiguity surrounding the way 'recall' has been conceptualized in Ley's work. We have also highlighted the assumptions in both models of a one-way model of communication in which the doctor or educator is dominant and has a monopoly of knowledge. In the case of the Health Belief Model we have also mentioned how a concern with subjective beliefs as valuable slid into a preoccupation with persuasion and propaganda.

The research findings of social scientists concerning the process of giving information may sometimes have been rather unclear and often been inaccessible. On occasion (and particularly in Ley's writings) they have, however, been described in a straightforward way. However, more important for communicating than clarity, we suggest, is the exploration and investigation of the underlying operational models and assumptions about a consultation that doctors and social scientists have. These models and assumptions are used by both parties to interpret each other's views but have not been shared between them. In the case of doctors, just like a patient in a consultation, they might be expected to 'fill in' and make sense of research results on the basis of their prior professional understandings and preoccupations. They may, therefore, have selectively perceived and interpreted those aspects of research which agreed with their stereotypes and concerns. It seems possible, for instance, that some doctors have unknowingly made sense of research findings, often at second hand, so that they could ease the pressures they felt under to give more information. Making sense of Ley's and others' findings in the way that has been done has the potential to ameliorate any blame and frustration that is likely to have been experienced when trying unsuccessfully to give information. Giving explanation and information adds to the many other tasks in the clinical encounter, is felt to be time-consuming, is a subject on which doctors have received little guidance, and one about which they can feel anxious and frustrated. If extensive efforts to give information are believed to be more or less impossible and the responsibility for this situation is placed on patients, it is not difficult to see that this may help to expiate blame or guilt – in much the same way that explanations about microbes as a cause of troubles feared to be personal or social, may help patients to deal with these same emotions. Certain of Ley's ideas and those of the advocates of the Health Belief Model seem ideal for such purposes (7).

In any case, the Ley and Health Belief Model traditions of research provide few warrants to support the widespread belief that most patients are too ignorant to share ideas with their doctors. Rather, the major barrier to improved communication in medical consultations appears to stem from the beliefs about patients that are part of the conventional stereotype used to describe them. There are echoes here to the conclusions of a paper exploring how children acquire language. The view reached was that in one sense there is no moment when the child first learns to speak. Rather there is a moment when the adults may first realize that is indeed what he is doing (Bullowa 1976). In the case of doctors and patients the richness and variety of the patient's thinking is long overdue for recognition. A change in the medical ethos which so easily devalues patients' contributions, long overdue from the days in which doctors fought to establish their status and economic power, will be one of the first steps necessary if communication between doctors and patients is to be improved.

Summary

Although patients very often remembered and correctly made sense of the key points their doctors made and were committed to them, it was also the case that in as many as half the consultations studied in detail patients either did not remember a key point, did not make sense of it correctly or were not committed to the view it implied. This level of communication failure seems to have been the result of the ethos prevalent in consultations which devalued the patient's contribution and so prevented an exchange of views. The ethos is part of an old stereotype of the patient which may also have been responsible for interpreting previous research findings in such a way as to blame failures of communication on the patient and his ignorance.

PART 5

Implications and conclusions

CHAPTER 11

Changing medical consultations

If medical consultations are to be used to share information more successfully than at present then according to our findings the main priority must be for doctors and patients to adopt different attitudes to the importance of the ideas a patient has. Doctors need to recognize the extent to which patients try to make sense of what is happening to them and to pay much greater attention to patients' explanations and ideas about what is wrong with them and what should be done. They need to encourage and welcome a patient's ideas when they are expressed and to aim their explanations directly at what a patient has said. At the same time a patient who wants to understand his doctor's views needs to state his ideas, doubts and questions in a more straightforward, open and articulate manner. One pre-requisite to changes of behaviour on the part of both doctors and patients is that they know why it is important to pay attention to patients' ideas. A second requirement is that they develop skills to do so.

As a final stage of our project we set out to communicate to some doctors and patients our ideas and suggestions for improving communication along the lines just indicated. One purpose of this activity was to explore how practicable the ideas and suggestions were. Another purpose was to discover more about the way doctors viewed their patients as part of the operational models of the consultation which they bring to their work. It followed from the theory of communication we have applied to consultations that if we wished to be successful in communicating our ideas it would be necessary to elicit and explore the ideas doctors had on the relevant issues. While some idea of 'official' models could be obtained from the medical textbooks and academic accounts on which we have drawn it was unclear how these might reflect the way practicing doctors actually worked or would react to our ideas.

The efforts we undertook to communicate our ideas to practicing doctors and their trainees included detailed case discussion, an intensive curriculum programme, a contribution to vocational training courses, small group discussions with General Practice trainers and trainees, a discussion group with hospital-based physicians and the development of a patient educational pamphlet (1). In the space available we shall describe three of these efforts starting with the detailed case discussions. Some conclusions will be drawn towards the end of the chapter.

Detailed case discussion

A starting point was the fact that most of the doctors we had studied (especially those in the Study group) were interested in the aims of our research and, therefore, in our conclusions. Without exception both Study and Comparison group doctors were dedicated to their work, mostly enthusiastic about it and hard-working. Many of them were keen to try to improve their communication and saw this possibility as a reason for trying to co-operate with our research requirements when we were collecting the main data. At a subsequent conference arranged to feed back some results of the formal study several of the doctors expressed the wish to understand more about and to experiment with our ideas. We, therefore, decided to start our educational efforts by sitting in with them in their consultations and talking with them about cases in detail. These efforts, like the others, were intended only as a preliminary exploration and, consequently, were not limited by the constraints of research.

Three of the research workers who had taken part in the main study (MB, CO, AW) began case discussions with several doctors each. We agreed between us that each research worker and each doctor should be free to develop ideas and actions in the way they thought suitable, the only proviso being the general objective to encourage a mutual sharing of ideas in consultations and the requirement that the research worker keep a detailed diary of events, observations and feelings (2).

Detailed case discussion began with sitting in with doctors on their consultations for one or two surgeries each week, tape-recording the consultations, and then analysing some of them with the doctor at a later time. By sitting in on consultations an opportunity was provided for short conversations, after each patient had left and before the next arrived, in which the general practitioner and the research officer made quick observations and comments on each consultation. Such short conversations were quite limited in scope. None the less, they allowed research workers several opportunities: to encourage doctors to seek a patient's ideas or to invite a patient to elaborate his ideas and to clarify with doctors what might be meant by these tasks; to ask a doctor to give a rationale for his approach; to query details of management and alternative forms of management; to be informed about alternate diagnostic hypotheses; or to find out about a patient's history. Often such conversations would continue for half an hour or so after the surgery was completed – while equipment was put away and before a doctor would have to 'rush off' to a home visit or other appointment.

The short conversations possible during and just after sitting-in on consultations were an important preliminary to the efforts to use case discussions for exploring and exchanging ideas with doctors about their operational models. They provided the doctor with instant feedback and clarification of our concepts (such as 'patient's views'; 'reactive explanation', etc.) and forced research workers to develop and specify ideas in the 'real' situation of having to make an immediate response to a patient. On the other hand, the conversations were also very limited because quite often the points at issue were deeply embedded in superficial queries made by one or the other which could not be explored within the time constraints.

Because of the limitations of the short conversations more detailed case discussion mainly took place in formal meetings between the doctor and the research worker arranged at a later date. When sitting-in, research workers made notes on the consultations recorded. After the surgery they would ask the doctor to choose which consultations he would like to discuss and would add to those choices ones they believed posed communication problems or ones which would highlight issues. A time was then arranged for a one or two hour meeting the following week. Meanwhile, research workers transcribed and had typed three consultations – the basis for discussion at the meeting. Having transcripts enabled doctor and research worker to look in detail at what happened in the consultation, to take note of pauses and non-verbal nuances, to look at what might have gone wrong and why, and to discuss what the doctor could have done differently. Mrs Robinson's consultation provides the basis for describing the kind of discussion that often took place in the early stages of work with a doctor.

Mrs Robinson

Mrs Robinson was aged nineteen and nineteen weeks pregnant. Her husband had a non-manual occupation. She presented with sharp pains which had occurred over the previous weekend when she went to the lavatory. She was visibly distraught. Her doctor responded by asking a series of questions related to the duration, frequency, location and quality of the pain. During this sequence of questions the patient added to one of her responses the comment: 'I was wondering if it might be muscles because I thought it could be that. It could be compared to a pulled muscle. . . .' Before she could develop this idea and finish what she was saying about her explanatory model, however, her doctor interrupted to ask if the pain was sharp or burning. She answered 'sharp' and was then told to lie on the couch. Her doctor examined her abdomen, asked if she could feel the baby move and then asked her to get dressed. When she was dressed again (and seated) the doctor said:

Doctor: Well, firstly let me say I don't think there's anything serious and it won't harm the baby.
Patient: It's still there and alive?
Doctor: The baby's still fine. So it's alright. It's one of two things. It's either muscle like you suggest or it might be infection of the water in the urine – which is quite common in pregnancy.
Patient: Yeah?

Mrs Robinson's doctor then suggested that she hand a form to the receptionist to enable a specimen of her urine to be checked. He then handed her a health education leaflet on cystitis and stipulated that she 'drink lots and lots of fluid so you're flushing your bladder through so that if there is a lot of. . .any infection it's being washed out. And to empty your bladder completely'. Handing over the leaflet the doctor indicated that the consultation was at a close. The patient began to gather her things and to get up. Stopping, she said:

Patient: The other thing I wanted to ask you if it's muscle or not, I don't know. I do some keep fit that I did before being pregnant and I do it twice a week. And what do you think I should do? They know I'm pregnant, and I'm doing less and less exercise, but more for pregnant women so I don't know, is it too much or. . .?

Doctor: (interrupting): No! It's a very good thing to do. It's quite safe for the baby. The baby's very well protected in fluid so there's no risk there at all.

Patient: So the pain I had, it had nothing to do. . .

Doctor: I wouldn't think so. And it's good for you. People who are fit tend to have better labours and things. So it's good to go on. Alright?

Patient: OK.

Doctor: So there's no danger from that at all.

Patient: (laughing) I'm so relieved!

Doctor: Now we'll have the results from that test at the end of the week, if there's anything abnormal I'll get in touch with you.

Patient: Thank you.

Doctor: Goodbye.

At the discussion of this consultation sometime later, Mrs Robinson's doctor remembered the consultation as straightforward and uncomplicated. He felt satisfied with his investigation, questioning and differential diagnosis. As in all the discussions, the research worker then began by discussing, what seemed to be, the more positive points of the consultation. For example, she pointed out that instead of presupposing why the patient had come the doctor had offered an open question ('How can I help?'). In addition, he had let the patient present the initial problem without interruption, although he had not encouraged her to go on. He had also managed a thorough history of the presenting symptoms. He had been courteous and enabling by letting the patient dress and be seated before telling her the results of his examination and had been well-mannered, concerned and empathic.

Doctor and research worker then turned to speculate upon potential problems in the consultation. First, the battery of history taking questions immediately following the patient's initial presentation was mentioned. It seemed to the research worker that this was potentially premature and might have inhibited the patient from presenting her explanatory model. It was noted that the sequence and speed of the questions appeared to have changed the nature of the patient's contributions. Whereas she started out forthcoming and elaborated her presentation she now became rather monosyllabic, answering in 'yes' and 'no' terms only. Second, it was noted that when the patient did volunteer her ideas about muscles she was interrupted in mid-stream. Perhaps the experience would 'educate' her to give monosyllabic responses and not to develop her ideas. It might convey to her that her explanatory models were not of interest. At this juncture, it was noted, the doctor had no real idea what the patient might mean by 'muscle' or about the worry that later emerged relating to her theories about the potential conflict between keeping fit and the health of her baby. Third, it was suggested that the reassurance the doctor gave immediately after Mrs Robinson's examination might not have been as effective as he initially supposed. He may have reassured himself that nothing was seriously wrong, but what about Mrs Robinson? At this point in the consultation the doctor knew little about the patient's model of understanding and might have been creating new worries (what, for example, would she make of a water infection?). In these circumstances it would not be possible to 'structure' Mrs Robinson's understanding of her problems, her worries could not be ruled out and she could not really be reassured. Fourth, doctor and research worker also began to speculate about what might have happened if the consultation had ended when the doctor handed over the form and the leaflet. The consultation, apart from reassuring himself, might have succeeded only in altering the patient's life for the worse. Only Mrs Robinson's willingness to resist dismissal and to ask a further question had prevented this outcome (although the doctor's general friendliness may have helped). Finally, (after noting how the doctor did respond to what Mrs Robinson said) doctor and research worker discussed how, once Mrs Robinson had mentioned her exercise classes, he could have encouraged her to elaborate further on how she believed the exercises might have caused the pain or harmed the baby, whether she believed the pain to have resulted from exercise or to have injured the baby, and in what way. If this had been possible, the explanation and reasoning given could have been fuller, clearer and more certainly related to the patient's ideas. In making each of the points doctor and research worker exchanged ideas about what could have been said, how it could have been said, in which order questions might be asked, etc.

Examining Mrs Robinson's consultation in the way described proved to be exciting. The doctor agreed that although from a diagnostic point of view the visit was routine he could now see that the assumptions underlying his view of the exchange were in fact problematic. He accepted the observations made by the research officer about the patient's explanatory thinking and the need to relate to it.

An intensive curriculum programme

Based on experience with case discussions, the starting point for trying to communicate ideas about the value of allowing a mutual exchange of views was in itself to try to facilitate and structure a mutual exchange of ideas between ourselves and the doctors. Attention would, therefore, have to be paid to eliciting and elaborating the operational models of consulting which doctors used and on checking their understanding of our models. The most thorough attempt to do this was a ten-week programme of discussion and practical exercises initiated by one member of the research team together with three general practice trainers and two trainees (3). It was envisaged as a programme which might form the basis of tutorial and practical work, about half a day a week, within ten weeks of the vocational training period of a year. Five tasks for the programme were devised focusing on exploring the processes influencing the cognitive outcomes of consultations and on developing specific communication skills. The objective, method of achieving and outcome of each task will be described in turn.

Clarifying the goals of the consultation

The first task was to start trainees thinking about the central question of what they were trying to do in the consultation. To do this they were asked to produce a list of goals and then to discuss them and their reasoning in putting them forward. Depending on time and interest background issues such as those mentioned in the first chapter of this book could be researched by reading.

In a meeting to discuss the goals of the consultation the trainees produced a written list of objectives. It was similar to those developed by others (for example, Pendleton *et al.* 1984) but it was the process of producing it, not the results, which were primarily important. The exercise forced trainers and trainees to clarify the aims and goals of the consultation and perhaps to consider broadening them. It also meant that all concerned felt committed to the goals because they were not imposed as goals they should have but drawn out as goals they did have.

Understanding the patient's part in the consultation

The second task was designed to enable the trainees to look at the extent to which the goals they had agreed were actually met in consultations and to explore some of the factors which would influence it. In particular, it was designed to stress that a consultation which appears straightforward and unproblematic from the doctor's point of view may appear very different from the patient's. By looking at the consultation from the patient's perspective, it was hoped that the trainees could gain insights into those factors which influence the cognitive outcomes of the consultation but which may not have been immediately apparent from their own perspective.

To achieve this aim one of each of the trainer's surgeries was tape-recorded and three patients presenting a new problem were asked if they would talk to a trainee about it, at home, in the following few days. Using an interview check list which focused on the patient's perspective, the trainees asked the patient what he and his family had thought was wrong before he went to the doctor, why he had thought as he had, what he remembered of the consultation, what he understood of the doctor's views on his problem, how he assessed those views and what comments on those views his family and friends had made so far.

One trainee had interviewed a young man who had presented with a sore and swollen thumb. The doctor had said it looked as if it had been knocked and prescribed Indocit tablets. When the trainee interviewed the patient a few days later, the young man said that his thumb had swollen the evening before his consultation, at which time, because several of his friends had dislocated their thumbs playing football, he thought he had dislocated it. In the consultation, however, the doctor had said only that the thumb was inflamed which the patient took to imply that it was not dislocated. He was very doubtful of the diagnosis and treatment. He felt that the doctor should have sent him for an X-ray to make sure his thumb was not dislocated. He had taken the tablets the doctor had given him, but as he had anticipated, they had not helped. This outcome supported his idea that the thumb was dislocated and reinforced his desire to seek more appropriate treatment.

After the interview, the trainee was very impressed by the fact that even in an apparently straightforward consultation, the agreed goals were not met. The patient's rejection of the diagnosis and his desire for different investigations and treatment undermined the value of the doctor's advice. Central to his rejection of the doctor's view, the trainee saw, was the patient's prior view, developed in the context of his family and friends, that his thumb was dislocated and required X-ray. These views were not dealt with in the consultation and so served as a basis for doubting the doctor's diagnosis and treatment when he left the surgery.

Recognizing the patient's views in the consultation
The third task was to help the trainees to look at their own consultations in terms of their knowledge of the factors which influence cognitive outcomes and to see how and where communication problems may arise. Since doctors cannot normally interview their patients after their consultations, they must learn to recognize a patient's lay theories, to see how they may influence the consultation and to speculate on their likely effects, on the basis of the face-to-face interaction alone.

The trainees were asked to tape-record their own consultations for two or three sessions and to select from these a 'good' and a 'not-so-good' consultation for analysis and discussion. These consultations were transcribed by the trainees, and the transcripts used in conjunction with the tape-recordings for analysis and discussion. The trainees were asked to identify the patient's theories in each consultation, to describe how they influenced the interaction (for example in the form of questions, doubts, etc.) and to speculate about the way they might have influenced the patient's subsequent understanding and evaluation of the doctor's decisions. Bearing these insights in mind, the consultation was then considered from the point of view of how far the trainees had met each of their goals.

In one consultation which was discussed a young man began his consultation by saying 'I've been having sinus trouble for years, and my mother keeps on telling me to get something done about it . . . And just lately, this cold, it's been getting really bad, it's been making my nose sore, I keep coughing. I'm getting a sore throat. . . . ' Later he repeated, 'I've always got a blocked nose, it's always running, and my mother reckons it's sinus trouble. She works at F. hospital.' After examining him, the doctor decided he had an Upper Respiratory Tract Infection, and said 'Your nose problem will never get better while you smoke.' The young man disputed this saying, 'Well, how come it was there before I smoked?' Doctor and patient argued along these lines until they ended the consultation.

In analysing the consultation afterward, the trainee pointed to the patient's theory that he had 'chronic sinus trouble' which he wanted 'something done about'. In the consultation itself, he had dismissed this theory as medically irrelevant and had tried to deal with the problem as a simple Upper Respiratory Tract Infection. Looking at the transcript, however, he saw how important the patients' theory probably was and how it seemed to have influenced the way the patient had acted in the consultation: for example, the symptoms he had presented, his concern for the underlying chronic problem rather than the current acute episode, his resistance to the diagnosis (repeating his own diagnosis and appealing to his 'medical' mother for support) and his questioning of the smoking advice. The trainee also felt that, since he had not addressed the patient's theories, he had not convinced the patient that those theories were inaccurate and that the patient would reject both diagnosis and treatment when he left the surgery.

Exploring patients' theories

The fourth task was to help the trainees to develop practical skills in recognizing and elaborating patients' theories in the consultation. By this point, they had understood the importance of patients' theories and could recognize and conceptualize their influence in consultations. It requires further skills, however, to recognize, to conceptualize and to elaborate relevant aspects of patients' theories while the consultation is in progress.

The trainees were asked to tape-record two surgeries in which they tried to elicit their patients' theories and to read some detailed notes on how to do so (4). To help them concentrate on this task, they were asked to write out, at the end of each consultation, the lay theories of each patient. A recording and transcript of two consultations (good and not-so-good) were then used for analysis and discussion. In discussion the trainees were asked to point out how they had tried to elicit their patients' theories, to assess whether they were effective in doing so and to consider the reasons for their success or lack of it. Where they had not been successful, they were asked to consider how else they might have approached the subject. Finally, the trainees were again asked to consider, in the light of this discussion, how far they had met each of their goals in the consultation.

One example concerned the consultation of a young man who had complained of 'sort of symptoms of a 'flu sort of thing' followed by a sore throat which had 'progressed to swell up' and a 'slightly dull' ear. The doctor asked him to clarify his symptoms and then asked, 'What did you think was going on in your ears?' The patient replied that his girl-friend had had a throat infection and 'I don't know whether she gave it to me but I've just got worse. I've never had anything like it before, not when it's gone to my ear.' After examining him, the doctor said 'You've got a throat infection which has spread up to your ear on that side and that ear is infected as well. I think the appropriate way to treat this would be with antibiotics.'

In the discussion, the trainee said that he felt his question had been useful in establishing the patient's views and concerns which he could then confirm or rule out. He could also see, however, that the patient's answers seemed to imply that he saw his problem as a 'not typical' earache, a view which appeared to be exactly contrary to that put forward by the doctor, and one which called into question the doctor's treatment. To clarify the patient's view, the trainee realized he should have followed his initial question with more detailed questions about what made the patient think his earache was different. He could also have tried to establish the patient's views on the way it might be treated, or his possible worries about catching things from his girl-friend and the implications of that.

Giving reactive explanation
The final task was to help the trainees to develop practical skills in giving reactive explanations. To achieve this the trainees were again asked to tape-record two surgeries. In these consultations they were asked, first, to explore patients' theories and, second, to give reasons for their own views which related to those of their patients. A handout providing detailed examples of such explanation was provided as guidance (5). Two consultations were again selected for transcription, analysis and discussion. In discussions the trainees were asked to say what each patient's initial theories were, what were their own views, and to show how they had related them together. They were asked to consider their degree of success and the reasons for it. Finally, they were, once again, asked to consider how far they had met the agreed goals.

A consultation in which a middle-aged woman consulted the doctor concerning a sore red eye, illustrates the discussion. The previous day, when she had been in her garden, the patient had 'turned round and a twig went into it'. When asked her views, she said 'it feels as if there's something in it but I thought it was probably just scratched'. The doctor examined her eye and said: 'Right, I can't see anything in it or see any obvious damage to the surface of the eye, so I think, as you suggest, it's a scratch across the eye, and that often feels as if there's something in it.'

When presenting this consultation for discussion, the trainee pointed to the patient's alternative theories about the nature of the problem and to the way he had couched his own diagnosis in terms of those theories: that is, he had responded to both the theories which the patient had presented, ruling out one (something in the eye) with one warrant (can see nothing in it) and providing reasons for his theory about her symptoms in terms of a warrant drawn from her description (scratched the eye). Although a very simple explanation, it appeared to have been effective in dealing with the patient's concerns and in conveying the doctor's understanding to her.

A patient pamphlet

The third effort to influence consultations was directed, through their doctors, at patients. Based on the findings of the formal study it appeared that many patients had ideas, questions and doubts which they would have liked to have mentioned in their consultation but which they often indicated only covertly or not at all. Two explanations for this state of affairs included the idea that patients felt it was improper or would be damaging if they expressed themselves more clearly and the idea that they might be unfamiliar with the appropriate communication skills to adopt. If, however, patients could be influenced to participate more directly and more skillfully this might be expected to improve the chances of their taking advantage of the information a doctor could give them in a consultation. To this end, therefore, the doctors in two health centres were approached and asked to co-operate in a project to influence patient's behaviour by giving them a pamphlet which would legitimate and encourage the activities of patients who expressed ideas, asked questions and expressed doubts and which would give them specific help in doing so.

The pamphlet was developed by two of the research workers after discussion with patients, doctors, and staff at the Health Education Council. It was entitled *Speak for Yourself: A Guide to Asking Questions of Your Doctor* and opened with a brief rationale which tried to indicate that doctors expected patients to have questions and doubts and would be unhappy if their patients were to leave the consultation with them unstated and unanswered (*Figure 11.1*). Designed to be read in the waiting room but then taken home after, one side of the pamphlet dealt with the issues a patient might think about before the consultation: 'what to tell the doctor'. The other side of the pamphlet dealt with talking to the doctor in the consultation itself.

The pamphlet encouraged patients to 'think through' beforehand the nature of their problem, what they believed it was, what they thought ought to be done, what they thought could be done to prevent it and what other more general problems it might be causing. A box with a space in which to jot down ideas and a list of prompts was provided under each of these headings. Under each box patients were reminded of the importance and rationale for mentioning their ideas on each issue (*Figure 11.2*).

Under the heading 'Talking To Your Doctor' it was suggested that patients think first of putting their doctor 'in the know' by communicating the ideas raised in

Figure 11.1 A guide to asking questions of your doctor

'One of the common complaints people make about visits to their doctor is that they come away with a lot of unanswered questions. Sometimes we forget the questions or ask them in a way that makes it difficult for the doctor to understand. Sometimes we don't ask questions in case the doctor may think us silly. Other times we don't ask questions because we feel the doctor is in a hurry, we feel it will waste his time or we think he may not answer.

Asking questions is a very important part of your visit to your doctor. Your doctor is not a mind-reader and wants you to ask questions. By asking questions he can clear up doubts, concerns or worries you may have about your problem. Getting information from your doctor means that you are more likely to understand the treatment, how it should help and what you have to do to carry it out. Asking questions may save you from having to make another visit and may help you get better quicker.

Your doctor hopes that this guide to asking questions will help you speak for yourself on your next visit.'

the previous paragraph. Their part, thereafter, the pamphlet stated, was the important one of making sure, by the end of the consultation, that they knew what was wrong and why the doctor thought so, what was to be done, why this was advisable and precisely how to carry out instructions (*Figure 11.3*). Under the headings 'Are You Quite Sure?' and 'Still Have Doubts?' they were advised of the need to ask questions or to express doubts and given examples of questions or doubts they might have (*Figure 11.4* and *Figure 11.5*). A 'final thought' tried to explain that they should not be put off if they thought the doctor was having difficulty explaining. Some hints about how to deal with various difficulties were also given (*Figure 11.6*).

Ideally, we thought that a pamphlet of this kind would be most effective if it could be given to the patient before the consultation and an opportunity could be provided to discuss it and the purpose behind it. Since resources were not available for this task, however, it was left to the receptionists of each of the three doctors with whom we piloted the pamphlet to hand it out when patients arrived at the surgery and it was left to the doctors to reinforce with the patients the importance and value of trying to present their ideas, ask questions and express doubts.

Some impressions

One objective of the three activities we have described was to explore the viability of the ideas and suggestions we have made about the value of trying to use consultations to allow a mutual exchange of views.

Overall, each of the three activities was appreciated by those who participated in them. The doctors who took part in the detailed case discussions and the

Figure 11.2 What to think about

Your problem

How am I affected by this problem?
How have things changed?
Do I have symptoms?
If so, what are they?
How long have I had them?
How long do they last?

Remember:
It is important to tell your doctor all about your problem and all symptoms you think you have. The details or symptoms you think may be silly or irrelevant may be important in helping the doctor make a diagnosis.

What you think it is

Am I worried about my problem?
Is it serious?
What do I think caused it?
How long will it last?
Am I worried it will come back?

Remember:
If you have your own ideas about what is wrong it is important to bring them into the open. Worry itself is bad for you. Unless your doctor knows about your ideas and worries it will be difficult for him to set your mind at rest. The doctor wants to know what you think is going on. Tell him and give him your reasons.

What do you think ought to be done?

What do I think can be done to help my problem?
What kinds of treatment do I know about and how do I think they will work?

Remember:
If you tell your doctor what you think ought to be done, he can tell you whether or not this is a good idea.

How can I prevent it?

Should I stop doing something?
Should I do something different?

Remember:
Sometimes one can avoid getting a problem again or stop it getting worse. Share these ideas with your doctor and he will tell you whether it might help.

Is my problem causing other problems?

Is my problem causing difficulties at work or home?
Will it affect my future?
Will it affect the way I feel or look?
What can I do about it?

Remember:
Sometimes one's problem can cause other problems in one's life. The doctor may
not know about these. If you tell him, he may be able to help.

---

intensive curriculum programme found that the way of looking at the consultation to which they had been introduced was valuable and rewarding. This was
particularly true of those who participated in the latter. The vocational trainers
thought that the experience had changed the way they both approached and behaved
in consultations despite thirty years of practice. The trainees thought it had been
one of the most valuable parts of their medical education. Together they have become
advocates of the approach (see Boulton *et al.* 1984).

The doctors who participated in the patient pamphlet project also valued the
exercise. Before it began they had agreed with the general proposition that patients
should say when they did not understand but at the same time had been very sceptical. They had doubts whether patients would read such a 'wordy' pamphlet.
They did not think it would be much use to patients from lower-class occupational backgrounds or from minority ethnic groups. They were anxious that it
would encourage neurotic patients and others to bring 'shopping lists' of complaints.

In the event the doctors agreed that only one of their expressed fears had proved
accurate. Patients from minority ethnic groups (to whom no special concessions
were made in the pamphlet) seemed to find the experience mystifying. Other patients
read the pamphlet, appreciated it, used it to jot down and organize their thoughts,
and found it clear and understandable. They did not bring the feared 'shopping
lists' and in some cases, apparently as a direct result of the pamphlet, seemed to
have opened up areas of discussion with their doctors which they had clearly held
back in the past. In this way they allowed their doctors to provide them with
important and needed information. Two consultations in which a research worker
was present after the patient had been given the pamphlet contained clear evidence
of this kind of development:

(1) 'I was going to ask you if it might be some kind of asthma because you
can get nervous asthma when you sort of lose your breath and I saw that operation

Figure 11.3 Talking to your doctor

First:

Put your doctor in the know at the beginning.
Tell the doctor:
What your problem is.
What your symptoms are.
What you think it might be.
Whether this worries you.
What you want done about it.

Remember:
If you tell your doctor not just your symptoms but also your ideas on what you think is the matter and why you think so, your doctor will be in a better position to know what your concerns are. Being clear and direct with your doctor helps cut down on guess work and saves the doctor time.

Second:

After your doctor has asked you questions and possibly has examined you he probably will tell you what he thinks is going on and what can be done about it. Your part is to understand what the doctor has said.
Do you understand what is wrong and why this is so?
Do you understand what is to be done and why this treatment is best?
Do you understand how the treatment works and how you carry it out?

Remember:
Patients who ask questions get better explanations of what is wrong and what has to be done. If you are uncertain, check with your doctor that you have got it right. Sometimes we can use the same word but mean different things. For example, if your doctor said, 'I want you to rest', should you go straight to bed or just take it easy? Use the following list to help you ask the right kind of questions.

---

on TV last night, 'Your Life in Our Hands'. I was going to say, perhaps I have cholesterol and it may be that is what's making me short of breath. Well, you gave me a questionnaire [the pamphlet] that says I can ask you all the questions, so I'm asking them.'

(2) 'That's why [because of the pamphlet] I asked about the tablets. I was reading it and I thought I'd ask about the tablets: what was the difference between the Navadrex and the Propanalol. You probably wouldn't mind. I think it [the pamphlet] is very good actually.'

The fact that both doctors and patients valued the experiences is not of course to say that they were completely or easily successful. A number of doctors and

Figure 11.4 Are you quite sure...

...about what's wrong?

Doctor...
Why do you think that is what I have?
How does this happen?
What is the cause?
How serious is it?
How long will it last?

Remember:
If you are not quite certain about what your doctor thinks is wrong, ask right away. If you are not sure now you will only be more confused when you get home. The best way is always to ask what is wrong and why this is so.

...about what to do?

Doctor...
What makes you think this treatment is best?
Could you tell me how this medicine works and how it will help me?
Are there any side effects?

Remember:
You have a right to ask and to find out what your treatment is and how it works. Your doctor wants you to understand. You cannot help yourself unless you know what is being done. And you probably will not be convinced unless you understand why it has to be done.

...about how to do it?

Doctor...
Why do I have to take all the tablets?
Should I take them on an empty stomach?
Can I drink alcohol or drive during this treatment?
Why should I change my diet?
Do I have to come back and see you?

Remember:
Instructions for treatment are often complicated. It's important to get it sorted out before you leave. If it helps, write them down.

---

patients remained uneasy to the end and most of them would need to practice and develop the new skills to which they had been introduced for a long while before they would become ingrained. Future work is needed to develop and test the approaches.

Figure 11.5 Still have doubts?

You still may not be convinced about what the doctor said and what is to be done. An open discussion of the pros and cons helps you have a say in what is best for you. It helps you understand the reasons why the doctor has made certain decisions. If you disagree about something, help your doctor understand why you disagree. You might say:

...about what's wrong

Doctor,
You said it was just muscular but I wonder if it isn't arthritis because it just comes and goes even if I have not been straining myself.

Doctor,
If there is nothing wrong with my heart why do I get these palpitations, because I thought palpitations and heart trouble were one and the same thing?

Remember:
These are only examples. But if you give your doctor a reason he will be able to understand why you disagree. If your reason is incorrect your doctor will be able to explain to you why this is so and why his advice is more appropriate.

...and what to do

Doctor,
I cannot take these antibiotics because I am allergic to them.
I don't think I can take these tablets because I am a driver or I work with machinery and I am worried they'll make me sleepy.
I cannot go to bed and rest because I have three children to look after.

Remember:
The doctor may not know about these things. By telling him, it will help him make the best decision for you.

Assumptions, affects and operational models

In the discussions which took place with them both doctors and patients revealed much ambivalence about what they were asked to do. Some patients were highly sceptical as to whether doctors were interested in what they thought or whether they had been prepared to listen to them when they tried to follow some of the pamphlet's suggestions. Alternatively some doctors and some patients considered that they already did what was suggested, despite the empirical evidence from observations of their behaviour that they did not.

As far as doctors were concerned the various discussions we had with them (especially the detailed case discussions) provided an opportunity to explore in some

Figure 11.6 One final thought

The causes of illness are often complex and so are the treatments. The doctor may not know all the answers as yet. Be prepared for occasions when there is no clear-cut answer. Don't be put off if your doctor interrupts you. Try asking the question again. Up to now your doctor has been used to asking all the questions and may forget that you have a few that you would like to ask yourself.

Sometimes you may want to know more. If you feel you would like a longer chat, ask your doctor if you could make another visit to talk in greater depth.

Remember:
Your doctor is there to help you. If you are not sure ask now. Check that you have got it right. So...

Speak for yourself

---

depth how they conceived communication in the consultation and how they understood our ideas about it. Aspects both of their ambivalence to the ideas and why they thought they already behaved in a way we thought they patently did not, became clear.

Initially, none of the doctors with whom we worked had any doubt about the general proposition that lay theories could advantageously receive more attention in their consultations. Essentially, this is why they agreed to take part. However, it soon became very clear that this general enthusiasm could mask a great deal of confusion and even anxiety and outright hostility about the proposition that lay theories should be explored. In early discussions we were often told that seeking patients' theories was for some 'other consultation' than the one being studied; had been informed that it had been achieved by throw-away remarks like 'What can we do for you, do you think?'; that it was not wanted by the patient under discussion; or that such activity should be reserved for consultations with patients whose problems the doctor did not know how to diagnose (especially patients with whom the doctor could find nothing wrong physically) (6). We often demonstrated that these warnings and doubts were difficult to substantiate – more like axioms than evidence. However, when we then tried to show that what we had in mind was a more meticulous and rigorous procedure of establishing the evidence for what patients' thought and anticipated, more complex assumptions and emotions began to emerge. Doctors expressed doubt and anxiety about the wisdom of letting patients 'prattle on'. They admitted to have curtailed their efforts because they felt foolish or felt embarrassed that they would appear patronizing or intrusive (7). They found themselves arguing that they knew what a patient was thinking without having to ask.

In fact, it soon became apparent that each doctor's initial understanding of the role of lay theories, although based on agreement with the brief outline of our findings which we had given to them, was usually very different from our own. Moreover, in most cases their view of the role of lay theories did not make the task of seeking them a very extensive or priority activity. To make progress we realized we would have to make the doctors' different assumptions about the role of lay theories and when they should be elicited clear to them, and then differentiate them from our own ideas (just as we would argue they have to deal with patients' understanding of what they say). In any case, we found that their ideas could be characterized as belonging to one or more of the following four theories.

First, some doctors recognized that patients had subjective knowledge about themselves and their own bodies which, if elicited, could help a doctor to arrive at the clinically 'correct' diagnosis. These doctors were led by their theory to pay some attention to what patients had to say insofar as it gave them clues to what was wrong. Some of them, adopting a particularly elaborate version of this approach to patient ideas, saw them as necessary to allow a 'whole' or 'complete' diagnosis of the problem – that is, one encompassing both physical, psychological and social aspects. Such doctors believed it was right to allow patients to talk about their ideas because in this way, for instance, they can help a doctor to be aware of 'real' or underlying problems.

Second (and not necessarily in conflict with the previous view), some doctors considered it was important to attend to lay theories because not to do so would be to appear superior or not interested in the patient's subjective reality. They considered, therefore, that it was both therapeutic and rapport-encouraging to listen to what patients said and to be empathic. Such doctors criticized themselves for interrupting a patient in many circumstances and would see it as their duty to appear interested. Patients allowed to talk, such doctors believed, could experience a cathartic relief and would feel helped by the experience of sharing their thoughts and feeling understood.

Third, some doctors saw patients' lay theories as providing a clue to the reassurance they might be given. Some patients, they considered, might have specific worries about serious conditions such as diabetes, heart disease or cancer. In this way the theory of these doctors was most like our own. But there was usually a crucial difference. Most doctors did not consider it necessary to construct a model of explanation from what a patient said. Rather, they seemed to consider that the patients used a very simple semiotic system. For example, the mention of sugar suggested diabetes; pain in the chest indicated a fear of heart disease; lumps on the body suggested cancer; aches and pains in the joints meant a fear of crippling arthritis; headaches implied the possibility of a high blood pressure or tumour. A consequence of this semiology was that once a patient gave the appropriate signal, the doctor gave the appropriate reassurance, examination or treatment, without needing to explore a patient's theories further.

Fourth, and finally, a few doctors found it very difficult to regard patient theories, like Brackenbury (1935), as anything more than indicators of ignorance and superstition. While they thought it might be polite or similarly necessary on some occasions, they really considered time listening to such ideas to be wasteful and thought that patients should be educated not to take up their time in this way.

The various theories doctors had about patients' ideas once they were elaborated and their implications appreciated, indicate, perhaps, why those in the main study so rarely explored them. Albeit in a different way, each of the views we have mentioned places a low priority on a careful examination of what a patient thinks. The first approach regards lay ideas solely as an aid to diagnosis. The second sees them as something to be tolerated. The third considers patients beliefs to be expressed in a simple code. The fourth considers them an irrelevance. Certainly, lay theories – specifically lay theories about diagnosis and appropriate treatment and prevention – were not seen as of the same order as biomedical theories: that is, as more or less structured and grounded attempts to explain problems and to indicate causes, probable treatments, and likely prognoses. Nor were they seen, usually, as emanating from a competent and responsible individual trying to make sense of and to act on his problems in a responsible way.

If the detailed theories doctors had about the role of patient theories were a barrier to their seeking them in a thorough way, the ideas they had about the purpose, content and method for explaining to patients, were equally inhibiting. Initial observations confirmed those of the main study. Many consultations contained what we recognized as attempts to make clear diagnoses or treatments or to provide reasons for them. However, these explanations were not 'reactive' to patients' ideas and were often communicated in a disjointed, *ad hoc*, discursive, and unnecessarily time-consuming way. When, in discussion, we sought to try to 'improve' explanations by suggesting how they could be more organized and systematic, as well as reactive to patients' ideas, it was once again clear that our view of the aims of a consultation and the role of explanation within it, and those of the doctors', were often quite different. Again these differences had to be drawn out and clarified. When they were, it became clear that there were a series of objections to giving explanations.

The first and foremost objection was time. More explanation, doctors seemed to assume, would require more time and this could only lead to them seeing fewer patients or diverting activity from other priority tasks. A second objection was that patients would not understand more explanation: 'Even when I explain things in very simple terms someone always gets it back to front' was a typical comment. A related objection was grounded in the research work of Ley and his colleagues, already mentioned at length in the previous chapter. Doctors would question the value of more explanation if so little was remembered: 'Here's a case! I spent fifteen minutes last week explaining to her what was wrong and she's back this week asking the same questions and none the wiser!'. The lesson this doctor had learned was that explanation was a waste of time. A fourth objection concerned the ethics of conveying bad news. It was specifically mentioned in the case of the medically more serious diagnoses. Rational explanations, the objection ran, do not often reassure anxious or phobic patients and in any case many ordinary patients 'don't want to know'. Some doctors implied that patients are unable to cope with the responsibility of knowing what is the matter with them or of making decisions about what should be done. Such patients were thought to want to leave the management of what information they should receive to the doctor. Finally, a fifth objection centred around the difficulty of providing information to patients when a doctor can never know for certain. Some doctors went so far as to make socio-legal arguments to defend their reticence. The general proposition was that if their explanation was subsequently proved wrong they could lay themselves open to charges of deception or incompetence. It would be better to say nothing.

The assumptions doctors made about patients' theories and the potential for explanation in consultations probably go some way towards explaining the pattern of communication we observed in the main study. Assumptions such as the ones we have outlined would militate against systematic attempts to obtain patients' views and systematic attention to explaining. In the main study we found few consultations in which there was more than an *ad hoc* approach to either patients' ideas or to explanation. Some of the reason-giving that was observed also appeared to have been motivated more by a need to control the consultation than to inform the patient.

However, once the way doctors and ourselves were conceiving the aims of a consultation and the role of explanation and lay theories had been clarified, considerable progress towards a shared understanding of the importance of a patient's ideas could be made. The ways patients' theories could differ from the doctors' and how they might function could be spelled out. Doctors could be shown how time was often wasted when, because of an absence of explanation or a failure to pursue the patient's ideas, a consultation was conducted at cross-purposes. They could also be shown, as the weeks of discussion proceeded, that some of their objections to giving explanation – whatever their validity in some cases – could more often be understood as 'excuses' or as ways of defending against feelings of anxiety, embarrassment or helplessness. For instance, they could be shown that they seemed to offer explanation to some patients and not others but could not really justify it to themselves. Or they could be shown that when they tried to explain or to ask patients to elaborate on their theories they became anxious and got into difficulties. When such clarification had been achieved, indeed while it was in process, practical skills in conceptualizing patients' explanatory models and asking appropriate questions could be developed (8).

Discussions with doctors also highlighted and helped to clarify some of the reasons why doctors, who often agreed with the research workers' aims in principle, did not use those ideas in practice. The 'common-sense' assumptions doctors made about both patients and the consultation process often distorted the way they made sense of and acted on our suggestions. For example, we have mentioned that some doctors would appear to agree with the idea that lay theories were important but then, in consultations, insist that they knew 'intuitively' what a patient was worried about and so did not have to ask. Thus, patients with sore throats were assumed to want antibiotics or patients complaining of pains in the joints were thought to be worried about arthritis and so reassured about it. One doctor learned the hard way about such a simplistic semiology. On one occasion he reassured an elderly lady complaining of aches in her neck and shoulders that she did not have a nasty spreading arthritis. But in the consultation the patient then let him know that she did not know what he meant. She said that she had not associated pains in the neck with arthritis and began to become very alarmed. The consultation soon deteriorated into a long and uncomfortable conversation at cross-purposes – the kind of case which, in other circumstances, could be held to prove the foolishness of trying to explain to patients.

Two assumptions, although they were not ones to which they had usually given much thought, often dominated a doctor's consulting behaviour and his assessment of priorities. One was that a doctor's overwhelming priority was to make a diagnosis and another was that he should always be 'in charge'. Mrs Robinson's consultation (above), as also Mr Nixon's (in the main study), are examples of the way the former assumption could distort the whole process. It will be recalled that in both consultations doctors became caught up in a kind of clinical 'catechism': a series of questions and procedures stemming from their wish urgently and precisely to elicit the clinical phenomena about which the patient was complaining and to obtain the information relevant to a proper differential diagnosis. In both cases their exclusive early preoccupation with the catechism led doctors severely to inhibit their patients from expressing their explanatory hypotheses and created a strong possibility that the entire consultation would be at cross-purposes. In both cases (as in most cases seen in virtually every medical consultation in or out of hospital) the majority of armchair observers would agree there was no pressing need to make the differential diagnosis in such a hurry. Yet, when we suggested to doctors that they might delay their catechism for a few minutes, until they had an idea what the patient thought he had come for and what explanatory theories he had in mind, they frequently became agitated. They implied that it was easy for us to say that, felt very unhappy about proceeding without knowing the exact diagnosis and felt that their job was above all to achieve it.

The potential conflict between the 'catechism' approach to making a diagnosis and allowing patients to present their ideas was tackled quite explicitly with three doctors. In case discussion we argued that an early priority on diagnostic issues inhibited patients from presenting their own ideas, inhibited their spontaneity, trained patients to use monosyllabic responses, trained them not to mention their own ideas or psycho-social matters, and generally created an artificial and stilted atmosphere in which a patient would feel 'inferior'. Several consultations were then carefully examined to show how, even ignoring the above points, taking a history before seeking patients' ideas, would often lead to a long, confused, repetitious and uncomfortable consultation, such as in the case of Mr Nixon. The result was that a consultation could both take longer and, even, lead to a detailed diagnosis of an irrelevant problem. In particular, using data from a small analysis of history-taking in the consultations in the main sample (9), we showed that general practitioners were simply unable to arrive at a thorough clinical picture in the time most consultations took. Whether they realized it or not they usually limited their inquiries to the subjective complaints patients volunteered and were selective in the detail they sought and the areas in which they questioned. Some potential subjects of inquiry might never be mentioned. To be effective history-taking was dependent on the patient and his theories.

One of the two doctors appreciated these arguments and was prepared to experiment with a more relaxed approach to history-taking. The two others remained unconvinced. As one put it 'I like to know what's in the front yard before I go exploring what's in the back yard. One needs to be convinced and not adapt new styles for the sake of exercising one's skill at adapting.' Both these doctors still retained extensive links with hospital medicine (in which a patient is seen after the presenting problem has been sorted out elsewhere) and it is interesting to ask whether this fact and their disagreement stemmed more from their difficulty dealing with their own anxieties about the clinical task than from any evidence in support of their view. None the less, despite their objections to the specific suggestion they experiment with their diagnostic approach, both doctors were very favourable about the overall value of the viewpoints put to them in case discussions and might be expected to be cautious about ignoring a patient's ideas in future.

The same two doctors (and many others) also had a second 'gut' anxiety about allowing patients to develop their theories: it threatened their sense of being a doctor and 'in charge'. When they tried to encourage patients to talk about their diagnostic and therapeutic theories they seemed to find it very difficult to listen to what they heard. They would often become uncomfortable about the passing of time and become very fidgetty. They seemed to find the looseness and uncertainty of the resulting situation almost unbearable.

In general, the observations made as a result of our various discussions with doctors both concur with and help to explain findings by those such as Byrne and Long (1976). They have suggested that many general practitioners conduct their consultations in a doctor-centred manner, preoccupying themselves with the data they require and finding it very difficult to see the consultation from the much more 'messy' point of view of the patient. It seems to us that the wish to avoid the discomfort of being passive and the lack of training in holding the anxiety of 'not knowing' were powerful influences behind some of the difficulties the doctors were having and also behind many of their assumptions and theories.

Summary

Three attempts to modify the behaviour of doctors and patients so that they would try to use consultations to allow a mutual exchange of views have been described. These attempts were appreciated by both the doctors and the patients and they have provided some further data with which to understand why doctors in the main study did not explore their patients' ideas. Essentially, the concept they had of their role and that of their patients was not very different from that implied in the conventional stereotype. Even when doctors thought that finding out about patients' views or explaining to them was important, their ideas about it were contradictory and confusing. Attempts to articulate and exchange the doctors' models and ours led to a very considerable understanding of the potential role of patients' ideas but not necessarily or quickly to dramatic changes in behaviour.

CHAPTER 12

Summary and conclusions

In the course of describing our study we have concentrated on what doctors and patients said to each other in consultations. Our interest has been in a rather neglected area of research: the spoken ideas of the participants and how far primary care consultations are used, and could be used more, to share thoughts and explanations. To examine the process we started by looking both at the information the doctors choose to give to their patients and the information they chose to seek from them. At the same time we looked at the information patients volunteered to doctors and at the information they chose to seek from them. Finally, we examined what patients could remember, the sense they made of what their doctors told them and and how they evaluated it.

The starting point was to direct our attention to the ideas doctors and patients shared with each other insofar as they talked to each other about four pre-defined topics: the diagnostic-significance of a patient's trouble, the doctor's treatment-action or preventive advice and the consequences of illness and its treatment. The idea was that if patient and doctor succeeded in sharing ideas on these topics doctors would have been able to use the consultation to give patients the benefit of their biomedical knowledge and patients would have been in the best possible position to choose what would be best for them.

The first finding we reported (Chapter 4) was that the doctors and patients in our sample very rarely talked to each other about the consequences of a patient's illness. Although both doctors and patients would talk about the other three topics they very infrequently (and then only very peremptorily) conversed explicitly (even in soliloquy) about such matters as the feelings a patient had about having a particular illness; the implications for family, work or plans; or the social consequences of or feelings about accepting treatment or preventive suggestions. The other three topics, on the other hand, were mentioned quite frequently. Moreover, doctors usually said enough to make it possible for a patient to be aware of their views, although what doctors said was often judged, by us, to be unlikely to be very clear to patients.

The second finding (Chapter 4) was that doctors usually shared with their patients some of their reasons for thinking as they did. In two-thirds of the consultations they gave some reasons which might have helped patients to understand why doctors thought they had a particular condition or would be advised to adopt a particular course of action. Although, our rating judgements suggested patients might find quite a few of these explanations unclear, it did seem that attempts to share information about what was wrong and what should be done was a normal feature of the consultations studied in detail.

If we found that doctors usually spent a fair amount of the time in their consultations sharing what they thought with their patients, it also seemed that they spent very much less time trying to share what patients thought. Indeed the third finding was that, in the main, the consultations studied were one-sided (Chapter 4). Doctors and patients did not manage to achieve a dialogue and so did not share or exchange ideas to a very great degree. Doctors did little to encourage patients to present their views, quite often actively inhibited them from doing so or evaded what patients did say, very rarely explored what a patient was understanding of what they said, and did not usually tailor advice and instructions to known details of the patient's life. Moreover, the few attempts made to establish the patients' ideas and explanations were brief to the point of being absent. These findings applied equally to the consultations studied intensively and to those studied in less detail.

Patients, in the consultations studied, also often limited the chance of dialogue. In this sense they did not make it easy for their doctors. Although as many as four out of five patients provided at least some indication in the course of their consultation that they had ideas and a viewpoint they could have shared with a doctor, we judged that only half this number actually made this explicit (Chapter 6). A small minority went so far as to make it clear to the doctor they wanted to know his reasons. A similarly small number made their reasons for disagreeing with what doctors thought, or the thinking behind their own explanatory theories, at all obvious. However, our findings also suggested some of the reasons why patients were relatively silent. First, it seems that when they did behave more openly (as people with ideas, questions and doubts) this increased their chance of experiencing a consultation in which disagreement was evaded and tension evident. Second, after their consultations, they quite often explained their silence by volunteering that they were frightened about their doctor's response, felt hurried or thought their doctor might think less well of them.

Because they neither made clear, nor were helped to make clear, their theories, patients could not receive explanations which were reactive to them (Chapter 4). Although some explanations were responsive to patients in a general way they could not be reactive in the sense of relating, precisely and in detail, to what patients actually thought. Because doctors did not know the details of what patients were thinking, the information they did give could not relate, in any precise or considered way, to the ideas patients themselves possessed. In short there was little dialogue and little sharing of ideas. In consequence, doctors could have no way of knowing whether the information they offered was being understood 'correctly' or not. Equally, patients could have no way of knowing whether their understanding of what the doctors said was 'correct'.

The assessments we made of the cognitive outcomes of consultations seem to have reflected what we observed to occur in them (Chapters 8 and 9). Just as the consultations themselves appeared to contain much information-giving so it seemed at first that there had been a remarkable communicative success. Contrary to some expectations, few patients among those studied were unable to remember the key points of what their doctors told them. Most were also able to make sense correctly of the key points of what they were told and usually evaluated doctors' advice favourably. The so-called 'competence' gap was thus in these ways distinctly bridgeable. We have argued that patients managed to remember and understand so much because in a sense they were already 'expert'. Their own prior ideas allowed them to pick out the important points to remember and helped them to 'fill in' gaps in what they were told. None the less, despite this success, half the patients studied also either did not understand a key point of what they were told or disagreed with it. In these cases what occurred could be likened to a divergence of expert views. When the prior ideas and theories patients had were in some way at odds with those of the doctor they 'filled in' incorrectly, or came to evaluate what had been said unfavourably. Moreover, even when there was a successful outcome, this could not really be attributed to the information provided in the consultation: broadly patients who understood or agreed with the doctor did so because they already knew what was wrong or what should be done and already agreed with the view the doctor would take. Viewed in this light, communication reflected the main conclusions reached while observing what happened in consultations: patients and doctors did not succeed in sharing their points of view. Consultations, therefore, did not usually lead to patients being more aware of their doctors' biomedically-based ideas than they were before they came. By the same token doctors were not in a position to amend or tailor their advice to the patients' individual priorities. They, therefore, had not succeeded in helping patients to make choices with the advantage of the biomedical expertise they possessed.

There are various ways in which the pattern of communication which has been described can be further understood. But before proceeding with this aspect of the argument it will be appropriate first to consider some aspects of the validity of the inferences being drawn and how far they can be generalized. We will then turn to the importance we think might be given to the findings and to the priority that might be given to the changes they imply.

Questions of inference and generalization

The design and methodology of the study (Chapter 2) placed a number of limitations on the inferences that can be drawn and also on to the situations to which they can be generalized. In the first place the data refer to only a single consultation in a probably ongoing relationship between a general practitioner and a patient. An intended strength of primary care consultations of the kind studied is that they are not meant to be seen as complete. General practitioners argue strongly that they provide continuing personal care and do not attempt to deal with every relevant aspect of a problem, or even every relevant problem, in a single consultation. On this basis, the study of the unfolding pattern of a series of consultations might provide a better basis for drawing inferences about the kinds of things that get said and do not get said and the kind of understanding that is achieved. Selecting individual consultations for study, it might be argued, may present a distorted view of a process. Data was also limited in other related ways. Consultations were chosen without reference to the day-to-day realities of practice, such as emergency determined shortages of time, 'off-days' a doctor may have, or the effects on doctors and patients of occasional busy surgeries, crises and long waiting times. In some cases it might be misleading to draw conclusions from what we observed.

A second limitation of the data is that it was based on a record only of the audible events which took place in the consultation. We could and did attend to what was said, to exclamations, to silence, to the tone of voice, to inflections, even to the sound of movements (such as of writing or of rustling papers), as we have mentioned in preceding pages. While, therefore, we were not limited to speech alone, we have paid attention to a limited range of communicative acts. Insofar as doctors and patients can share the information on which we have concentrated, by means of gestures, facial expressions and other visible but not audible signs, the study is limited.

Third, but perhaps most important, the inferences we have drawn depend on the series of subjective rating judgements that form the main data: assessments of what information was given, how it was given, what questions or doubts were expressed, what understanding was achieved, etc. We have tried to make clear in the opening chapters that if one is to say anything about the process of sharing ideas in consultations judgements of this kind are inevitable. If explicit, judgements make it a great deal easier to draw inferences than if they are implicit. In the past, it will be recalled (Chapter 2), to assess how much information was given or remembered, statements have been counted indiscriminately. We have also tried to set out the basis on which judgements were made and to present evidence that rules for judging were applied consistently. Nonetheless, each of the various judgements may or may not indicate what we have argued. Moreover, we have yet to show that our definitions of 'clear', 'moderately elaborate' or 'overt' (etc.) actually assess useful concepts. There was evidence that the measures we developed to describe how patients behaved had some of the hypothesized effects on the information they were likely to receive (Chapter 6). There was also evidence that the different measures of outcome were influenced in hypothetically expectable ways. But, as yet, several of the measures are not of proven value. The relative uniformity of the way doctors behaved in respect to patients' ideas, made it impossible to test the hypotheses for which the measures were designed. We do not know if behaviour such as 'reactive' explanation would have improved commitment or if efforts to 'check' patients' ideas would have improved the chance they would make correct sense of what doctors said, etc.

Most important, our 'third-party' judgement of key points, the critical yard-stick against which we determined patients' recall and the sense they made of what doctors said, depended on a number of disputable assumptions. Essentially, we have taken the working diagnoses or actions (based on what doctors said to patients) as the basis for judgements of what doctors hypothesized or advised. We have imposed a meaning on them. Yet, there are now studies which suggest that the working models used by doctors in practice are often idiosyncratic and significantly different from those in textbooks (Bloor 1976; Katon, Kleinman, and Rosen 1982). The explanatory models adopted by doctors to account for the problems they encounter in their practice are often as inconsistent and contradictory as those developed by patients, perhaps especially in the case of more 'minor' or 'emotional' illness and in the one-third to one-half of cases where there is 'nothing physically wrong' (Katon, Kleinman and Rosen 1982; Helman 1981; Higgins 1983). Sometimes the assumptions we made about the diagnostic-significance of a hypothesis the doctor mentioned or about the value and purpose of a treatment he had advised, may have been quite erroneous. The doctors may have been using the terms differently or inconsistently and may even not have fully realized it. Moreover, it might be argued, by observing only one consultation in a possibly on-going process, we may have distorted such judgement even further.

Fourth, there are problems of external validity mentioned in the second chapter. How far did the research itself (for instance because we tape-recorded consultations and made doctors self-conscious) influence the findings? How far is data based on the particular selection of doctors and their consultations which we chose generalizable to others?

Limitations of some kind are inevitable in any research effort. Throughout the text and the notes we have mentioned the various steps taken to guard against problems of validity at each stage of the research. None the less, there can be no doubt that a second study of the kind we have conducted could improve on what we did. We have mentioned how third-party judgement could be improved and checked, for example (Chapter 7). We have also mentioned the rather marginal way in which we estimate video-recordings would have helped. It would also be most interesting to repeat the study in an experimental context – comparing a group of doctors and patients who did succeed in 'sharing' ideas in the ways indicated with another group who did not. Also, studying a sequence of visits over time, were it practicable, would also be fascinating. At present, however, the critical question is how far can the limitations just mentioned (or others) be considered to undermine the conclusions we have reached. We have presented the data in detail to help readers make such judgements for themselves. For ourselves we are satisfied that the main conclusions probably apply to most consultations, at least in the UK. We shall try to support this argument.

As far as conclusions about how information was shared in the consultations are concerned, we would point to the overwhelming pattern of findings that we have reported: findings about 'first' consultations in a series and subsequent ones, findings about the consultations in the main sample and the 5 per cent (unselected) sample, findings which were remarkably uniform across consultations for patients given different diagnoses, consultations for patients from different social backgrounds and consultations conducted by different doctors. Even the tutors and university teachers selected for the Study group and those chosen to be more representative in the Comparison group did not differ markedly as far as the extent to which they shared information was concerned. Moreover, the same pattern of observation was repeated during the efforts we made to try to change doctors and patients and have reported in the last chapter.

As far as the understanding patients developed after the consultation is concerned, there is clearly room for argument about whether our assessment of when patients made correct sense are valid. It is possible that what might be considered 'errors' were made when meanings were assigned to what individual doctors meant when they gave advice or mentioned diagnostic hypotheses. If made, however, such errors would merely underline the problem for the patient. They would also underline the basic conclusion we have reached: what is important is that sense has to be made by filling in what doctors say on the basis of lay theories. If doctors had left fewer gaps and uncertainties to be filled in, or, more importantly, if they had checked that their patient's understanding was correct, it would have been a great deal easier for research workers to observe the process! In fact, we doubt if we have overstated the degree of communication difficulty in the consultations we studied: because we took steps to be conservative when attributing errors to patients. For example, we operated a rule that in cases of doubt patients should be rated 'correct'. Also, of course, the general practitioner working group we used to check some of our judgements arrived at very similar conclusions to ourselves (Chapter 7).

The study was designed mainly to explore how to investigate the various issues quantitatively while trying to retain some sensitivity and clarity in the concepts used. It was intended to make it possible to analyse statistically the effect on understanding of sharing ideas with patients in different ways. However, the general uniformity of results restricted such analyses considerably: sharing ideas in a way that related to a patient's model of explanation was not very evident in the consultations and so its effects could not be assessed. Bearing in mind other findings, based on more developmental studies (1), research evidence suggests that the basic pattern that we have described is probably generalizable to most consultations in the UK and probably very many elsewhere. The very frequency of the experience we are describing means that most readers will be able to analyse the consultations in which they take part as doctors or patients and to test the applicability of conclusions for themselves.

Because the pattern is so overwhelming such problems as how to make allowances for doctors having 'off-days', or difficulties with individual patients, or the 'ambivalence' between a doctor and some of his patients, etc., all of which must exert an effect, seem to us of secondary relevance.

Of course, just because the pattern of results is so overwhelming and because this might have been expected, both from smaller qualitative studies and from the enormous difficulty we had when trying to establish what doctors advised each other about explaining and sharing information, it might reasonably be asked whether it was necessary to conduct such an elaborate project. Such a view neglects several important findings which we have reported.

First, we would argue, the study has shown, more clearly and systematically than hitherto, that what we have called the traditional stereotype of the patient (someone who is often too ignorant to remember or make sense of what he is told (Chapter 10)) is grossly misleading. Patients could remember nearly all the 'key' points made in 328 consultations. This particular finding, together with the detailed and systematic evidence we have presented to show how patients came to make sense of and evaluate the key points of what their doctors say, was worth all the effort. It seems to us to change fundamentally the traditional justification for making explanation a 'cinderella' area of practice and to undermine, beyond recovery, the grosser paternalism that went with the stereotype. The argument, with which we had some sympathy, that earlier findings were based on unrepresentative or particularly articulate patients, no longer has the same force. Attention must now be focused not solely on the patient's competence to understand and remember what his doctor says but on the doctor's competence to recognize and conceptualize what he is saying.

Second, although it may seem obvious in retrospect (even to the doctors we studied) that we might have expected to find that doctors paid little heed to their patients' ideas, this was by no means so clear when we began. A textbook used by most of the doctors in our study group stated the need for the general practitioner to obtain 'an extended range of information' including 'the patient's view of his illness' (Horder *et al.* 1972: 29). Likewise the doctors we worked with in the educational phase mostly agreed that to obtain the patients' ideas was part of their task. The problem, as we tried to illustrate in the last chapter, is that there seem to have been nearly as many ways of making sense of this imperative as there are doctors subscribing to it. A similar problem exists in regard to promoting self-reliance and self-care (Abel-Smith 1981). The demands and discipline of a quantitative study forced us, even as social scientists working with the ideas for some time, to be a great deal clearer about what constituted seeking or elaborating patients' ideas, giving information, being reactive, etc. It took eighteen months of intense discussion, comparison and examination of consultations to become at all clear what we meant when we thought a doctor had or had not begun to do one of these things in the wide variety of situations which the doctors encountered.

Only after this activity could we be precise about the way doctors did not seek and elaborate patients' ideas, did not explain in a reactive fashion, or did not check how patients understood them. The value of some of this conceptualization was that it specified the original hypothesis and thus our conclusions. Moreover, it clarified our thinking sufficiently to make the educational work possible.

The question of priorities

How far do the communication failures we have described and the absence of effective sharing of ideas in consultations that we have found, actually matter? How far should consultations be devoted to talking to patients and, therefore, to sharing ideas with them?

We started in the first chapter by rehearsing some of the reasons why some physicians and health care specialists, as well as some patients, have argued that doctors need to define their job as to help patients to make decisions, rather than to aim to impose them on them. They have emphasized that it is patients who chose whether to take advice and who have to live with the consequences of illness and its treatment. Moreover, in the case of many modern approaches patients' motivation is vital. Great gains could be envisaged, therefore, if patients can formally be treated as competent. These arguments, moreover, can be evaluated within the framework of other debates: about changing health care priorities; the proportion of medical effort to be devoted to chronic illness; the increasing intrusiveness of treatment strategies; a growing awareness of the socially defined context of health and illness; doubt about the effectiveness and efficiency of technology; and so on.

We have argued that, in practice, patients are not treated as competent 'experts' in their own health care – at least to nearly the degree that might be possible. Their ideas, explanations and opinions are not sought in any systematic or thorough way and tend to be devalued as not useful or relevant. Moreover, insufficiently precise attention is paid to explaining to patients. In consequence, we have suggested, in so far as increased biomedically inspired understanding might be an objective of consultations, there is a great deal of room for improvement. The consultations we studied were largely redundant from the point of view of sharing information and ideas. We have implied this was so not because patients cannot or could not appreciate the niceties of biomedical thinking, but because patients were not given the opportunity to do so. The consultations did not provide patients with the opportunity to make decisions based on the best biomedical knowledge their doctors could give them. In itself, we suggest, this is an important shortcoming. But the absence of an exchange of ideas is also likely to be disadvantageous in other terms. First, treatment outcomes will be less likely to be successful if, as with many conditions, success depends on being aware of patient's priorities which have not been established. Second, patients will be less likely to be well motivated and more likely to ignore advice, vary treatment and, therefore, waste resources of time and money. More generally consultations cannot be part of the wider educational process, called for as part of the WHO strategy for health for the year 2000 (Mahler 1981), in which a population is encouraged to participate with professionals in the setting of health care priorities and policies.

While the arguments we have just mentioned ought to be one source of pressure making the improvement of communication a major priority in medical consultations, there are several objections. One line of argument, for instance, makes what we have suggested seem impractical. It is suggested there is no time for more communication or that patients (especially in the UK) are simply not interested and not educated enough to use more biomedical information. It is also suggested that to give more information more precisely (especially in the USA) is impossible because the doctor himself often does not know what is wrong or what to advise and lays himself open to litigation the more he says. Finally, it is suggested that consultations have much higher priorities to attend to than sharing ideas – among these might be making the right diagnosis, giving the right treatment and empathizing with patients non-verbally. A second line of argument doubts the wisdom of devoting much more time to sharing ideas with patients. It is suggested that patients may be better off with their lay ideas than with biomedical hypotheses. The latter, it can be argued, have a life of about five years before becoming dated and inaccurate. Some also argue that the goal of patient autonomy implied in our approach is simplistic and evasive of important moral issues. It is said that many patients want to leave the thinking, understanding and deciding to their doctors and that it may do more harm than good to give them information or to warn them about risks which are very remote. Patients may also be less interested in information than in action. They may want their doctor to do no more than to support their definition of the situation, perhaps by repeating some prescription, diagnosis or advice, which legitimates their means of coping with personal or social stress. Such arguments may throw doubt on the priority to be attached to an exchange of ideas intended to allow a patient to achieve an improved and more appropriate biomedical understanding of his situation.

The two lines of argument just mentioned were ones which we encountered in one form or another in the educational efforts we made towards the end of the study and which we have discussed in the last chapter. It seems important to state that they all represent lines of thinking which can increase the subtlety and precision of managing the process of sharing ideas with patients. As such they are valuable. It is certainly axiomatic to the way we think that there are a wide variety of individual situations in medical practice which cannot be handled in any pre-packaged or stereotyped way. 'Horror' stories about unthinking, failed or insensitive and persecuting attempts to inform patients are a feature of many discussions on this subject and certainly point to the need for caution and consideration. However, it must also be asked how far many of the arguments, like the stereotypical view that patients will forget most of what you tell them (2), are used to evade rather than confront the underlying issues.

In the consultations which we have studied (whether in the pilot, the main study or the educational work) time has frequently been wasted by not discovering patients' ideas or not trying to share points of view. Second, the hints patients have given about their theories and capacities for thinking and understanding have often been missed. In this way patients' behaviour may have appeared more ignorant or incomprehensible than it was. Third, while doctors have not always known exactly what was wrong, this would rarely have precluded them ruling out a great number of possibilities. Often the worries patients themselves actually have can be ruled out without making a final diagnosis. Fourth, alternative more urgent priorities than that of sharing ideas were not often that evident in many of the consultations we studied. The clinical content of the great majority of them (as represented by the various extracts quoted in the book) might suggest that in the large majority giving education, information and reassurance might be considered as the priorities. Indeed, it was often the *raison d'être* of them.

Neither are arguments doubting the wisdom of exchanging ideas overwhelmingly convincing. For example, the view that changes in medical knowledge make it not worthwhile to explain is a *reductio ad absurdum*. Biomedical theses might properly be treated with caution and lay theories respected and valued. But this does not mean going to the extreme of regarding biomedical theories as not worth knowing. Likewise, it seems that the argument that the pursuit of patient autonomy has gone too far is all too easily based on extreme situations and bizarre cases (3). While, no doubt, there have been times when patients have been persecuted by information and responsibility this was hardly evident in the consultations we studied. Moreover, what can be discerned in such arguments against sharing ideas is a familiar and poorly considered paternalism. Once again reasons are being found to permit doctors to control scarce knowledge and to act omnipotently.

Most of the arguments we have been discussing seem to us either to avoid paying rigorous attention to the need to exchange ideas with patients or to run the risk of prejudging the issue: doctors, whatever their good intentions, were frequently creating arguments to justify doing anything but having a dialogue with their patients. In this way they are acting out what might be considered a special example of Balint's 'Apostolic' function. He wrote:

'It was almost as if every doctor had revealed knowledge of what was right and what was wrong for patients to expect and endure, and further, as if he had a sacred duty to convert to his faith all the ignorant and unbelieving among his patients.' (Balint 1964: 216)

For many, the crucial question to ask of themselves will still be that posed by Szasz and Hollender (1956) nearly thirty years ago and which we quote for the second time: 'Do we take the patient's word for it (what is best) or do we place ourselves into the traditional parental role of "knowing what is best"...?'

(1956: 588). Without exploring a patient's diagnostic hypotheses and treatment ideas (including his arguments about causality) it is impossible to know with any certainty what he wants to have done or what he wants to have explained.

Concepts and emotions

As we have mentioned in the first chapter a traditional sociological preoccupation is to explain why doctors tend to limit the exchange of ideas in consultations by pointing to the way information is controlled in the interest of maintaining professional power and authority (Freidson 1970a; West 1976; Waitzkin and Stoeckle 1976). By cultivating an aura of superior expertise doctors in the past have sought to establish and maintain their economic and social position. As part of the process lay ideas and expertise have been devalued and the creation and maintenance of a hierarchical relationship between doctor and patient has been established as a norm. Several observations made in our review of medical ideas about information-sharing are pertinent to this point of view. The aims and methods of explaining to patients have been rarely discussed in medical literature and then only in a haphazard way. Until recently teaching about the tasks of explaining to and sharing understanding with patients have been virtually absent in medical education and they still have a very low priority. Patients are often conceived of as having inadequate knowledge or low intelligence. If such general observations support the idea that doctors have paid little attention to patients as thinking individuals, the findings we reported about the educational phase of the study were illustrative of the same phenomenon. Many of the doctors with whom we worked were uncomfortable and unwilling to give up 'being in charge'. They were noticeably anxious about the implications of promoting to an important place in their routine what patients had to say. They were also uncomfortable about sharing information with them, rigorously and precisely.

The pattern of consulting we have observed (and some of the reasons given to justify it) may, in part, be the product of more or less conscious attempts to maintain hierarchical relationships. But these in turn may result from still more fundamental causes. Virtually all of the doctors whom we studied and with whom we later worked gave us the impression that they were very devoted to the welfare of their patients. In recent years medical practitioners, especially in the UK, have devoted an enormous amount of time and effort to self-evaluation and self-criticism. Many doctors also spend a great deal of their time voluntarily trying to improve their skills. Moreover, as Hughes (1982) has argued, some of the supposedly controlling behaviour noticed by some observers of medical consultations may reflect a doctor's attempts to cope with the lack of communicative competence in his patient. Patients often do not find it very easy to know what to say or when to say it. This was particularly noticeable when some doctors in the educational phase reported their patients' difficulties in dealing with new and unfamiliar behaviour by the doctor, such as asking a patient for his views. In the uncomfortable atmosphere that followed doctors very often became very directive.

The need to maintain or create hierarchical relationships can be caused by other factors than the pursuit of power. For example, the innate conflicts and anxieties built into being a doctor may all too easily produce the need to stay in control. The doctor's consulting role carries special responsibilities and anxieties and is inherently difficult. He must deal on a day-to-day basis with his own and his patients' uncertainties, experiences of disaster, failures, helplessness, blame, panic, and anxieties, as well as with the unconscious feelings that go with them (Parsons 1978; Balint 1964). Actions must sometimes be taken quickly and routinely without adequate knowledge and with the awareness that a mistake can be fatal. Inevitably decisions will sometimes be hard to justify in cooler moments. The role also involves conflicts arising from social reality: for example, the doctor must mediate the demands of different patients, allocate scarce resources, mediate between the patient and his family and social network, mediate between the needs of his patients and those of himself, etc. (Tuckett 1976: 193 ff.). To cope with the role both institutional and personal methods of coping have been developed: including, perhaps, tunnel vision, emotional withdrawal, being busy, being obsessed with one or more technical aspects of medicine and being omnipotent in his behaviour. The 'Apostolic' function is a similar defence. Whether these defences help rather than hinder and whether in the end they make life more difficult for doctors (and their patients) is an open question. Nevertheless, it should never be forgotten that it is with this fraught background that the already inherently difficult task of mediating potentially divergent explanatory frameworks must be conducted. We are arguing in fact that the emotional aspect of medicine to which Parsons (1951, 1978) has paid so much attention is more important for understanding the behaviour of doctors than of patients.

One aspect of giving explanations is that it means being able to think through and justify to oneself one's ideas, suggestions, and evaluations of priorities (4). It also requires a clear view of relevant matters to provide an organized and unambiguous explanation to a patient. Such clarity may involve facing difficult and worrying ideas and feelings which it sometimes may be tempting to 'fudge'. Similarly, listening to and being aware of patients' theories, worries, questions and doubts is likely to increase a sense of losing control. This might be considered especially likely if conceptual models for understanding and elaborating patients' ideas are inadequate or muddled, as among the doctors described in the last chapter, or if patients themselves find the process difficult. Moreover, noticing what patients are thinking and feeling may often increase personal doubt and uncertainty, increase unwanted feelings of emotional involvement, and increase a sense of helplessness. It seems possible, therefore, that the contributions towards sharing ideas that patients made in their consultations, bearing in mind that they more often hinted than were explicit about what they thought, were ignored because of the discomforting complexities and feelings they introduced for the doctors. Uncertain conceptualization and relative lack of skill is unlikely to have helped matters. Moreover, although we are arguing, strongly, that patients should never be regarded as 'not competent', this is not to imply that they have the same competence and expertise as the doctor either in their knowledge or their communicative ability. Very real skills are needed by a doctor both to understand and conceptualize a patient's thinking and to understand and conceptualize relevant aspects of his own biomedical thinking with which to explain. To achieve the kind of skill at elaborating patient ideas and explaining what we envisage is likely to be a long process. The skills are likely to be mastered only after much practice and self- and peer-criticism – as is the case with diagnostic and therapeutic skills. Moreover, as an added difficulty, patients are likely sometimes to make the process difficult. They will sometimes have many of the same reasons not to confront the emotions and difficulties as their doctors: as has been described in a slightly different context by means of the 'truce' concept in regard to repeat prescriptions (Marinker 1970). They may also be unskilled at communication. In providing doctors with detailed notes on how to obtain a patient's ideas we have made the suggestion that 'meta-level' questions may help in this regard. Such questions clarify the communicative context for the patient and ought to reduce conversations at cross-purposes (5).

The maintenance of hierarchical attitudes and behaviour (as in the conventional stereotype of the patient) seems to us, therefore, to be as likely to be caused by the inherent difficulties of the situation as by any motive on the part of a doctor to maintain economic and social status. In some ways, if this is so, it would be encouraging. In the first place, although it is not widely admitted, it seems to us that the discomfort and evasion implicit in the present experience of consultations exacts an unnecessarily high emotional cost for doctors and that this could provide a motive to change. One might see the defensiveness and tension evident among many doctors and, perhaps, the development by some of interests in anything but consulting, as indicators of this evasion. Other negative indicators might be patient non-compliance, growing (if still muffled) criticism of doctors, and, perhaps, growing interest in fringe medicine (6). Once concepts are appreciated and skills are learned, consultations organized as sharing experiences could be less uncomfortable. The educational work we described in the last chapter showed that consultations could be made more pleasant experiences for doctors and patients and that doctors could find them much more interesting. Similar optimistic reports have been experienced using approaches allied to our own (Lazare, Eisenthal, and Wasserman 1975; Good and Good 1981; Katon and Kleinman 1981; Pendleton *et al.* 1984). It is also to be hoped, although it is not yet proven, that such consultations can be more effective in terms of all their various outcomes as well.

It is, perhaps, asking a great deal of doctors to make what amounts to a fundamental alteration in the detailed way they think about and routinely conduct their task. Until now communication skills have usually been treated in a haphazard way and have been seen as relevant mainly with problem cases. However, the challenge to improve is one to which the 'true' professional might be expected to respond with vigour. As a profession, doctors have been willing to be self-critical and evaluative (for example, Cochrane 1972; McKeown 1976). Few social scientists or other occupational groups have indicated the same inclination. It is not our impression that the doctors we studied and worked with were primarily 'shop-keeper-type' professionals intent on bolstering their economic and social self-interest. A test of this view, of course, will be to see how they respond to the challenge of the future, especially if the growing demand for involvement by patients which has been noted by some general practitioners (Marinker 1981; Metcalfe 1982; Pendleton *et al.* 1984) is confirmed.

Patients as 'experts'

At the risk of being repetitive we would like to end by summarizing what we have meant when arguing that patients should be treated as the experts we believe they are.

We conceive of the consultation as a meeting between one person who has, by his training and experience, access to scarce and specialist knowledge and another person who has, by experience, immersion in his culture and past discussion, a set of ideas about what is happening to him. Both parties form models of what is wrong, what should be done, what are the consequences of the problem, its treatment and so on, based on their own reasoning and background knowledge. These models may involve a degree of inconsistency and uncertainty. A major aim of the consultation, then, is the initiation of a process of explicit sharing of models, so that the patient is placed in a situation, as far as he wants to be, where he can choose to take advantage of the specialist biomedical ideas and skills his medical adviser can offer. We have described in the previous chapter some ideas about how to achieve this.

Successful shared understanding will have taken place if, following a consultation, a patient can remember the key points of what a doctor said, make correct sense of them, and be aware of the points of conflict and difference, if any, between himself and his doctor as well as the reasons for these differences. For this to happen several things are necessary:

1 Doctor and patient must both agree on the problem they are seeking to understand.
2 The doctor must use his biomedical expertise to establish in his own mind what is going on, what the options are and what the consequences may be. He develops an explanatory model.
3 The patient's explanation of his problem (and to some extent his reasoning behind it) must be verbalized and elaborated together with his ideas and

reasoning about what should be done and what consequences there may be. This will involve piecing together, elaborating and conceptualizing the hints about their ideas that patients will drop. It may also require the doctor to comment on the value his patients' ideas have for him.

4 The doctor's understanding (together with his reasoning) must be made clear to the patient and related to the patient's own way of thinking, as it has emerged in the consultation. Sometimes a doctor's advice will include options and an effort to indicate the costs and benefits of them.

5 In the process of the doctor communicating his understanding and the patient being encouraged to communicate his, opportunity must be allowed to explore questions and doubts either side may have and to check and clarify what is being meant and understood. It is equally important to clarify the terms and ideas being used and the reasoning behind them.

In conceiving of the patient and the doctor as experts we have said that we do not see them as having the same expertise. In our model the patient has come to see the doctor to consult him for his advice. He, therefore, needs to integrate the biomedical way of thinking with his own. Nor are we advocating an erosion of the traditional diagnostic side of the doctor's task. The doctor's advice can be no better than the quality of his diagnostic skill and his knowledge of therapeutic remedies.

In referring to a 'consultation' when explaining how patients should be treated as experts, we are not necessarily advocating that everything can be done at a single meeting. We have expressed doubt about how far studying only one consultation has misled our conclusions but this should not be understood as an argument against sharing ideas over a series of meetings. Indeed, it seems likely that the process of demonstrating to patients that consultations are available to be used to share ideas can go on over several consultations for different problems. The most mundane consultations, when urgent diagnostic business is least likely, might be particularly appropriate times at which to give sharing a priority. There are plenty of consultations with this potential. Nor are we advocating the need to force the sharing model on an unwilling patient. How far a patient wants to share ideas in a consultation is an important matter to explore with him. A dialogue needs to take place about it. What we have been sceptical about are claims that patients do not have ideas or do not want to share those of the doctor, based on inappropriate or non-existent efforts to establish that this is so. Without words, and probably also the ability to discuss directly and openly with patients what is happening in the consultation, a dialogue is very unlikely.

Finally, we are emphasizing that our purpose for establishing a patient's ideas is to help the doctor to know what to explain. There are other important reasons for talking to a patient and listening to him (such as to encourage a sense of mutual understanding and caring). Some of these purposes may be met unobtrusively by following some of the suggestions we have made. But the purpose we have in mind for exploring a patient's ideas is specific and finite. The idea is to be able to conceptualize key elements of the patient's way of thinking: the diagnostic-significance he attaches to his problem, his ideas about action and his ideas about the consequences and implications of his illness or its treatment. Such knowledge should allow a doctor to adjust his ideas and explain to the patient so that he can understand the biomedical way of looking at what is happening and what should be done about it.

The interview checklist

The interview checklist

1 **Background story**

I expect you know that your consultation with Dr was tape-recorded. Well, I haven't listened to it. Since we are trying to see how far doctors are successful in trying to communicate to their patients I would not want my memory of things muddling it up. I don't know anything about you.

So, can we start by your putting me in the picture a bit. How is it that you came to be seeing Dr......on......?

2 **The problems**

So, as I understand it your doctor paid attention to ......? (problems clearly attended to so far) Is that right?

Any other problems he paid attention to?

Did he think you needed help with anything else at all?

Note
Throughout investigators are expected to link questions to the detailed story obtained at the beginning.

Note
Be careful to establish the exact symptoms a patient is complaining of (*not* hypertension, high BP, cancer) and locate the problem in the body with care. ALSO get information about how long each problem was discussed, what proportion of consultation on each.

He saw that as a problem you wanted help for?

Keep probing
Any others?
(until you get a negative)

For example
Other symptoms/problems
job, housing,
relationships,
monotony of daily routine,
the way you feel in yourself?

Probes
You wouldn't have liked him to concentrate on anything else? (mention specifically any problem hinted at so far)

Probe for any problems that come up
These were problems he addressed on......?

Were these the problems you wanted him to address?

3   Understanding the significance of symptoms

For each *symptom* cluster explore:

When you saw Dr on . . . . . .what did he think was wrong with you?

On . . . . . .did you get an impression from Dr that there was any chance that what you have might be serious?

Interpretation
Rate what impression patient had as to *how likely Dr thought* the problem was serious.

Be careful to question on all possible symptom clusters and hypotheses mentioned in the consultation. Check what was mentioned.

You've mentioned he thought it could be . . . . . ., is there anything else you got the impression it could be?

Did you gather how likely he thought it was, this could turn out to be one of the serious possibilities?

Were there any differences in emphasis
between you and Dr? As to what
problems needed attention?

You were quite satisfied on that? You
agree you needed help for......?

Nothing else?

Probe
What does he mean by that?

Probe
In what sense?

Probe
I mean by serious something like:
heart disease,
cancer,
stomach ulcer,
thrombosis,
serious arthritis

You know, something dubious or
worrying?

Something which could:
kill you,
maim you,
make you an invalid,
cause you trouble in future?

Check
you had that impression on......

Could be caused by something serious?

Probe for all alternatives doctor mentioned

Are they serious?
What does that mean?

How likely is it?
What are the chances?

If insist they have no idea
Would you say then that the doctor
thought there was no chance of
something serious, or do you just have
no idea?

Recall
Can patient remember Dr specifically
stating the chances?

What gave you that impression? Did he
actually tell you the chances of it being
serious or did you just gather that?

Detailed understanding
Does the patient understand, in his case
in his own terms, the supposed potential
seriousness of what information is
needed (supposedly) to resolve any
uncertainty about it.

I'm interested not only in what you
learned from your doctor on . . . . . . but
also in any other medical knowledge you
may have, you know – from the doctor
on other occasions, from TV, books,
radio, friends in the know, etc. NOW . . . . . .

Can (the symptoms you have) ever be
serious? What are the chances? What is
the worst thing that can happen?

Well then, how sure can one be that
what you have is/is not the serious kind?

Did the doctor examine you? What
would that be supposed to tell him?

Are there any tests? Can the hospital
help one to know?

Commitment
Does the patient agree with the doctor's
assessment of the chance of seriousness?

Now, you got the impression from your
doctor that what you have is/is not
likely to be serious. How convinced are
you that's right?

Either
I've had to mention things like cancer
and heart disease, what makes you so
sure that it's not (a dubious alternative)?

Which?

Check
You had that impression on......?

If no recall probe satisfaction
Should he have told you?

In the sense we were talking earlier?

What do you mean?
How do you understand that?
Get exact details of course of
illness/vulnerability, etc.

How do doctors tell if you've got X or
Y?

Can you explain?
How does that work?

How's that supposed to work?
How is one supposed to be sure about
this?

Can you explain?

Check
This is what's supposed to be the case,
as far as you know?

Remember: If the patient admits to any areas of ignorance, explore own role in requesting explanation/justification

Do you have any doubts?
Does he go into it enough?
Do you agree there's a high/low chance?

How would you convince a friend that's
not so?

Doctors can't always be right,
Isn't it likely it is/is not serious?

Or

Your doctor says its......and you think
this means......but what makes you so
sure it's not really just......?
(nothing/really serious)

Right, so to sum up you got the
impression from Dr on......that what
you have has a no/low/high chance of
being something serious. And you tend
to agree/disagree with that judgement?

What are your reasons? What makes
you agree/disagree with your doctor?

---

4   Understanding treatment-action

Interpretation
Rate package of actions patient
attributes to Dr's decided strategy.

Did you get any idea from the Dr when
you saw him on......whether there is
anything that can be done to cure this
problem(s) now?

Be careful
to establish which actions are desired to
effect which symptom clusters.

Anything else? (Keep probing)

Cover for all problems–it is the package
of actions that matter.

Did you get any idea from him if
anything can be done to help (i.e.
alleviate at all)?

Be careful
to establish actions are viewed as cure or
alleviation or investigation and not
prevention.

Anything else? (Keep probing)

Are you supposed to see him again?
Did he give you that impression?

*If patient has no idea or once he runs out of
recall ask*
Nothing else at all?
I wonder if you got any idea on......
what Dr thinks the value of any of these
things would be for your case:
Taking something from the chemist?

Remember: If any doubts are expressed probe: own role doubting, satisfaction

Why do you think that?

Can you explain?

Why should that convince you?

Probe
Get rid of this?

That's what you gathered on......?

Probe
Ease the pain/make things
a bit better/stop symptoms

For all actions
Did you get the impression that's
something you'll always have to do, or is
just to get better now?

Is that a cure? Or just for relief?

Will that stop you having this again, or
is it just for now?

Keep checking
This is something you gathered
on......?

Aspirin?
Panadol?
Rennies?

You, changing your routine?

Letting (it) get better on its own?

Taking help/advice from someone else?

Having an operation/more powerful drug?
Doing something more to find out what
the trouble is?

If still no idea
Would you then say your Dr thinks
nothing is appropriate, or do you just
not know what he thinks?

Recall
Does patient actually remember Dr
mentioning each action, or did he just
gather these were the actions?

So you got the impression Dr thought . . . . .?
Can you remember him actually
mentioning each of these things, or were
they just things you gathered?

Detailed understanding
Does patient understand the range of
actions that could be utilised in his case
and what is involved and how effective
these actions are?

Again, I'm interested not just in what
you learned from Dr on . . . . . ., but in
your own medical knowledge – what
you've learnt from books, TV, radio,
other Drs.

How are these thing(s) the Dr has
recommended meant to help in your
particular case?

Be sure to ask these questions

Well, these are the things your Dr has
recommended this time. Is there
anything else that can be done as far as
you know, for someone in your
situation?

Work?
What you do every day?
Doing nothing?

Another Dr?
Hospital?
Social Worker?
Psychotherapist?
Osteopath?
Someone like that?

X-ray?
Tests?
Specialist opinion?

Probe each item of package
How good is that supposed to be?
What difference is that supposed to make?
What is supposed to happen if not done?
When will you see the benefit?
Will it help for ever?
Are there side effects/disadvantages?
What will be gained by doing this?

Keep probing
Exactly what do you mean?
Can you say more?

How does that work?
That's what Dr thinks?

Suggest possibilities and then probe each item as above
What about some of the things I mentioned
earlier?
(chemist/routine/nothing/other
help/operation/investigation)

Exactly what do you mean?
Can you say more?
How does that work?
That's what Dr thinks?

Is there anything you are *not* supposed
to do?
Any side effects?

If no ideas
Does that mean it's supposed to make
no difference what you do?

Commitment
Does the patient agree with the package
of actions Dr recommended *and* can he
reject alternatives we suggest?

So, as I understand it your doctor
thought . . . . . .was the thing to do.
How effective do you think this strategy
will be? Will it work?

Do you have any doubts about it?
Doctors can't always be right.

What it is that makes you think
that . . . . . .(some of the alternatives I
asked you about) wouldn't be better for
you?

So really you tend to agree/disagree with
Dr? Can you give me some reasons for
that?

---

5   Understanding preventive action

Interpretation
Rate actions patient gathered Dr
thought appropriate.

Did you get any idea from Dr, when
you saw him on . . . . ., whether there
was anything that could be done to
prevent you getting this trouble again in
future?

Anything else at all?

Nothing else at all?

What about smoking/eating/drinking
etc?

Really doesn't matter?   Doctors would say so?

Remember: if patient expresses any ignorance, ask own role
Did you ask Dr......Why not?

How much difference will it make?   That's what you really think, yourself?
Does it really matter?
What will happen if not done?

Wouldn't you be as well off letting it
get better on its own?
What about some of these new
treatments they have nowadays?

Remember: if any doubts, check own role
Why didn't they ask?

Why do you think that?
How does that work?
Is that a good reason?
Why should he be right?
Doctors can't always be right.

Probe
Stop you getting this again in future?   *Keep probing*
Any causes that can be prevented?
Or at least make sure it's not as bad in
future?

Probe   *Check*
Anything else?   That's what you gathered on......?
(until get a negative)

Did you get any idea on......whether the Dr thought there was any value in any of the following:

Making changes in what you do every day?

Changing where you live?

Other people behaving differently towards you?

Do you smoke? Would stopping/cutting down help according to Dr?

Eating or drinking differently?

Taking more exercise?

If no idea

Would you then think Dr thought there was nothing that could be done, or are you just unsure?

Recall
Does the patient recall doctor talking about appropriate prevention?

So, you got the impression Dr thought......?
Can you remember him actually saying this, or was it something you gathered?

Detailed understanding
Does the patient understand the range of preventive actions that could be utilized in his case *and* what is involved and how effective these actions are likely to be.

Again, I'm interested not just in what you learned from Dr on......, but in your own medical knowledge – what you've learnt from books, TV, radio, other doctors.

How are these things the Dr has suggested meant to prevent you getting trouble in future, in your particular case?

Well, these are the things your Dr suggested this time. Is there anything that can be done to stop you having this trouble again in future?

That will stop this happening again?
Or at least make sure it's never as bad?

Probe
Housework
Work
Leisure

Probe
Spouse
Friends

Which?

You just got that impression?

If no recall
Remember satisfaction

Probe each item of package
How good is that supposed to be?
What difference is that supposed to make?
What is supposed to happen if not done?
When will you see the benefits?
Will it help for ever?
Are there any disadvantages?
Suggest possibilities, then use above probes

Keep probing
Exactly what do you mean?
Can you say more?
How will that work for you?
That's what doctors think?

Exactly what do you mean?
Can you say more?
How will that work for you?

What about some of the things I suggested earlier?

Also try and ask
Do they know what can be done for someone like......

If no ideas
Does that mean it really doesn't matter what you do, it'll make no difference, as far as you know?

Commitment
Does the patient agree with the package of preventive actions attributed to Dr and can he reject alternative?

So, as I understand you got the impression from your Dr on......that......was the way to avoid getting this trouble again in future? And I think you tend to agree/disagree?

How effective do you think......will be?
Will it work?

Are there no better things to do? What about some of the possibilities we've been discussing?

What is it that makes you think......(an alternative) wouldn't be better than what your Dr has suggested?

So I get the impression you tend to agree/disagree with your Dr on this. Can you give me some of your reasons?

Smoking/eating/drinking/change in
everyday life/change in others/exercise?

That's what doctor think?

Doctors would say so?

Remember if patient expresses any ignorance, ask own role
Did you ask your Dr......Why not?

Make sure it doesn't happen again?
What difference will it make?
Does it really matter to do......?
What will happen if not done?
Do you have no doubts?

Smoking/eating/drinking/routine/change
in others/doing nothing?

Wouldn't you be better off/as well off
doing nothing?

Remember: probe any doubts, disagreements with own role:
Did you tell Dr how you felt......Why not?

Why do you think that?
How does that work?
Is that a good reason?
Why should he be right?

Chapter 1. Sharing ideas and its importance in medical consultations

[1] 'the sick person is not, of course competent to help himself. . . He is not only generally not in a position to do what needs to be done, but he does not "know" what needs to be done or how to do it. It is not merely that he, being bedridden, cannot go down to the drug store to get what is needed, but that he would, even if well, not be qualified to do what is needed, and to judge what needs to be done. There is, that is to say, a "communication gap"'' (Parsons 1951:441). Parsons goes on to demonstrate the empirical validity of this view by pointing out how laymen always say their doctor is the best and so demonstrate that they have no proper criteria for judgement.

Chapter 2. A study of general practice consultations and their outcomes

[1] In fact, as will be explained below, only 1,302 consultations were actually analysed. By surgery sessions we refer to periods when doctors saw anything between ten and forty patients in stints of one and a half to two and a half hours in a morning, afternoon or an evening.

[2] The usual distinction that is made between quantitative and qualitative research is one we find potentially misleading and so we are comparing 'quantitative studies' with 'developmental' ones. By quantitative studies we refer to those in which formal measurement and statistical analysis are used. It is because this is not, in principle, incompatible with developing the kind of sensitive indicators of concepts more often to be found in what is usually called 'qualitative research' that we have preferred to refer to research not using formal measurement and statistical techniques as 'developmental'.

[3] The work to which we refer is that of authors like: Davis (1960); Zola (1973); Stimson and Webb (1975); Hayes-Bautista (1976); West (1976); Danziger (1978); Sharrock (1979); Alexander (1981); Katon and Kleinman (1981); Silverman (1981); Drass (1982); Hughes (1982).

[4] The studies to which we refer are those of authors like Milton Davis (1968); Freemon et al. (1971); Korsch, Gozzi, and Francis (1968); Lucas (1978); Pendleton (1982a); Pendleton and Bochner (1980); Joyce et al. (1969); Ley et al. (1973, 1976); Stiles et al. (1979). While looking in great detail at various aspects of the style with which doctors manage consultations these studies have not looked at the meaning of what doctors and patients said to each other. An exception, bridging aspects of qualitative and quantitative traditions is the doctoral study by Svarstad (1974). As we will argue below she was able to show that the content of what was said in consultations was a crucial influence both on patient's subsequent understanding of the medication they should take and on their compliance with

instructions. Essentially, Svarstad showed that very often patients were not given the information they would need in order to comply.

[5] All the doctors whom we observed in the pilot and main studies, together with those that advised us throughout, attended a meeting to discuss our provisional findings in October 1981. At the meeting it was clear that the meaning of the term explanation varied a great deal between them. One argued that a facial expression he made in a consultation, giving a patient negative feedback because he had sought help with a cold, was explanation. Others selected comments like 'this is diabetes', 'don't smoke', and 'you should avoid lifting unless your back is straight', as examples of explanations they had given. Two poles of opinion are illustrated by the following comments:

Doctor A: Now I frequently snort, to some effect, and this is an example of non-verbal communication. One does not need to gild the lily; simply pursing the lips can be effective education.

Doctor B: I would find it difficult, skilled as I am in non-verbal and para-verbal communication, in body posture and with a detailed knowledge of my patients, to explain by the flick of an eyebrow why it is that the patient should, for instance, put cold compresses–if indeed one should–on an injured ankle in the first stage and hot ones later.

Some aspects of the medical literature on the topic of explanation are reviewed below.

[6] A crucial part of the process is that disagreements over the interpretation of data should take place within the rating team in the early stages of the project. A process rather similar to that we followed has been described by Hollingshead and Redlich (1958) in their classic account of how they developed a measure of an individual's social class.

[7] Mainly because we had been overambitious about how many things we could measure the work of rating scale development was still incomplete after eighteen months of pilot work. At that time, however, institutional constraints dictated that the selection of the study sample had to begin. This eventuality was dealt with as follows. In some cases, in which scales were still not easily agreed, they were made the joint responsibility of several investigators. In these instances two or more investigators rated every case independently but then discussed their judgements in a formal meeting before reaching an agreed view. Eventually, we considered we could rate reliably all the main scales. At that moment each scale became the responsibility of one of the four investigators (DT, MB, CO, AW) who made the ratings for all remaining cases. The reliability (or consistency) of the ratings was then determined by arranging for a second investigator to rate a random sample of the cases independently.

[8] The practice has been followed in the text whenever case material is reported with an identifying case number. The few exceptions to this rule were selected so that a particular point could be illustrated economically or where a whole series of points have been made on a single case. Cases drawn from the work conducted after the study proper was over could not be selected at random because no formal measurement was undertaken.

[9] Several reported studies are based on tape-recording (using audio or video) parts of the consultation only. For example, Larsen and Smith (1981) report that they video-recorded the 'interview portion only' (apparently when patients were sitting down and talking). Pridham and Hansen (1980) based their reliability study on an audio-tape of the whole consultation if it was less than fifteen minutes. If it was longer they divided a consultation in half and then worked with either half chosen at random. In the present study the whole consultation was tape-recorded from the patient's first entry into the room

until his final dismissal by the doctor. In some cases this meant the microphone being taken by the doctor to an examination room.

[10] The actual question used by Ley and his co-workers is not published in any of the various articles. The question reported in the text is one suggested by one of Ley's collaborators, John Kincey, in a personal conversation. It reflects the kind of question asked and is of the 'free recall' type.

[11] Among consultation studies Larsen and Smith (1981) analysed the consultations of 34 patients who were new to the doctor. The doctors were volunteers from the author's own department. No information was given as to whether any patients refused to take part. Ley *et al.* (1973) based their results on 40 consecutive attendances of 'lower working-class patients' with a new illness. They attended one doctor. Information was not made available on these definitions or on how or why the particular doctor was chosen. Ley *et al.* (1976) based their study on the consultations of four doctors from one inner-city practice. Patients included children, adults and the 'elderly'. Forty-six per cent of patients invited to do so returned the questionnaires on which conclusions were based. Stiles *et al.* (1979) based their study on 52 consultations conducted by several doctors at a local hospital. Patients were attending on a 'walk-in' basis and no information was given about selecting consultations or rates of refusal. Korsch *et al.* (1968) studied 800 consultations. Some of these were not tape-recorded but no reports about the effect of tape-recording were present in published papers. Most of the data is based on 285 patients attending a 'walk-in' pediatric clinic. The clinic was local to the university and doctors were mostly junior. No information was given about refusal to be tape-recorded. Finally, Inui *et al.* (1982) studied 143 consecutive new patients attending their 'main management visit' at a local hospital. After refusals, tape problems, and pre-test exclusions, data was based on 95 cases.

[12] It seemed likely that only about 400 patients could be both interviewed and systematically studied in depth. It also seemed desirable to compare the effects of different potential styles of consulting. A sample of about 400, given about 25 patients per doctor, meant limiting the number of doctors to sixteen.

[13] In one case the doctor chosen was the 'third' name selected and in the other the 'second'. The previous doctors selected had been invited but refused to take part.

[14] We arranged to tape-record further surgeries until at least 25 of the doctor's patients we had selected for study had agreed to be interviewed at home. If a situation in which 32 patients had agreed was reached while recording a surgery the investigator monitoring the consultations stopped his activity before waiting for the end. The number of patients a doctor might see in a surgery varied from as few as seven to as many as thirty. As a result the number who were selected and agreed to be interviewed at any given surgery session varied substantially: between none at all and ten. The variation explains, hopefully, the reasons for what may have seemed, but was not, a haphazard selection process.

[15] Patients could tell the doctor if they did not want to be recorded and in a few cases the doctor himself made this decision. Discussion with the doctors about the kinds of cases missed in this way did not reveal any striking pattern. For instance, among the cases not recorded were patients with strained muscles as well as emotional or sexual problems (as among cases recorded).

[16] The exact numbers of patients attending the various surgeries we recorded, attending a recorded surgery for the second time, refusing to be recorded, not being recorded due to technical problems, selected as suitable for study, refusing a home interview, not keeping a home interview appointment, etc., for each doctor, can be seen from *Table 2.1n*.

Table 2.1n

Dr	Tp	En	Ert	Etec	Ttr	Ti	Ri	Rf	Sc	Si
A	116	2	33	2	79	43	16	3	24	19
B	84	0	4	2	78	39	10	6	23	18
C	110	0	6	4	100	45	10	13	22	18
D	62	0	1	2	59	38	6	2	30	24
E	103	0	12	1	90	40	8	7	25	18
F	97	2	2	1	92	36	8	4	24	18
G	63	0	2	3	58	42	11	6	25	19
H	111	2	6	4	99	44	20	3	21	16
I	67	0	4	2	61	39	10	3	26	20
J	68	0	4	6	58	32	4	4	24	19
K	87	1	3	2	81	37	8	3	26	22
L	117	1	7	7	102	41	11	6	24	19
M	71	2	5	2	62	32	1	3	28	22
N	102	2	3	2	95	39	7	1	31	24
O	98	4	8	3	83	31	5	0	26	27
P	114	2	6	1	105	41	9	6	26	25
total	1470	18	106	44	1302	619	144	70	405	328

Key:

Dr Doctor

Tp Total consultations taking place in surgeries

En Number excluded because attending more than once while recording in process

Ert Number excluded because recording was refused

Etec Number excluded because technical problems occurred

Ttr Total consultations tape-recorded

Ti Total after investigator excluded cases not suitable for study

Ri Number refusing interview

Rf Number failing appointment

Sc Total in consultation sample

Si Total in interview sample

[17] These were consultations in which patients were presenting problems already discussed with the doctor and in which no change of view or strategy took place. They included consultations concerning repeat prescriptions, routine follow-up, check-ups, and problems or queries with past treatment or with relationships to specialist services.

[18] Consultations of an administrative nature were mainly consultations concerned with giving patients health certificates: for a short- or long-term absence from work and handing out birth control prescriptions or giving vaccinations without discussion of the underlying issues. They were also consultations in which time was mainly devoted to discussion of how to get a new doctor when the patient moves, how to register someone else with a doctor, and to the requirement that a doctor sign a patient's passport or stamp a form

for a local education authority, etc.

[19] Consultations for coughs and colds in which only a prescription was given very often overlapped with administrative consultations–about half these consultations were associated with a certificate.

[20] The fact that nothing much seemed to be decided or communicated in such consultations is not meant to imply there might not have been all kinds of underlying communication problems or that it might not be interesting to study them. It seemed to be a higher priority, however, to examine consultations in which speaking did take place.

[21] We chose to study consultations after we had excluded those in which there was very little likelihood of much talk because we felt that other more obvious criteria, such as restricting analysis to new patients or patients presenting new problems, were less suitable for obtaining a picture of communication in primary care. Although consultations with 'new' patients might be more likely than others to contain information-giving (how else could a doctor know that his patient knew what he was thinking and advising?), in general practice they are very rare and, in many ways, at odds with the continuing and ongoing nature of the work. Another option would have been to select patients who doctors could define as presenting 'new' or 'self-initiated' problems rather than 'old' or 'doctor-initiated' ones (Morrell, Gage, and Robinson 1970). Although attractive and apparently more systematic than the method we eventually adopted, the difficulties of using such a distinction soon became apparent in the pilot phase. We discovered that classification systems adopted for appointments purposes in working surgeries were by no means a reliable guide for research purposes. For example, although one group of doctors actually distinguished their appointments in terms of doctor- or patient-initiated (using different coloured inks), when we analysed the clinical content of these consultations, let alone how much information was given, we found it very difficult to guess which consultations were which. 'Doctor-initiated' consultations, for example, did not stop a patient introducing something new and 'patient-initiated' consultations often included patients who had made an appointment to follow up an earlier one. The 'errors' in either category, as a guide to clinical content, were simply too many. It certainly did not seem worth trying to persuade other doctors whom we would study to instigate such a system.

[22] The three categories ((1) administrative; (2) coughs and colds; (3) little new) were defined in a way to be a guide rather than definitive criteria to the investigator monitoring consultations. In all cases, if an extended discussion or explanation of issues transpired the investigator could include the case. The following are seven, randomly selected, consultations which were not chosen for detailed study (the number in brackets after the case number indicates which of the three criteria were used to exclude):

1195 (3): Patient with infection reporting back. Brief examination, virtually no talking; issues presumed clarified before.

1328 (1): Patient arrives for a continuation of a disability certificate and a discussion of how to get a doctor when he moves; no discussion of clinical type issues.

1536 (3): Patient arrives for routine blood pressure check and a repeat prescription. Beyond single word comments and pleasantries no discussion.

1788 (1,2): Patient arrives with heavy cold and wanting a certificate. The consultation included pleasantries and lasted as long as it takes to write out a certificate.

2020 (1): Patient arrives for family planning repeat prescription. Blood pressure is taken and prescription issued with no explanation save 'that's fine' and no other clinical comment.

2227 (3): Patient with chronic backache; given repeat prescription and brief examination without much comment – issues presumed to have been clarified in a previous consultation.

2432 (3): Patient visiting (with husband) on routine check for epilepsy; no clinical comment or new decisions; issues presumed clarified before.

[23] Patients attending on behalf of someone not present in the consultation or on their own and under the legal age of consent (N = 18), or with obvious severe mental disorder (N = 2) or those with obvious language difficulties (N = 52) were not eligible for selection due to the obvious complications for interviewing that their cases would involve.

[24] The 5 per cent sample was a 5 per cent random sample of the 1,302 consultations tape-recorded and, therefore, a selection of consultations designed to be statistically representative of all those observed, not just those studied in detail. It was selected by first choosing, at random, 26 surgeries (one-fifth of the 108 surgeries recorded). Then, again selecting at random, every fourth consultation in the 26 surgeries was chosen for analysis, resulting in a sample total of 69 consultations (5.3 per cent of the 1,302). The tape-recordings of these consultations (which included several consultations already analysed in detail in the main sample) have been analysed to describe the problems patients presented, the status of their visit, diagnoses and advice given by doctors, efforts made to discover patients' ideas and explanations, and any reason-giving explanation patients received. Data from this sample thus describes, in a representative way, the range of problems presented in the 108 general practice consultations we studied, the topics on which doctors gave information, the efforts made to explore patients' ideas and the kind of reason-giving explanation attempted. In this way the data provides background against which to interpret the results based on the more intensive study of a smaller number of consultations.

[25] The exact period of time between the recorded consultation and the interview varied according to several practical considerations–essentially the availability of the respondent, the 'success' rate in obtaining patients for interview in a given surgery, and the day on which the consultation took place. In general, surgeries were recorded on the first three days of the week and interviews took place within the same week. On some occasions a gap of up to ten days elapsed. It was also the case that in less than ten cases interviews were conducted elsewhere than in a patient's home, for the convenience of the patient. No systematic analysis of the effect of the length of time that elapsed between the consultation and a patient's subsequent recall or understanding was undertaken.

[26] A fourth (male) interviewer left the project and emigrated from the UK so that reliable analysis of the 77 cases assigned to him was not possible.

[27] Fortunately, presumably because cases were assigned to interviewers in no special way, the absence of 77 interviews does not appear likely to have influenced results in any way. None of the consultation variables deemed important in the subsequent analysis varied in a statistically significant way as between cases assigned to different interviewers.

[28] The only investigator of whom we are aware who has not taken this view is Hughes (1982). He argued that since several medical students, nurses, and visiting doctors were routinely present in the consultations (in an out-patient clinic) and because Hughes, himself, was there and could make notes without asking permission, it was acceptable to record the consultation first and ask permission afterward.

[29] Given that a trial comparing situations where doctors and patients did not know they were recorded was unacceptable, we had to fall back on relatively soft ways of investigating possible effects. In the pilot study, when we recorded and interviewed in one health centre over a period of several months and were, therefore, very much more obtrusive than in the main study, we regularly asked doctors and their reception staff about noticeable effects. We also included a routine question at the end of our interview with patients. Each doctor in the main study was also asked, when recording was complete, whether he felt he had behaved 'differently'.

[30] Some doctors had sometimes obviously altered their consulting behaviour because they were being studied. In a few instances they actually told jokes in their consultations for the benefit of research workers. However, just because they were aware of being observed and changed some aspects of their behaviour it does not follow it made a difference to the issues with which the study was concerned. Average consultation times were reported to be much as usual and doctors seem to have seen the usual selection of patients (few surgeries were organized so that any very thorough pre-selection could have been conducted). Some patients reported that they sometimes felt doctors had explained more or 'tried harder' than usual and there was also clear evidence, later admitted by the doctor, that one doctor told far more patients than usual to give up smoking (perhaps because our study was known to be funded by the Health Education Council). As we intended, it is possible to consider that doctors gave slightly more information than usual, but not to consider they gave less. As far as patients were concerned, many with whom the effect of recording was discussed seemed to have been relatively unaware of the tape-recording and some, because they could not see a recorder, even reported that they had assumed recording was off for their consultation and therefore that their permission had been sought unnecessarily. Some patients did refer during consultations to 'those listening in' but no doctor in the main sample gave us the opinion that patients had behaved noticeably differently. In general, it seems, as far as doctors were concerned, that the obtrusive effect would tend only to amplify the main conclusions to be reported. In the case of patients, it seems that the potentially intrusive tape-recorder was, at worst, one small factor among many other features of their consultations which (as we shall show) inhibited them from a full and frank exchange of views with their doctors. The fact of recording was not something mentioned to us as a reason for withholding doubts or questions and, in the light of the overall findings, seems to us, in retrospect, an irrelevance.

Chapter 3. The problem of information

[1] Although our measurement approach was developed quite independently it is in fact similar in logic to that created by Svarstad (1974). She studied the extent to which a series of patients attending a New York clinic followed the treatment instructions their doctors gave them. To test the hypothesis that those patients who got more information would be better at following instructions, Svarstad considered what physicians *could* cover to help patients to know exactly what they would have to do. Using this method to study consultations she reported that subsequent compliance with instructions (as measured by patients' reports and detailed bottle checks for each drug at interview) was strongly related to how much doctors told them (and also wrote down) about the length of time they should take drugs, the dosage, the regularity and the name of the drug: whereas 54 per cent of those who received 'high' instruction on all or most of these points followed instructions correctly this was true of only 29 per cent of those who received little or no such information. She concluded that a substantial proportion of incorrect drug-taking derived from unclear instructions.

Svarstad's approach can be considered another application of the general principle we followed. If the purpose of giving information and the topic on which it is given are defined theoretically, then it is possible to develop clear and reasonably generalizable criteria to determine if one set of information statements is more illuminating than another.

[2] The distinctions are similar to those made by the Oxford English Dictionary (Murray *et al*. 1933) and by the educationalist Brown (1978). The OED distinguishes three principal meaning for the verb 'to explain': to unfold (a matter); to assign a meaning; and to account for. Brown, discussing the construction of university lectures, distinguishes mainly between describing, interpreting and reason-giving. We have taken the view that assigning a meaning and interpreting involve stating the doctor's view. Accounting for and giving reasons are clearly reasoning (which like Brown we distinguish from providing 'causes' (Brown 1978:9)). Unfolding and describing are the methods by which stating or reason-giving are achieved.

Chapter 4. The information shared with patients

[1] The judgement of the view a doctor took was made in association with those to be described under the heading 'Third-party judgement' in Chapter 7. Whether a doctor took a preventive view depended on whether any of the advice he gave was considered relevant to the prevention or at least control of future episodes of the trouble the patient had. There were 123 examples among the 405 consultations. They included 14 cases where the preventive action involved modification in the social sphere; 41 where habit change or attempts at personality change were involved; and 61 where the advice involved medical intervention or relatively minor changes in behaviour.

[2] The results reported in this chapter are based on an analysis of the 405 consultations. Judging by comparison with the 69 cases forming the 5 per cent random sample of all the consultations tape-recorded, these results slightly overstate the amount of information patients are given in an 'average' consultation (*Table 4.1n*).

[3] Examining the 405 consultations we found that in only about one in eight was there any obvious awareness of implications of the kind mentioned in Chapter 3 and that even then discussion was usually limited to a chance sentence or comment: for instance a comment about the impact of the patient's emotional problems on his college studies (1131); one phrase recognizing that a patient's condition meant she could not go on holiday for the time being (1238); or a statement that in the case of a patient with persistent vaginal irritation she must be 'pretty fed up with it' (1093). Similar limited interchanges took place in one in ten of the consultations in the 5 per cent sample. The conceptualization and discussion of 'implications' or consequences with patients appeared to be an area of undeveloped potential.

[4] Ratings of how clearly doctors had stated diagnostic-significance and treatment- or preventive-action ideas to patients could be made reliably. Agreement between two independent raters, after comparing a one in four random selection of cases rated by the main rater and a second investigator, shown both in percentage terms and by means of the weighted kappa coefficient (Cohen 1968), was as follows:

scale	% agreement	weighted kappa
diagnostic-significance	91	0.78
treatment-action	98	0.90
preventive-action	100	1.00

(N = 48)

Table 4.1n *Information-giving in two samples*

no. of consultations in which:	main sample		5 per cent sample	
		(%)		(%)
1 topics mentioned				
diagnostic-significance	369	(91)	58	(84)
treatment-action	405	(100)	69	(100)
preventive-action	124	(31)	16	(23)
implications	47	(12)	7	(10)
2 reasons given				
(a) diagnostic-significance				
more elaborate	85	(23)	9	(16)
minimal	134	(36)	10	(18)
none	150	(41)	37	(66)
(b) treatment-action				
more elaborate	48	(12)	2	(3)
minimal	142	(35)	17	(27)
none	215	(53)	43	(69)
(c) preventive-action				
more elaborate	19	(15)	2	(14)
minimal	33	(27)	5	(36)
none	72	(58)	7	(50)
(d) at least one topic				
more elaborate	128	(32)	10	(15)
minimal	177	(44)	20	(31)
none	100	(25)	35	(54)
(3) patient views explored				
some active effort	54	(13)	2	(3)
passive or ambiguous efforts	118	(29)	9	(13)
none	233	(58)	58	(84)
total (N)	405		69	

[5] Because a doctor could state his view in so few words we found that either he did so or he did not. Gradations of how clear he was were not really necessary and a two-point scale only was used.

[6] The main task of the rater was to examine any jargon used by the doctor and to decide if it was likely to be understood by a patient of the background of the one in question. The task could mostly be achieved reliably. Agreement between two independent raters (tested as before), shown in percentage terms and by means of the weighted kappa coefficient (Cohen 1968), was as follows:

scale	% agreement	weighted kappa
diagnostic-significance	89	0.74
treatment-action	88	0.75
preventive-action	85	0.44

(N = 48)

[7] The main task of the rater was to identify the warrants the doctor used and to decide if they supported his views or weakened alternatives (this could be a complex matter if several problems were given diagnoses or treated). The rater then decided if reasons for and against were detailed. By following prearranged steps it proved possible to undertake this task reliably. Agreement between two independent raters (tested as before), shown in percentage terms and by means of the weighted kappa coefficient (Cohen 1968), was as follows:

scale	% agreement	weighted kappa
diagnostic-significance	89	0.85
treatment-action	92	0.77
preventive-action	85	0.86

(N = 48)

A four-point scale was used but kappa was weighted to penalize most severely any disagreements between moderately elaborate and minimal, minimal and none (the distinctions used in the text).

[8] The doctor actually said:

'If you don't have a mattress (then) if you imagine that's your bed there, when you lie on it it goes down a little bit. Then, if you are lying on your side, your spine gets that shape, or if you are on your back, and you are forced to lie with your head there, there are your shoulders, the small of your back there then lies off the bed and you retain the shape of the small of your back. Whereas, if your bed isn't flat, your spine can droop there. It is worth trying and it can often work.'

The key point about descriptive explanations of this kind was that raters should be satisfied that the relevance of the description to the patient's presenting complaint could be established: it had to describe reasons for a view about the diagnostic-significance of the complaint or reasons why advice would help the complaint.

[9] Our method followed the logic of the approach to communication implied by the 'Flesch' formula (Ley 1979). It depended on an 'average person' approach. Raters were instructed to assess whether an 'average' person in the patient's circumstances, taking account of their educational and occupational background, would have difficulty. Individual idiosyncrasies were not considered. The approach means that some technical terms used, for instance, to a nurse, might be considered comprehensible. To another patient the same terms might not be so. The measure was not a prediction of whether the patient *would* understand but of whether the message was broadly comprehensible in a 'one way' situation, that is without further clarification and exchange. By following prearranged steps it proved possible for raters to judge the probability a patient would understand the reasons

given in a reasonably reliable way. Two independent raters were able to agree their ratings (over 48 randomly selected cases as before) on four-fifths of the ratings they made (82 per cent), giving a weighted kappa coefficient (Cohen 1968) of 0.64. (Comparisons were made across ratings of all topics because the total number of cases compared was less than ten.)

[10] The ratings depended on (1) establishing how much a doctor knew about a patient's ideas and (2) how far his reasoning related to them. So few doctors appeared to try to exchange ideas in any detail (let alone to relate explanations in a reactive way) that precision in developing the scale was never achieved. As a result it was not possible to demonstrate that these ratings could be made consistently. One of the 48 cases compared was judged to be minimally reactive by one rater but not by the other. From the point of view of the point made in the text, however, what matters is that with this one exception raters agreed there was no reactive explanation in every case.

[11] Agreement between two independent raters (tested as above), for ratings of how far doctors checked their patients' understanding, shown in percentage terms and by means of the weighted kappa coefficient (Cohen 1968), was as follows:

scale	% agreement	weighted kappa
diagnostic-significance	98	0.83
treatment-action	98	0.90
preventive-action	92	0.67

(N = 48)

[12] The first consultation has been selected at random from all those consultations in which 'moderately elaborate' reasoning was present. The other two consultations have been chosen to illustrate themes established by the statistical data.

[13] The doctor asked: 'That's all? What's all? What's happening in your world?' But he did not get a reply for several minutes because of various interruptions by the child. The doctor tried to help, saying 'They do go through this. Just let her take this hand, take that hand and give it to her–let her wave it around, let her get the feel of it.' The child eventually calmed down and the doctor could address himself back to the mother.

[14] What was actually said was as follows:

Patient: My mum
Doctor: How are you and she hitting it off?
Patient: Well, we get along fine.
Doctor: Are you?
Patient: Yes. I just feel absolutely fed up at the moment.
Doctor: I can see it luv.
Patient: Yeah. I work.
Doctor: Terribly wearing isn't it?
Patient: Mmm.
Doctor: Do you think she misses you when you are at work?
Patient: Well, I don't start till five. No.
Doctor: And what time do you get back?
Patient: Ten o'clock.

Doctor: Do you?
Patient: She goes to bed.
Doctor: Yeah. She's getting her fair share of you isn't she?
Patient: Well I'm with her all day.
Doctor: Yes.
Patient: Then the weekend I have with her.
Doctor: How do you see the future?
Patient: Alright I suppose. Alright.
Doctor: Do you. Had disappointments?
Patient: It's not as good as I'd like it to be, but while she's alright I'm not really bothered.
Doctor: No.
Patient: No.
Doctor: How do you feel about going on living with your mum?
Patient: Oh alright, I don't mind.
Doctor: Are you girls together. Has it very much got to be her way?
Patient: Oh no, no. It's all my way.
Doctor: Is it (laughter).
Patient: She spoils me.
Doctor: Does she?
Patient: Yeah. I do whatever I want to, you know.
Doctor: (child, who had gone quiet, is crying again) Is she missing your dad?
Patient: No, I don't think so. Now and again I'd watch her and I think she's thinking about him, but...
Doctor: It was really a mercy wasn't it in the end? And how about you. Do you miss him badly?
Patient: Yeah I miss him terribly. (Child starts crying louder)
Doctor: When's the anniversary?
Patient: Yesterday.
Doctor: Does this come, has this been very much in your mind for the last couple of weeks?
Patient: No. I've just felt down lately.
Doctor: Yeah.

[15] In this way the consultation illustrates some of the issues described by Hughes (1982) who argues that the fact that patients do not get their views on the agenda is caused by their inability to communicate them when given the opportunity. In a sense they are communicatively incompetent. We shall return to this issue in later notes to this chapter and again subsequently.
[16] Unfortunately we are not in a position to know what this patient thought of her consultation. It was one of those 77 cases for which interview material was not available.
[17] The consultation continued as follows:

Doctor: No, you had got something there and it does seem to be quite clear from the X-ray report and as I say, I'm afraid that once you get this scarring it does produce pain from time to time.
Patient: Yes.
Doctor: Now there are some ways of trying to reduce it and you know, since your father had a duodenal ulcer, I'm sure you know a lot about diet.
Patient: Yes, I do, yes.

Doctor: But I think the most important thing is to have small frequent meals.
Patient: Yes. 'Cos I don't have anything fried. If I have bacon it's grilled or sausages grilled or fish. I don't eat fried fish.
Doctor: Yes.
Patient: Um, I haven't done for quite some time because I know how it plays me up.
Doctor: Yes. But as I say the important thing is to have small frequent meals.
Patient: Yes.
Doctor: That's every couple of hours just have a sort of small snack of a non-acid food.
Patient: Yes.
Doctor: And you can have a cup of tea and a biscuit or you can have a sort of glass of milk.
Patient: Mmm.
Doctor: Something like that.
Patient: Yes. Egg whipped up.
Doctor: Yes. I wouldn't have too many eggs actually.
Patient: No I find...
Doctor: Funnily enough...
Patient: I think that eggs do sometimes tend to make you um get this aggravate it a bit but I love eggs. I'd sooner have eggs than meat so, and cheese, I like cheese. Would that be aggravating it, cheese, I find it does sometimes?
Doctor: They do tend to be a little fatty.
Patient: Yes.
Doctor: ...and its the fatty foods that might disturb you as well. I'm giving you some medicine to take and I would have, when you get a sort of bad bout, have a couple of teaspoonfuls before meals.
Patient: Yes.
Doctor: Now the timing is important. Take it about half an hour before the meal.
Patient: Yes.
Doctor: Now you know most of these medicines are given after the meal.
Patient: Afterward, yes.
Doctor: This should be given before the meal about half an hour.
Patient: Mmm.
Doctor: OK?
Patient: Yes.
Doctor: And do that two or three times a day if you get a bout of pain and you'll find after a short time it will subside.
Patient: Yes.
Doctor: But it will come back.
Patient: Yes, yes.
Doctor: Now it's not a neurotic thing.
Patient: No.
Doctor: Neither, you're not a hypochondriac. There is something there and it will produce pain from time to time.
Patient: Yes.
Doctor: OK?
Patient: Yes.
Doctor: Are there any questions?
Patient: No. I mean normally I feel pretty, I've been feeling pretty well. I was thinking,

oh, you know, oh I've got all I have is a bad chest. But since I've had, um, bronchitis earlier this year I don't seem to have picked up at all. But, er, you know, normally I don't really, I'm not a person that's had a lot of ill health.

Doctor: How's your weight going?

Patient: Well, I think I'm a bit on the heavy side. I mean I am trying to lose a bit, I go, I tend...

Doctor: Well, we won't deal with that just yet. I'd like you to see how you go with the medicine...

Patient: Yes.

Doctor: and taking it before the meal...

Patient: Yes.

Doctor: and having small frequent meals...

Patient: Yes.

Doctor: and then if you settle down fine. And if you don't come and see us again.

Patient: Yes. Right ho. And mostly bread, I have wholemeal bread so I mean that doesn't um...

Doctor: That's alright.

Patient: If I eat that or if, say, if I knock out eggs, I don't know what I could replace that...

Doctor: I won't be so cruel as to say knock out eggs...

Patient: Just cut them down.

Doctor: (laughing) Just reduce them.

Patient: ...and I love salads but you see there again, cucumber and things like that really...

Doctor: Undressed as well. If...

Patient: ...really kill you.

Doctor: you like a nice salad dressing with vinegar in that's not too good for you.

Patient: No, I don't worry about that with salad.

Doctor: All right.

Patient: Thank you very much indeed.

Doctor: Bye, bye Mrs Jones.

Patient: Bye, bye.

Mrs Jones' consultation lasted for just under nine and a half minutes.

[18] In fact he interrupted (Who's they?) at the beginning and so cut off her understanding of what had been established in the past. Also, he did not try to understand why the discussion about eating became so tortuous. There was clearly something in the patient's mind but it was never established. In fact at one point she stated that she believed eating made no difference (p. 59) which suggests a belief system which will interfere with his advice.

[19] This, it may be thought, is already suggested in the rather confused discussion about eating. In any case, when interviewed later, Mrs Jones, despite being very positive about the caring and understanding received from her doctor, had little clear understanding of the basic elements of her condition and was considered not to have made 'correct sense' (see Chapter 8) of the doctor's advice to her as to how to modify her future experience of symptoms. (It is interesting that the main information she received was that her condition was chronic. Yet she already knew this when, early in the consultation, she volunteered 'it's just something they told me I've got to live with'.) Some further details of Mrs Jones' case are discussed below in Chapter 6.

[20] The examination 'sounded' as follows:

Doctor: Do you smoke?

Patient: Er, yes. Not a lot though. I've just had my annual chest clinic. I go every year.

Doctor: Oh Yes. They're happy are they?

Patient: Yes, yes.

Doctor: Um, you're not a heavy smoker? How much do you smoke?

Patient: Well, I suppose about ten a day. I roll my own.

Doctor: You roll your own.

Patient: Yes.

Doctor: Mm I just want to feel the pulse here. Your toes don't go blue or anything like that?

Patient: No (pause) I'm rather, if to say, rather active on the feet, so to speak workwise, you know. . .

Doctor: Yes?

Patient: There's nothing sort of tenderish in the foot, just the sort of outward skin.

Doctor: Stand back. Let's have a look at those veins.

Doctor: (after pause) You don't ache at all?

Patient: No.

Doctor: Take a seat will you Mr Nixon. (Pause) This is where you get it, is it?

Patient: Oh yes, right on the round there sometimes, round the ankle type, you know, I've um, while it can be annoying it's eh. . .

Doctor: When I'm touching you with cotton wool, you feel that alright do you?

Patient: Eh, just a . . .

Doctor: (interrupting) Let's have you on the couch. Probably be easier. Alright?

Patient: (indistinct)

Doctor: You feel that alright do you? Can you feel that?

Patient: Yes I can.

Doctor: Feel the same on both legs?

Patient: Yes.

Doctor: Mm. (Pause) It feels the same everywhere does it?

Patient: Yes. There's nothing I mean . . .

Doctor: You feel that as a pinprick do you?

Patient: Eh, yes. Just the same. (Pause)

Doctor: That feels the same everywhere? Um . . .

Patient: *I don't know whether it might be diet?*

Doctor: I think probably it's just to do with a dry skin but I'm not too clear in my mind whether you're describing a nerve irritation or a skin irritation.

Patient: Yes you know . . .

Doctor: (interrupts) I'll check for you. (Tapping) Now, you're kidding me there. That was a false one!

Patient: Yes that was, that was.

Doctor: (laughs) You were just trying to help me, weren't you. Close your eyes, close, just shut your eyes and tell me does your toe point upwards or downwards now?

Patient: Upwards.

Doctor: Now?

Patient: Down.

Doctor: And now?

Patient: Upwards.

[21] In fact the pseudonym applied to this patient, Mr Nixon, provides the clue to his theories. He revealed in his interview, within the first two minutes, that his theory was that he suffered from *flea-bite-us (sic)*, an itching and taut condition of the legs, caused by a circulatory condition–hence his emphasis on diet and sugar seen by Mr Nixon as precursors of cardiovascular troubles. In biomedical language he thought he had phlebitis, like the ex-president of the USA and a friend of his at work, who had been hospitalized for the condition not long before the consultation. Interestingly enough, his consultation caused him to drop this hypothesis to second place behind the hypothesis his troubles were nervous, not neurological but caused by 'nervous tension' due to upsets at work and over his daughter's marriage. Bearing in mind Blumhagen's (1980) 'Hypertension' there might even be a further theory there, although this did not emerge in the interview. Mr Nixon's theories emerged rapidly in the interview, undoubtedly because the interviewer did not need to interrupt him to ask for details of his symptoms. In fact, in answer to the initial questions (tell me what you went to see your doctor about) the patient had replied: 'Well, er, the reason being, er that I get a sort of skin aggravation on the legs, you see, and on and off it's playing me up from time to time not over-alarming but enough, um, you know here. . . . It comes and goes, um. I'm not one to analyse these things eh, but, eh, I rather, eh, had the impression it was a bit of flea-bite-us (sic) or something like that. . . .' The interviewer asked him two minutes later, when there was a pause, what he meant by flea-bite-us. The patient explained easily and quickly.

Another of Mr Nixon's theories was also hinted at in the final part of the consultation and again ignored by the doctor who was clearly preoccupied by his own routine and thoughts. The last part of the consultation went as follows:

Patient: Um Yes.

Doctor: But I think that's purely a skin problem. I'll give you, er, some cream.

Patient: Yes, very kind of you. Thank you very much. *Oh, I sort of thought it might possibly be a nerve itch, you know, rather.*

Doctor: Mmm. (writing) Are you on your feet a lot?

Patient: Yes. I am rather active, so to speak, at work. The shop I'm in charge of, moving here, there and everywhere, like, you know. Anyway, it's very nice to see you. Haven't seen you. . .

Doctor: (interrupting) Haven't seen you for a long time. Is your hearing getting worse?

Patient: Er, I do get, er, rather poor hearing on that, er, side. The hearing's dying down, you know, rather.

Doctor: Mm. I'll just have a look in your ear. Make sure you haven't got any wax or anything. It's getting worse, is it?

Patient: Er, No, er, Not er. . .

Doctor: (interrupting) As far as I remember you always were a little hard of hearing.

Patient: Yes, it, er. . .

Doctor: What about your parents? Your father hard of hearing?

Patient: Er, yes, yes.

Doctor: Mm.

Patient: But eh, it's been a very soft hearing, you know, if sometimes at work people perhaps you know, notice, and er. . .

Doctor: (interrupting) Is it getting worse?

Patient: Er, Well if it is, it's very slowly.

Doctor: Uh, uh.
Patient: But, now, I think sometimes they do tend to be a little waxy, you know.
Doctor: I think it's true deafness you've got here. If you think it's getting worse, let me know and we'll get an ear man to have a look at you.
Patient: OK fine. Thank you.
Doctor: I'll leave you to think that one over and come back if you want to.
Patient: Yes. Thanks very much.
Doctor: OK.
Patient: Anyway, nice to see you.
Doctor: Nice to see you again.
Patient: Bye, bye for now.
Doctor: Bye bye.

Mr Nixon's consultation lasted just over ten and a half minutes.

[22] Bearing in mind patients' reluctance to volunteer ideas (Chapter 6) and also their probable uncertainty about exactly when and how to contribute to consultations (Hughes 1982), we thought the most effective type of question to discover a patient's ideas would be 'meta-level' i.e. a question which included a comment about why it was being asked. No examples of questions of this kind were found among the consultations. However, the various rating distinctions mentioned could be made reliably. Comparisons (made as before over 48 cases) between two independent raters showed agreement of 98 per cent and a weighted kappa of 0.95 in the case of doctors' attempts to discover both patients' treatment-action ideas and diagnostic-significance hypotheses.

[23] These ratings could also be made reliably. Comparisons (made as before over 48 cases) between two independent raters showed agreement of 96 per cent and a weighted kappa of 0.89 in the case of doctors' attempts to elaborate patients' diagnostic-significance hypotheses. Raters agreed in every case about efforts to elaborate patients' ideas about treatment-action.

[24] These ratings could also be made reliably. Comparisons (made as before over 48 cases) between two independent raters showed agreement of 87 per cent and a weighted kappa of 0.76.

[25] To be rated as 'inhibited' a consultation had to contain evidence either that the patient had no chance to develop his own ideas or was actually interrupted when trying to do so. The kind of situation described by Hughes (1982) in which patients simply 'ran out of steam' and a silence developed or doctors had to change the subject (rather like the beginning of Mrs Cumberland's consultation, above), would not be rated as inhibited.

[26] This was a simple rating scale by means of which we recorded every instance in which doctors gave any prediction about the future of a patient's symptoms. For example: 'I think it will take a few more days to go, even although it has already dragged on for a fortnight' (1394); or 'Once you've taken the tablets for a few days you will start to feel better' (1304); or, at a more detailed level 'You may find it (the rash) worsens over the next week and then gradually starts to get better....it will burn itself out' (1148).

[27] A similar scale to the last (26). In this case the rater noted any mention of a subjective effect that might be expected from a treatment. For example 'They are likely to make you sleepy' (1374) or 'Don't worry, there are no side effects' (1079).

[28] Another simple scale in which we tried to assess whether attempts were made to relate instructions to practical aspects of a patient's life. For example, one doctor prescribed anti-depressants and then said: 'You might feel drunk for the first two or three days. Do

you drive?'. When the patient explained that she drove her child to school the doctor modified his instructions: 'Well, probably wait until you get to school to take one, then. Then one in the afternoon and two at night.'

[29] See *Table 4.1n* above.

[30] All relationships reported in this chapter and subsequently (unless otherwise indicated) were statistically significant at the 5 per cent level or better. The chi-squared statistic has been applied to all situations in which nominal scale assumptions are appropriate. Kendall's Tau[b] or Tau[c] (as appropriate) has been applied to ordinal data and the 'T' test applied to interval data. Following the argument put forward by Fienberg (1981:22) Yates correction has not been applied to the chi-square test. Relationships which were statistically significant but of marginal strength have also not been reported. Lambda (asymmetric), gamma, and Pearson's R, as appropriate, have been used as measures of association.

[31] Using lambda (asymmetric) as a guide, knowledge of which doctor a patient saw gave a less than 10 per cent chance (lambda 0.10 or less) of predicting whether a doctor would state his views clearly, give reasons, explore patients' views or inhibit and evade them–in other words the variation between doctors was not greatly different to that within the consultations of one doctor. The only exception was checking a patient's views. Knowledge of which doctor a patient saw in this case gave one a 20 per cent chance of knowing whether the doctor would check his understanding or not.

[32] The gamma coefficients were as follows: stating views clearly 0.20; exploring a patient's ideas 0.11; taking a view on prevention 0.22; checking a patient's understanding 0.54; inhibiting or evading a patient's ideas 0.24; giving reasons 0.07.

[33] The Hope–Goldthorpe classification of occupations (Goldthorpe *et al.* 1978) was used so that the occupation and employment status of the head male of the respondent's household determined their social class. Women's occupations were, therefore, the determinant only if they lived alone and were employed. If they lived alone and were not employed the occupation of their husband (if divorced or separated) or father was used. In this way it was possible to classify respondents into 36 occupational categories and to combine these into a two or three class model. Both the two and three class models have been used to test all results.

[34] See *Table 4.2n.*

Table 4.2n *The effect of gender on doctors' reactions to patients' ideas*

	female (%)	male (%)	total (%)
patients' ideas evaded:			
yes	39 (15)	9 (7)	48 (12)
no	230	127	357
total	269	136	405

chi-square = 5.37 1 d/f p < 0.05
gamma = 0.41

[35] The diagnoses given to patients were determined from their consultations (in which they were often mentioned to them) and from the case notes. They were then coded into the 378 categories of the International Classification of Health Problems in Primary Care (WONCA 1979) and one additional residual category. To make a statistical analysis possible with 405 cases the 379 categories could be combined in various ways, for example into the seventeen major diagnostic category headings (I to XVII). Using assymmetric lambda to examine any resulting associations that were statistically significant the coefficients were as follows: mentioning prevention 0.05; stating diagnostic-significance views clearly 0.07; giving reasons 0.02; exploring a patient's ideas 0.005; inhibiting or evading a patient's ideas 0.10.

[36] Patients with diagnoses of hypertension (WONCA 1979: 120, 121), ulcer and related stomach complaints (151, 153, 155, 156), osteoarthritis, etc. (229, 234, 237, 238), anxiety and depressive disorders (70, 71, 77, 84)) were included in this category of 'Special Conditions' mentioned in the Royal College of General Practitioners (1981) reports.

[37] The basic purpose of this rating was to distinguish 'good' and 'bad' diagnostic news. Patients were considered to have a 'diagnostically-significant' condition if the problem they presented implied the kind of condition mentioned in the text or if he diagnosed a pre-existing condition as responsible for new ongoing nuisance or disability. Where the situation could be characterized by a phrase like 'Oh don't worry about that, that's just a bit of your old . . .' then, provided what was complained of was not an important source of discomfort or degeneration, it could be considered 'not significant'.

[38] The correlation coefficient (lambda asymmetric) between the main ICHHP categories into which a patient's illness fell and diagnostically 'significant' or 'not significant' categories was 0.09.

[39] An attempt to construct an index combining the variables which influenced whether patients were given information or not did not improve the chance of predicting who would get it.

[40] Following Cartwright and O'Brien (1976) the length of consultations was measured in two ways: first, from the moment a patient walked in until he left (total time); second, during all periods of conversation within the total time (conversation or speaking time). In those consultations in which patients were sent to a different room, or if the doctor left the room, the time taken was when both parties were in the same room. Average consultation times were as follows:

	total time	conversation time
mean	8.10	6.96
SD	4.55	3.84
median	7.11	6.15

[41] The correlation coefficient Pearson's R between total time and conversation time was 0.93.

[42] Patients with menstrual disorders were either given a consultation lasting less than four minutes or one lasting more than nine. They never saw the doctor for an intermediate duration.

[43] We are referring here to the results on the sample of 405 patients only.

[44] In fact the doctor who conducted the highest proportion of short consultations was observed during recording to spend an inordinately long amount of time waiting for his next patient.

Chapter 5. The importance of the part patients can play

[1] This has certainly been one of the authors' experiences (DT) over a wide range of clinical teaching situations. Many physicians, whether young and hospital-orientated ones or eminent members of the profession, will cite example after example of the frustrations they experience with patients. Alternatively, they will give examples of the patients they have experienced who have been very unhappy about being asked about their ideas or have wanted the doctor to make all the decisions for them. Above all, few doctors are able to conceptualize what patients say as forming a coherent body of quasi-biological thinking. It seems that these objections can only be overcome by a careful process of unravelling the thinking and assumptions on which they are based (see Chapter 11).

[2] Using a schedule method at the end of the *interview* we had arranged with them we asked about any symptoms they might have experienced, any self-treatment behaviour in which they might have engaged and any social and psychological problems and reactions they could report. Every patient was asked to volunteer the symptoms he had experienced in the two weeks before his consultation and was *also* taken through a short checklist of aches, pains and physical sensations, medications, reactions to symptoms and basic aspects of their mental state, life-style, housing situation and social relationships. They were asked:

In the last two weeks have you:
a. Had any pains or tenderness anywhere at all?
   (Probe: chest, arms and legs, joints, stomach, when sitting, when working)
b. Had any lumps or swelling anywhere?
c. Had any bleeding at all?
   (Probe: nose, bowel, in sputum, cuts)
d. Had any trouble sleeping (pause), or with tiredness (pause), or with your sex life?
e. Been breathless or puffy at all?
f. Had a headache or felt dizzy?
g. Been constipated or had diarrhoea or indigestion?
h. Felt nauseous or vomited?

The following questions were asked to find out about medications, possible reactions to symptoms, life-style, and possible crisis events and social difficulties:

In the last two weeks have you?
a. Taken any pills or tablets?
   (Probe: none? no others, no aspirins, no indigestion tablets, no sleeping tablets?)
b. Used any ointments?
c. Taken any mixtures or tonics?
   (Probe: cough mixture, something for an upset tummy?)
d. Missed any of your usual activities?
e. Taken any advice about your health at all?
   (Probe: other than from your doctor, from relatives or friends?)
f. Seen any other doctor, specialist or someone like an osteopath?
g. Taken any particular care about your diet?
h. Taken any regular exercise?
i. Drunk any alcohol?
j. Smoked tobacco, a pipe or cigars?
k. Moved house, had any problems in the home?

(Probe: Such as?)
l. Changed job, had any problems at work?
(Probe: Such as?)
m. Had any crises?
(Probe: Such as? For example with spouse, lover, parents, friends?)
n. Had any other troubles in your life?
(Probe: for example, accidents, unexpected happenings, bad news?)

The earlier question about sleeping (Had any trouble sleeping (pause), or with tiredness (pause), or with your sex life?) was considered a potential lead to psychiatric symptoms. But the specific question asked was:

> Have you in the last two weeks, the two weeks before you saw the doctor, felt miserable, unusually unhappy, or tense and worried?

[3] To make this rating it was necessary to define what comments a patient made could be considered as volunteered by him and what comments, as it were, were a response to a doctor's questions. The latter could hardly count as information volunteered. This problem was solved by considering only ideas introduced by a patient which had no antecedents in what a doctor said as potentially relevant. In this manner whether patients presented any diagnostic hypotheses and, if so, whether they indicated their reasons for hypothesizing in that way, was rated on a three-point scale. Agreement between two independent raters for this rating (tested as before over 48 cases), in percentage terms, was 88 per cent. By means of the weighted kappa coefficient (Cohen 1968), it was 0.82. Kappa was weighted equally between the three distinctions.

[4] The questions patients asked could be classified in several ways. First, raters determined whether a question overtly asked for reasons on a topic, whether it might appear to do so (covertly) whether it was a question mainly seeking further interpretation, or whether it was a question solely concerned with how to follow instructions. If questions appeared to be aimed at seeking reasons, raters then asked whether they sought the doctor's reasons *for* a particular view and/or *against* another one. Finally, they judged whether questions were part of a clarifying process (a sequence of questions) or just 'one-off'. Questions could be adjudged to ask for reasons, to seek clarification and to seek details of instruction, if it seemed appropriate. The result was three rating scales with varying number of scale points. It was not possible to test agreement for questions concerned with prevention, due to the small number of cases. Agreement between two independent raters (tested as before over 48 cases), on the other topics and for each scale point, shown in percentage terms and by means of the weighted kappa coefficient (Cohen 1968), was as follows:

scale:	*number of scale points*	*% agreement*	*weighted kappa*
seeking details			
of instructions	4	93	0.81
seeking clarification			
treatment-action	3	90	0.81
diagnostic-significance	3	98	0.97
asking for reasons			
treatment-action	7	90	0.70
diagnostic-significance	7	98	0.98

Where relevant kappa was weighted to penalize errors in assigning cases to overt, covert, or none distinctions.

[5] Some patients might express doubts which indicated the reason why they were doubtful. This seemed a further important distinction. In the event of a patient explaining his reason for doubt he might make it easier for a doctor to understand the cause of his doubt and perhaps encourage an exchange of information. Doubts given with reasons, it was thought, might be less likely to create an atmosphere of frustration.

[6] Whether doubt was expressed could also be rated reliably (tested in the same way).

scale	number of scale points	% agreement	weighted kappa
treatment-action	4	81	0.73
diagnostic-significance	4	79	0.62

Kappa was weighted to penalize errors in assigning cases to overt, covert, or none distinctions. As part of our concern about the influence of using audio- rather than video-based assessments of consultations, we also arranged a small exploratory trial to test the influence of sound-based as opposed to visually-based ratings. Comparing 46 consultations (recorded by the MSD Foundation) one rater coded video tape recordings with access to sound only, another rated with sound and picture. Results suggest that audio ratings (which can take into account pausing, intonation, pitch, loudness, even loud fidgeting, rustling of papers and inattentiveness) were no less accurate than video-based assessments in the case of 'overt' expressions of doubt. As might be expected video-based ratings did, however, appear to increase the proportion of consultations containing covert expressions of doubt by about one-fifth. It seems likely that higher agreement on this rating (which depended on tone of voice and other more subtle signs) might be achieved with a visual record.

Chapter 6. The way patients played their parts and its consequences

[1] The proportions of patients estimated to keep facts to themselves does not include those who reported that they had not told their doctor because they believed him already to know. When patients responded that they had experienced a symptom (etc.) they were asked (1) whether they had told the doctor in the consultation; (2) whether they thought he was aware of the information and (3) (if relevant) why they had not told him. Only those patients who reported symptoms (etc) which they believed they had not told him are included in the estimates.

[2] A small pilot study of the doctor's history-taking confirms this dependence further. In practice the doctors relied on patients to present the problems for which they needed help and did not usually go 'fishing' for other difficulties. Doctors' questions would focus on what the patient volunteered and on elucidating clinical signs and symptoms relevant to that complaint. This at least was the conclusion reached by applying a scheme to assess history-taking based on determining how thorough was questioning in five areas (*Table 6.1n*). The scheme took account of what patients volunteered (as if it had been asked for by the doctor) and questions in an area were rated 'more thorough' if the doctor had made any attempt to establish he knew about the range of relevant phenomena falling in the particular area. For example, he would have covered 'general health' in a 'more thorough' way if he had checked (Is that all? Is there anything else? No other troubles at all?) that the patient had told him all he wanted. If there was any question at all,

Table 6.1n *History-taking in five content areas*

| | extent of questioning: | | | |
	more thorough (%)	attempt only (%)	none (%)	total
areas:				
presenting symptoms	65 (58)	41 (36)	7 (6)	113
general health	22 (19)	41 (35)	54 (46)	117
pill-taking	11 (9)	34 (29)	72 (62)	117
reactions to symptoms, mental state, and life-style habits	5 (4)	38 (33)	74 (63)	117
consequences of symptoms, work, housing, and relationships	32 (27)	24 (21)	61 (52)	117

conceivably directed at one of the areas of information, this constituted an attempt. *Table 6.1n* demonstrates how doctors were most likely to focus on the presenting complaint and most unlikely to be 'more thorough' in other areas. If patients had problems they would be unlikely to obtain discussion of them if they did not volunteer them.

[3] *Table 6.2n* shows that the frequency of questioning and doubting did vary somewhat for the different topics.

[4] In this example, part of the exchange includes a question, rated here as an expression of doubt, which would also be an indicator relevant to patients' questioning behaviour. Some questions can be doubts, others may not be. The rating principles that were used allowed any patient behaviour to be rated as an indicator of more than one type of behaviour, if this seemed appropriate in terms of context, tone of voice, etc.

[5] Mrs Edwards (1397) was an example of a patient who indicated some aspects of her explanatory model which was then picked up and elaborated by her doctor. She offered her doctor the following explanation:

> 'And, I did finally see the doctor at the end of November, for seven weeks I've walked around with *fluid on my knee,* and I was in terrible pain really, and I eventually had the fluid taken off by the ice-packs around my knee and I went on for, well, I went back and forward...*I don't think it's all arthritis because I get this hard lump at the back of my knee, and it gets tighter and tighter and tighter...I think it is something or other, because I don't think arthritis would fluctuate to that degree...* And this is why I've come to see you, to see if I can come to any better understanding with you.'

After examining her knee, Mrs Edward's doctor explored her ideas further asking 'You say you don't think that its shooting arthritis?' and 'What do you think it might be?'.

[6] Asking for clarification of treatment was related to whether (and how) doctors interpreted treatment-action recommendations. Similar relationships were not found between asking for clarification of diagnostic-significance hypotheses or preventive-action recommendations and doctors being clear as to their view on these topics.

[7] An example of a consultation in which a request for clarification of treatment action

Table 6.2n *Patient activity on different topics*

| | information topics | | | |
	diagnostic-significance (%)	treatment-action (%)	preventive-action (%)	any (%)
requests for reasons				
overt	5 (1)	7 (2)	2 (2)	14 (4)
covert	130 (35)	89 (22)	16 (13)	185 (46)
none	234 (63)	309 (76)	106 (86)	206 (51)
requests for clarification				
overt	88 (24)	58 (14)	11 (9)	137 (34)
covert	47 (13)	38 (9)	7 (6)	62 (15)
none	234 (63)	309 (76)	106 (85)	206 (51)
requests for instruction details				
overt	–	11 (3)	2 (2)	14 (4)
covert	–	163 (40)	18 (15)	177 (44)
none	–	231 (57)	104 (84)	214 (53)
expressing doubts				
overt	52 (14)	57 (14)	17 (4)	109 (27)
covert	89 (24)	59 (15)	9 (2)	116 (29)
none	228 (62)	289 (71)	379 (94)	180 (44)

apparently led a doctor to state more thoroughly what the treatment was is that of Mr Eaton (1824). Referring to the prescription handed to him by his doctor the patient asked, first, 'What is this for?' and, later, 'Will that stop the buzzing I get at night time?'. This led the doctor to clarify that he was prescribing ear drops to help to remove the wax from Mr Eaton's ears. He also mentioned that this would improve his hearing and make it easier to see what was happening, but was unlikely to stop the buzzing.

[8] Patient activity was also associated with some differences in the length of time spent speaking in consultations. Consultations took slightly longer if patients presented explanatory models, asked questions, or aired doubts. Whether this was cause or consequence is uncertain.

[9] This is the same measure as that described above (Chapter 4, pp. 64–5).

[10] Examining all those cases in which patients asked directly for reasons, it was apparent that most often their doctor responded by trying to provide them. Among the 14 cases which contained a direct request for reasons, half, like those of Mrs Lane and Mrs Lawn, were ones in which doctors subsequently gave their reasons in a 'more elaborate' way. Direct questioning about reasons in the context of disagreement and evasion, as in Ms Anchor's

consultation, occurred in 3 of the 14 consultations. In one other the consultation contained both reason-giving and evasion. In the remaining three consultations neither evasion nor reason-giving were present, but the same processes were evident. In one consultation the patient's question (which he did not repeat) occurred immediately prior to a telephone interruption and seemed to get 'lost'–perhaps otherwise it might have been answered. In another consultation the doctor did not answer the question but was very restrictive on the patient's subsequent initiatives. The patient was kept in virtual silence–precluding any probable disagreement and therefore evasion. The third consultation was an extremely confused one in which the patient's question appeared to have been lost in the welter of problems he presented and the quantity of statements he kept contradicting.

[11] The 98 patients were selected at random from the 328 patients interviewed. All patients were interviewed about their attitude to asking questions (etc.) but it was possible to analyse only the sub sample of responses.

[12] Two examples may illustrate the way this data was actually collected.

Mrs Warner (2216) volunteered during her interview that she would have liked to know more about her daughter's complaint (pneumonia). She was asked why she had not told her doctor she wanted to know more and replied: 'I don't know, I don't have any medical knowledge. That's why we go to the doctor. I don't like going because you get a lot of pressure that you're being neurotic and you shouldn't keep going to the doctor and wasting their precious time.'

In Mrs Allan's case (2436) her ideas again started from a comment she made. The following is a direct transcript of the relevant part of the interview:

Patient: We've had epidemics around here a couple of summers ago and because she (her child) hasn't been vaccinated (against whooping cough) there's always that chance. So I've got that worry at the moment.

Interviewer: Did you mention that to him (the doctor) actually?

Patient: No I didn't. No, because I thought it was measles and not whooping cough. She didn't actually have that bad a chest.

Interviewer: And you never thought of asking him?

Patient: No, because, as I said, it seemed to me so quick, the consultation I mean. I would have liked to have a bit more time.

Interviewer: You felt conscious did you that there wasn't enough time?

Patient: Yes, yes.

Interviewer: It wasn't forgetting to ask?

Patient: No, no.

[13] Education was measured on the basis of information, obtained at interview, about each patient's school, college and vocational or professional training history. With guidance on the level of possible qualifications (HMSO 1970) respondents were assigned to one of three groups. 'More highly' educated was coded if a respondent had completed university or professional qualifications (including radiography, LAMDA, art college two-year diplomas, SRN, etc.). 'Intermediate' education was coded if respondents had 'A' or 'O' level or HND (etc.) type qualifications or had completed certain types of training (City and Guilds, Pitmans, RSA, OND, NNEB, one-year art college diplomas, apprenticeships, etc.). 'Basic' level education was coded for those who left school at the minimum relevant age. This measure of education was only moderately correlated with the two measures of social class – 0.53 with the Hope–Goldthorpe two-class model and 0.56 with the three-class model.

[14] See *Table 6.3n*.

Table 6.3n *The influence of the significance of patients' diagnoses on asking a doctor to give reasons*

	significance of diagnosis:		
	significant (%)	not significant (%)	total (%)
asking for reasons:			
overt	8 (7)	6 (2)	14 (4)
covert	59 (49)	126 (44)	185 (46)
none	54 (45)	152 (54)	206 (51)
total	121 (30)	284 (70)	405

chi-square = 6.65 2 d/f p < 0.05
gamma = 0.20

[15] See *Table 6.4n*.

Table 6.4n *The influence of gender on expressing doubt*

	female (%)	male (%)	total (%)
expressing doubt:			
overt	84 (31)	25 (18)	109 (27)
covert	77 (29)	39 (29)	116 (29)
none	108 (40)	72 (53)	180 (44)
total	269 (66)	136 (34)	405

chi-square = 8.86 2 d/f p < 0.01
gamma = 0.25

[16] Lambda (asymmetric) = 0.08.

Chapter 7. The problem of patients' understanding

[1] We have, therefore, restricted our review of empirical studies to those in which patients' accounts have been compared with what (is supposed to have) occurred in a consultation. Studies of patients' general medical knowledge or memory in hypothetical situations, etc., were not our concern.

[2] Blumhagen emphasized that they certainly did not consider tranquillizers an appropriate remedy. In fact, the diagnosis and, therefore, the condition, often helped them to justify difficult social circumstances and/or ways to avoid them.

[3] Svarstad (1974) reported that patients recalled 326 out of the 347 drugs prescribed (94 per cent) and that over seven out of ten patients, told how long to take the drugs, recalled what doctors said correctly (1974:80-4); Bain (1977) reported that nine out of ten patients knew the name of their condition correctly, over six out of ten remembered the names of the drugs they were prescribed, and nearly eight out of ten could recall, 'within acceptable limits', the advice received. Larsen and Smith (1981) reported that patients, on average, understood five-sixths of the information given (this is an interpretation of the report that, on average they scored 24.6 out of a 30 maximum understanding score). Such rates contrast with the estimates produced by Ley, Joyce and others in which patients were reported to recall just over or under half of what a doctor said.

[4] Crohn's disease is a complex, chronic, and possibly psychosomatically influenced, disease of the large intestine.

[5] Third-party judgements (and some other assessments) were also made on the 51 consultations selected at random from among all those who refused an interview or who subsequently did not keep an interview appointment. The consultations of these patients contained somewhat less efforts by doctors to provide their rationales and somewhat more inhibition and evasion of patients' ideas than might have been expected. It is possible that the inclusion into the interview sample of these patients would have reduced rates of recall, interpretation and commitment for reasons suggested by our main findings which will become clear in the next two chapters.

Chapter 8. Remembering and making sense of medical ideas

[1] The details of the interview schedule, which should be understood as a checklist and a guide to interviews, not a rigid document, are in the Appendix.

[2] Our reasons for choosing this approach to interviewing were discussed in Chapter 2.

[3] The rating scales that have been described depend on two sets of judgements: those made by the investigator responsible for the third-party judgement of the 'key points' of a consultation (described in the last chapter) and those made by the interviewers when they had to compare the third-party judgement with a patient's account of his consultation. For most of the cases assessed in the study, ratings of recall were first checked by all three interviewers meeting together. Every case in which the patient was rated as 'not correctly recalling' was discussed as well as cases at the margin and some randomly selected cases. Each interviewer had to justify his ratings in detail and in writing so that a standardized discussion could take place. The interviews had been tape-recorded and could be played back in the meetings. Discussions resulted in some ratings being changed and in the clarification or modification of rating criteria.

By the time it came to rate the last 51 cases in the series of 328, it was possible to put the reliability of interview ratings to a formal test. Pairs of raters listened separately to tape-recordings of the interviews and, with the third-party judgement to hand, independently made the relevant assessments. Results, which were satisfactory, were as follows:

scale	% agreement	weighted kappa
diagnostic-significance	94	0.92
treatment-action	92	0.70
preventive-action	96	0.90

[4] This approach to rating was particularly important in the case of consultations in which doctors' comments were markedly confused, full of technical jargon, or ambiguous, so that patients inevitably had difficulty making sense of them even if their memory of events was precise.

[5] A four-point rating scale, used separately for each topic, was employed to quantify the results of the comparison and to rate how biomedically correct was the patient's interpretation of the 'key points': the patient could be judged as making essentially 'identical sense' of the 'key points'; as making 'different sense of relatively unimportant aspects'; as making 'different sense of relatively important aspects'; and as making 'largely different sense'. Aspects were important or otherwise depending on how far they led to misleading conclusions about the 'key points'. Patients who made 'different sense of relatively important' aspects and 'largely different sense' were regarded as not making sense correctly.

[6] Ratings were made and reliability tested in the same way as described earlier for recall. Results of the formal test, which were satisfactory, were as follows:

scale	% agreement	weighted kappa
diagnostic-significance	78	0.79
treatment-action	86	0.75
preventive-action	82	0.84

Weighting was designed to penalize errors across the 'correct', 'incorrect' distinction.

[7] See Chapter 4.

[8] The data available to make comparisons consisted of the tape-recorded consultations and the tape-recorded research interviews. Both could be examined in detail to explore several hypotheses about how the process of remembering and making sense took place although interview material was not ideal for the purpose for two reasons.

First, interviews had been conducted *after* patients had attended their consultations and so had been potentially influenced by their doctors' ideas. We would argue that this restriction should make it more, rather than less, difficult to show the importance of the role of the initial theories patients had before the consultation. Second, interviews were not designed to collect comprehensive details of the lay theories and explanatory models patients had. Each patient was, however, asked at his interview for his understanding of what *might* be the possible diagnoses to test in his case, what might be the possible treatments and what might be possible ways to prevent the condition in future. The questions covered quite explicitly any ideas the patient might have derived from newspapers, radio, friends, and so on. They also indicated that interviewers were interested to know about patients' general medical knowledge.

[9] More cases were taken for diagnostic-significance than treatment-action because there were twice as many instances of patients unable to remember or make sense correctly of a doctor's ideas on this topic.

[10] Among the 20 patients who correctly made sense of a doctor's view on diagnostic-significance 10 had been given the diagnosis before and saw nothing problematic about it; 4 had minor common conditions; 4 presented lay theories (like Mrs Cecil) and had them dealt with and only 2 had new and unexpected (by them) diagnoses. In contrast among the 20 patients who had not correctly made sense there were 7 who had been to the doctor about the problem before but who in all cases had not yet reached an understanding consistent with the doctor's (in 3 cases doctor or patient changed the diagnosis from the previous time and in 4 the patient had misunderstood it from the previous occasion).

Seven patients had minor but unusual complaints, 6 had new and unexpected complaints and 3 had the lay diagnosis they offered rejected without discussion. Similarly, among the 10 patients correctly making sense of a doctor's treatment views 4 were given a repeat prescription, 1 had a treatment recommended by another doctor confirmed and 3 received referral to the hospital. Among the 10 patients who did not correctly make sense of treatment-action only 2 received a repeat prescription and 6 were given new advice. In the sub sample patients who did not make correct sense were about twice as likely to receive ambiguous and contradictory information and more than twice as likely to have views ignored.

[11] These questions were asked of all the patients whom we interviewed and who saw the last two doctors in whose surgeries we tape-recorded. There were 51 patients in all. Four were ex-smokers, 21 were non-smokers and 26 were smokers. Results are presented for 24 smoking respondents, the interviews of 2 of the 26 were incomplete on this subject. Patients were asked these questions whether or not they had a smoking-related disease and whether or not the subject had been mentioned in the consultation (a rarity in the sample as a whole).

[12] We have taken the views of the Royal College of Physicians (1971) as an indicator of medical views. They suggest that smoking is one of the highest risk factors for cardiovascular disease and for lung cancer as well as prejudicial to general health.

[13] The argument that our 24 smokers emphasized the benefits of smoking or the risks of other behaviours might be considered to derive from their need to justify their behaviour. Our point would be that biomedical understanding is intrinsically interconnected with moral issues of a cultural and social, as well as of an individual kind, at every stage. This complicates but does not avoid the fact that patients have a range of ideas and explanations on many topics.

Chapter 9. Evaluating medical ideas

[1] See Appendix for an idea of the way questions were asked.

[2] The ethics of appearing to place doubts in patients' minds may seem controversial: the interview might leave patients in a considerable state of anxiety and confusion. We developed our approach after a pilot study in which we found that patients normally evaluated what they were told, did not usually seem to find the questioning difficult and often relished the opportunity to talk about their doubts (also see Stimson and Webb 1975). In any case we were careful to warn that questioning was hypothetical and, as an extra precaution, to discuss with every patient we interviewed, at the end of the interview, the possibility that they were experiencing doubts. If they were, they were strongly advised to go back to their doctor and to tell him of their doubts. In a few cases patients were helped by the interview to feel confident enough to return to their doctors to have their doubts discussed. In some other cases they were very critical of their doctors but had not resented the interview.

[3] In fact one-third of those unable to reject diagnostic alternatives put to them were also unable to do so for action alternatives. Less than a third of those weakly rejecting action alternatives also weakly rejected diagnostic alternatives.

[4] The exact way a rating was made was, first, to determine if a patient had any doubts about the doctor's view (on key points). Patients were judged to exhibit no significant doubts, to have some doubts, or to be mainly doubtful. This was basically a measure of the patient's feelings about the doctor's ideas. The second step was to decide if, when presented with ideas which conflicted with those of the doctor, patients rejected such

theories unequivocally, were doubtful or unsure, or could not reject the alternative or even accepted it as better. Patients were considered 'not committed' (1) if they were mainly doubtful about doctors' ideas and, either, were doubtful about rejecting alternatives, could not reject them or actually accepted them; and (2) if they expressed some doubts about doctors' ideas and could not reject or even accepted conflicting alternatives. Alternatives were considered only important if they undermined or conflicted with what doctors said. Parallel alternatives, as it were, were not considered evidence of lack of commitment.

[5] Ratings were made and reliability tested in the same way as described earlier for recall (Chapter 8). Results of the formal test, which were satisfactory, were as follows:

scale	% agreement	weighted kappa
diagnostic-significance	87	0.77
treatment-action	89	0.92
preventive-action	86	***

Weighting was designed to penalize errors across the 'committed', 'not committed' distinction. In the case of prevention less than five cases were available for comparison.

[6] The number of cases in which patients were not committed to what doctors said on the prevention topic was too few for a reliable analysis.

[7] How to obtain the appropriate level of fear arousal in any given message has come to dominate much of health education. (See for example Leventhal 1971; Becker and Maiman 1975.) The view of the doctor–patient consultation as characterized by innate conflict has a long history in sociology (for example: Freidson 1961; Lorber 1975; Waitzkin and Stoeckle 1976).

Chapter 10. Stereotypes and the process of sharing medical ideas

[1] This statement was made at an invited conference held, to discuss the preliminary findings of our study, at the Royal College of General Practitioners on Friday 16 October, 1981. The doctor concerned said:

'Most of us have been conned by Ley that, if we give six statements, only four will be remembered, and this is what is done in hospital outpatients but not in general practice. We may have been consciously trying to economize on the number of statements that we give to patients on the grounds that if they are only going to remember a few of them, the more you give the fewer they remember. The implications of your research...mean that we have to change our whole concept of what we are up to in giving information...the actual fact, that you say patients have good recall of what we say, this is quite a new idea to me and it would change my behaviour considerably if it were true... (it) is terribly important, because you are not going to tell him the science behind it if he is merely going to forget most of it. But if he is going to remember more, then one can tell him, if one has time.'

[2] In fact at the beginning of the programme of work Ley and Spelman (1967:9) discussed the need to prepare patients to counter opposing propaganda and seemed to have a much more dynamic view than Ley subsequently emphasized.

[3] The difference between Ley's findings and our own could be explained in one of two ways: there could be something radically different about the patients we have each

studied (arising from the samples used), or there could be something different about the way recall was assessed. Only a further study allowing a comparison of methods on the same sample could clarify this matter for certain. There are, however, no obvious grounds for believing the sample of patients we studied was likely to have been very different from those in earlier research or is likely to be unrepresentative. In the first place, Ley and his colleagues have reported rather uniform rates of recall despite the different samples and situations they have studied. Second, differences in the recall achieved by individual doctors, even in past experimental studies, have been less than the differences between all previous studies conducted by Ley and that we have reported. Moreover, it does not seem likely that the present study was based on a sample in some way 'not representative' of the other samples: the sixteen different doctors were chosen to ensure as wide a variation in practice as possible and the proportion of patients recalling correctly did not vary significantly between the patients of different doctors.

Since there are no strong reasons for believing differences arise from sampling, it seems likely the results we obtained, when compared to Ley's, are the product of two methodological differences. First, restricting assessments to which 'key points' were remembered (in our study as in that of Pendleton 1982b) may have reduced estimates of how much patients forget, because patients remember 'more important' information better. Second, the methods of interviewing may have had an important effect. The standardized non-schedule approach used in the present study was designed to make clear to respondents the meaning of questions asked and to overcome the uncertainty we felt existed in schedule approaches such as those of Ley (see Chapter 2).The results of the present study probably provide evidence that this was so.

[4] See for example the discussion of Kirscht (1974) and King (1982). Investigators have reported, for instance, that individuals' beliefs in their susceptibility to specific diseases correlated with their participation in screening programmes (Fink, Shapiro and Roester 1972; Kegeles 1969; Haefner and Kirscht 1970), obtaining immunization (Leventhal, Hochbaum and Rosenstock 1960; Ogionwo 1973), taking children to preventive health clinics (Becker *et al.* 1977), and adhering to medication and life-style modifying regimes (Kirscht and Rosenstock 1977; Maiman *et al.* 1977; Becker *et al.* 1977; Kirscht *et al.* 1978). They have also reported that beliefs about the severity of symptoms and disease states and the relative value of action, taking account of its costs and benefits, have tended to correlate with such things as obtaining preventive dental care (Kegeles 1969; Tash, O'Shea and Cohen 1969), following preventive suggestions and seeking medical care (Suchman 1967; Battistella, 1971; Becker *et al.* 1977).

[5] The Health Belief Model is based on three principles that are the hallmark of utilitarian positivism: that is to say the theory's leading characteristic is 'atomism', it acknowledges the possibility of 'free' individual action, and it assumes (subject to differential motivations and features of heredity and environment) that social actors follow the rational norm of efficiency (Parsons 1937:60). According to the Health Belief Model departures from a 'rational' norm of behaviour, for example to following a doctor's instructions, are considered to be associated with an actor's knowledge falling short of adequacy. 'Ignorance' or 'error' are, therefore, conceived as the source of 'irrational' behaviour, correction of these states is the antidote. However, although a utilitarian positivist theory of this kind appears to describe social processes quite serviceably (Parsons 1937:57), it nonetheless also contains logical flaws. Even given perfect knowledge, action cannot be atomistic, 'free' and based on the rational norm of efficiency, *and* result in the achievement of given ends

(i.e. biomedically advisable behaviours). Logically, the only condition under which it is possible to imagine every free individual with perfect knowledge arriving at the same 'given' end is if they really had no choice at all – termed by Parsons the utilitarian dilemma (Parsons 1937:64). Like other theorists in their tradition Health Belief workers have had to avoid the dilemma by resorting to explanations of social behaviour in terms of chance or of its conditions–heredity and environment (Parsons 1937:67). Health Belief theorists have explained deviations from rational behaviour (where knowledge is 'adequate') by 'chance' – cues to action – or a combination of heredity and environment – anxious personality, loss of control, etc.

[6]   That is the pursuit of rational efficiency within a means–ends schema (Parsons 1937).

[7]   In fact, they are so congruent that one wonders if there has not been unconscious collusion between the architects and interpreters of the research. Interestingly, in pointing out the failure of utilitarian theorists to analyse the lacuna in their model, Parsons made a comment which may also apply to the research we have been discussing:

> 'The great majority of the social thinkers responsible for the development of the ideas under discussion have been at least as much, generally much more, interested in justifying a course of conduct of policy which they have considered ethically right, as they have been in an objective understanding of the facts of human action.' (1937:53)

Chapter 11. Changing medical consultations

[1]   In the UK it is now no longer possible for qualified doctors to enter general practice without participating in a vocational training scheme during which at least one year is spent in general practice (and into which the intensive curriculum programme was set). These doctors, although licensed and fully qualified, are 'trainees' and those general practitioners with whom they train in a special kind of apprenticeship are 'trainers'. Depending on the regional training scheme in different parts of the UK, there are vocational training courses for trainees taking up to a day or so per week. Some trainers meet together to develop skills and these meetings are sometimes referred to as trainers' workshops. Trainees also form groups to meet and discuss issues that concern them.

[2]   These notes were discussed regularly with each other and the project director (DT).

[3]   This programme has been more fully described in a publication by the participants (Boulton *et al.* 1984).

[4]   The following information (somewhat abridged here) was given to trainees:

Eliciting patient theories

a. What to elicit
In order to understand the way the patient makes sense of his symptoms, it is necessary to push beyond the superficial statements of his views on diagnosis, treatment, prevention and so on, and to establish what they *mean* to him. This may entail exploring the following sorts of issues which lie behind the simple view of diagnosis and treatment.

(i) *Diagnosis:* What does the patient think it is?
Why does he think it is that?
What does he think happens to people with that diagnosis?
(ii) *Investigations:* What can the doctor do to find out for sure it is that diagnosis?
How can you rule out other possible diagnoses?

(iii) *Treatment:* What can be done for that diagnosis (i.e. can it be cured or just alleviated or controlled?)

What treatment is best? Why is it best?

How does it help the symptoms/diagnosis?

What are the drawbacks/disadvantages of the treatment?

(iv) *Prevention:* What does the patient think caused it?

Can it be prevented/prevented from worsening?

(v) *Implications:* What problems does he anticipate in coping with his illness and its treatment?

It is important to remember that the patient may have a variety of different theories about his symptoms and that each of them may be more or less well elaborated in his mind. In addition, his ideas on diagnosis, treatment and prevention may be linked into a coherent 'explanatory model', so that his understanding of what is wrong with him logically implies how the diagnosis can be confirmed or ruled out, how the problem will develop in future, what the treatment should be aimed at and how it works and how it can be prevented or controlled.

Finally, if the diagnosis or treatment which the doctor eventually decides on are ones which the patient has not mentioned himself, it may be necessary to explore the patient's ideas about those as well. Terms like asthma, bronchitis, eczema, ulcer, hiatus hernia, virus, dermatitis and so on, may have connotations for the patient which they do not have for the doctor, and may mean very different things to him than the doctor intends. One researcher has listed five ways in which the use of terms may differ. (Harwood's (1981) ideas mentioned in Chapter 7 were set out here.)

As a result of these differences in meaning and connotation what the patient understands the doctor to mean when he conveys his decisions on diagnosis and treatment, may be very different from what the doctor understands himself to mean. By establishing what the patient's ideas are, however, the doctor is in a position to correct any important errors in the patient's understanding.

b. How to elicit?

Since patients usually feel diffident about challenging or contradicting doctors, the doctor may find it most effective to elicit the patient's views before stating his own. There are no set questions that should be asked each patient, although a few 'sample' questions are listed in the next section. Instead, the key to 'eliciting' is to understand what it is you want to know and why, and to use whatever questions are appropriate in a given consultation to get that information. Put in its briefest form, you want:

(i) To find out the various theories/explanations/diagnoses the patient has considered *in order* to rule out all the theories he has which challenge your own theory and which may leave the patient unconvinced or disagreeing with your decisions; to do so without wasting time by ruling out alternatives irrelevant to the patient or by giving unnecessary explanations; and to reassure the patient by ruling out his 'worrying' theories while not creating worries by discussing alternatives the patient has not considered.

(ii) To find out what makes him think it's that or how his 'theorized' diagnoses could produce his symptoms *in order* to rule out his theories/explanations/diagnoses convincingly, by dealing with the reasoning underlying them: that is, by showing how their links are incorrect and how you can link your hypothesis to the symptoms.

(iii) To find out what the patient understands by his 'theorized' diagnoses and what he sees as its significance or prognosis *in order* to ensure that you and the patient mean the same things by the terms you use, and to correct any important misapprehensions or to alter any incorrect ideas the patient has which may affect his response to your diagnosis (e.g. worry, rejection of diagnosis or alteration of the way medication is used).

Similarly, with regard to investigations, treatment, control and prevention, you want:

(iv) To find out how the patient thinks you as the doctor can rule out the various explanations/diagnoses he has considered (e.g. what tests, examinations, etc., he can do) *in order* to carry out the procedure which will effectively reassure the patient or to explain why it is not appropriate (and so to help to stem patient dissatisfaction when the desired tests are not done); and to avoid carrying out a procedure which both doctor and patient might agree is unnecessary.

(v) To find out what actions the patient has considered appropriate to cure/control/prevent/ the problem *in order* to rule out the patient's ideas which conflict with your own and which may give rise to patient disagreement and noncompliance, and to do so without raising other ideas and wasting time ruling out irrelevant options.

(vi) To find out what the patient thinks actions will do and how they will help his problem *in order* to rule out inappropriate ideas convincingly, by showing the error in the patient's reasoning and with regard to ideas of treatment which are *appropriate*, to correct any incorrect ideas about how the treatment works which could influence the way in which the patient carries out the treatment.

Finally, once the doctor has made his own diagnosis and made his own decisions about treatment, it is important for him to check the patient's understanding of those decisions if it has not already been done. That is you want:

(vii) To find out what the patient understands by your diagnosis *in order* to ensure that you and the patient mean the same things by the terms you use; to discover and deal with the meanings and connotations the diagnosis has for the patient which may undermine his acceptance of that diagnosis, and to correct any incorrect ideas the patient may have which could affect his response to the diagnosis and the way he uses the medication given.

(viii) To find out what the patient thinks the treatment will do and how it will help his problem *in order* to correct any incorrect ideas he has about the treatment which might influence the way in which he carries it out.

(ix) To find out what the patient thinks are the advantages and drawbacks of the treatment *in order* to correct any incorrect ideas which may alter the way the patient carries out his treatment.

c. Some examples of questions

(i) Opening questions:
What do you think it is?
What sort of explanations have occurred to you?
What sorts of ideas have crossed your mind?
What did you make of it yourself?

(ii) Clarifying questions:
(Sometimes there will be no response to the opening questions or patients will be brief or confused. In such circumstances try explaining to the patient what it is you are trying to find out.)
Most patients have considered some sort of explanation about their symptoms – what sort of things have crossed your mind?
Most people have some sort of ideas – what has crossed your mind?
I asked you this because it's useful to me to know what you have considered yourself, so I can explain to you better.

(iii) Elaborating questions:
(Once the patient presents some ideas try to elaborate them to get the information you need.)
What do you mean by. . .?
What makes you think you've got. . .?
What does. . .mean to you?
What else?
Tell me more?
What do you think happens to people who get. . .?
In what way?
How do you think (causal factor) causes you to get (symptoms)?

(iv) Additional reminders:
(Don't give up too easily.)
What else has crossed your mind?
Any other ideas?

[5] This was a handout similar in design to that for eliciting (another one, not reproduced here, explained the topic of implications). It set out what might be meant by an explanation, purposes for giving explanations and the distinction between giving factual information (stating) and giving reasons. The handout also pointed out that there was no set or easy way of giving explanation. Some guidelines were then given (here in an abridged form):

a. Stating the view or decision

An essential precursor to any explanation is the stating of a view in simple, everyday, language, whether it be the diagnosis, the treatment, the preventive action or the implications of the problem. Although this might seem obvious, it has been not uncommon to find consultations in which at least one of these central decisions is not explicitly stated by a doctor, or is stated in a muddled, roundabout, obscure or jargonistic way.

Under diagnosis such factual statement needs to include what is wrong, whether or not it is serious, what the prognosis is and possibly what caused the problem. Thus a patient presenting with a painful back would need to be told that it is, for example, a muscle strain brought on by heavy lifting, that it will heal up with rest and will not have done permanent damage.

For treatment such a statement should include the name of the treatment or investigation being proposed and its purpose, i.e. what it is meant to achieve. For example, a patient with tonsillitis should be told that an antibiotic is being prescribed to kill the bacterial infection and so speed recovery. Or a patient with suspected cystitis should be told the purpose of giving a urine sample for a laboratory test.

b. Justifying or giving reasons

This is the second aspect of explanation in which the doctor gives reasons for taking a particular view and/or reasons against taking a view. Bear in mind that even if you explain the reasons against a view you still leave open the chance the patient will not be convinced by the view you favour, that may need to be justified as well, and vice-versa. Either type of reasoning can be done in different ways:

(i) Classes of reason
We can distinguish between simply advancing a lot of reasons on a single theme and giving reasons that belong to different classes. Arguably, explanations that incorporate different classes of reason are likely to be more convincing for the patient. For example, a patient who was overweight could be told that weight-reducing tablets are inadvisable not only because they have potentially damaging side-effects (specified) but also that in the long run they do not work and even possibly cause more weight to be put on. Or a patient with chest pain might be told that incipient heart attack is unlikely because the pain is in the wrong place, because the physical examination revealed nothing wrong and because the pain does not relate to exertion.

In each of these examples the different reasons advanced draw upon different types and sources of knowledge and if an explanation draws on more than one type or class it may be considered more weighty.

(ii) Mechanisms and causes
A different kind of explanation to one that simply assembles different reasons (albeit of a different class) is one which explicitly demonstrates cause and effect relationships by spelling out the causal processes, for example, why a viral throat infection can lead to pains elsewhere in the body; how an antacid or alternative gastro-intestinal treatment influences an ulcer.

(iii) Vocabulary
It is widely agreed that jargon should be avoided but what constitutes jargon is a subject of debate. The issues raised in the paper on eliciting (note 4 above) are relevant here.

(iv) Reaction to patients' ideas
Fundamental to our idea is the principle that the explanations given relate to the theories the patient has. Eliciting is thus the precursor and guide to what to explain and how.

[6] One impression gained very strongly in this work concerned the considerable anxieties and difficulties for doctors surrounding their consultations with patients with emotional difficulties. These were patients who were not mentally ill in any psychiatrically definable sense but ones who created feelings of excessive anxiety and helplessness in their doctors. They are, essentially, the kinds of patients described by Balint (1964) and Balint et al. (1970). Trainees often brought these patients to discussions which, because of the nature of the underlying problem, were often abortive. We would want to emphasize that patients of

this kind require special and complex attention over and above the general approach we are advocating. Yet any practical programme of teaching rapidly has to grasp the nettle. [7] As one doctor put it: 'Too much eliciting from the doctor may make the doctor look pedantic, over-inquisitive or worse yet, make the patient look stupid. Intelligent patients don't want to be patronized or bamboozled into sifting every assumption with a fine tooth comb.'

[8] For example, a number of questions were selected to approach the theories of a patient with pre-menstrual tension (PMT). 'What do you understand by PMT? What do you think happens inside you when you get it? Is that permanent? Have you any ideas about what should be done?' What was then stressed was that questions be developmental, trying to sort out what significance a patient attaches, why she does so, and how her understanding of the mechanics can link to her ideas about treatment or long-term consequences. [9] See note 2 (Chapter 6).

Chapter 12. Summary and conclusions

[1] For example Stimson and Webb (1975); West (1976); Hughes (1982).
[2] A view which sits uncomfortably side by side with the view that what you tell them can have devastatingly negative effects.
[3] An example is Komrad (1983) who uses the following 'Typical example' to argue that medical paternalism is a complex question:

> 'Consider this typical example. A physician discovers a 1.5cm breast cancer in a 30 year-old woman without swollen axillary lymph nodes. He plans a total mastectomy instead of local excision of the mass followed by radiation therapy, which is controversially of equivalent efficacy. The patient requests her doctor to do 'whatever he thinks best'. Can the physician accept this invitation?'   (Komrad 1983:40)

[4] It can be argued that the clarity required would aid 'traditional' skills – such as making an accurate diagnosis. A diagnosis which must be thought through and justified may also be more accurate.
[5] See note 22 (Chapter 4).
[6] In the UK, both private medicine and fringe medicine often live off the problems of NHS medicine. In many cases, what the private or fringe practitioner may provide is the feeling of time to talk.

REFERENCES

Abel-Smith, B. (1981) Health Care in a Cold Economic Climate. *The Lancet* I, 373–76.

Alexander, L. (1981) The Double-Bind Between Dialysis Patients and their Health Practitioners. In L. Eisenberg and A. Kleinman (eds) (1981) *The Relevance of Social Science for Medicine*. Dordrecht: D. Reidel.

Anderson, J.L. (1979) Patients' Recall of Information and its Relation to the Nature of the Consultation. In D.J. Oborne, M.M. Gruneberg, and J.R. Eiser (eds) *Research in Psychology and Medicine, 2*. London: Academic Press.

Bain, D.J.G. (1977) Patient Knowledge and the Content of the Consultation in General Practice. *Medical Education* 11:347–50.

Balint, M. (1964) *The Doctor, his Patient and the Illness* (2nd edn). London: Pitman Medical.

Balint, M., Hunt, J., Joyce, D., Marinker, M., and Woodcock, J. (1970) *Treatment or Diagnosis*. London: Tavistock.

Bales, R.F. (1950) *Interaction Process Analysis*. Cambridge, Mass.: Addison-Wesley Press.

Baruch, G. (1981) Moral Tales, Parents' Stories of Encounters with the Health Professions. *Sociology of Health and Illness* 3(3): 276–95.

Battistella, R.M. (1971) Factors Associated with Delay in the Initiation of Physicians' Care among Late Adulthood Persons. *American Journal of Public Health* 61:1348-361.

Becker, M.H. (1974) The Health Belief Model and Sick Role Behavior. *Health Education Monographs* 2:409–19.

Becker, M.H., Drachman, R.H., and Kirscht, J.P. (1972) Predicting Mothers' Compliance with Pediatric Medical Regimens. *The Journal of Pediatrics* 87 (9): 852–62.

Becker, M.H. and Maiman, L.A. (1975) Sociobehavioral Determinants of Compliance with Health and Medical Care Recommendations. *Medical Care* 13 (1): 10–24.

—— (1980) Strategies for Enhancing Patient Compliance. *Journal of Community Health* 6 (2): 113–35.

Becker, M.H., Nathanson, C.A., Drachman, R.H., and Kirscht, J.P. (1977) Mothers' Health Beliefs and Children's Clinic Visits, A Prospective Study. *Journal of Community Health* 3:125–35.

Beeson, P.B. and McDermott, W. (1975) *The Cecil and Loeb Textbook of Medicine* (14th edn). Philadelphia: W.B. Saunders.

Bertakis, K.D. (1977) The Communication of Information from Physician to Patient, A Method for Increasing Patient Retention and Satisfaction. *Journal of Family Practice* 5:217–22.

Blackwell, B. (1976) Treatment Attendance. *British Journal of Psychiatry* 129:513–31.

Blaxter, M. (1983) The Causes of Disease, Women Talking. *Social Science and Medicine* 17 (2): 59–69.

Bloor, M. (1976) Professional Autonomy and Client Exclusion. In M. Wadsworth and D. Robinson (eds) (1976) *Studies in Everyday Medical Life*. London: Martin Robertson.

Blumhagen, D. (1980) Hypertension, A Folk Illness With a Medical Name. *Culture, Medicine and Psychiatry* 4:197–227.

Boreham, P. and Gibson D. (1978) The Informative Process in Private Medical Consultations, A Preliminary Investigation. *Social Science and Medicine* 12:409–16.

Boulton, M., Griffiths, J., Hall, D., McIntyre, M., Oliver, B., and Woodward, J. (1984) Improving Communication, A Practical Programme for Teaching Trainees about Communication Issues in the General Practice Consultation. *Medical Education* 18:269–74. Oxford: Blackwell Scientific Publications Ltd.

Brackenbury, H.B. (1935) *Patient and Doctor*. London: Hodder and Stoughton.

Brown, G. (1978) *Lecturing and Explaining*. London: Methuen.

Brown, G.W. and Harris, T.O. (1978) *Social Origins of Depression*. London: Tavistock.

Brown, G.W. and Rutter, M. (1966) The Measurement of Family Activities and Relationships, A Methodological Study. *Human Relations* 19 (3): 241–63.

Browne, K. and Freeling, P. (1976) *The Doctor-Patient Relationship*. 2nd edn. London: Churchill-Livingstone.

Bullowa, M. (1976) From Non-Verbal Communication to Language. *Linguistics* 172:5–14.

Bulmer, M. (1979) Concepts in the Analysis of Qualitative Data. *Sociological Review* 27 (4): 151–67.

Byrne, P.S. and Long, B.E.L. (1976) *Doctors Talking To Patients*. London: Her Majesty's Stationery Office.

Cartwright, A. and O'Brien, M. (1976) Social Class Variations in Health Care and in the Nature of General Practice Consultations. In M. Stacey, (ed) The Sociology of the National Health Service. *Sociological Review Monograph No 22*. Keele: University of Keele.

Cartwright, A. and Anderson, R. (1981) *General Practice Revisited, A second study of patients and their doctors. London: Tavistock*.

Cassata, D.M. (1978) Health Communication Theory and Research, An Overview of Communication Specialist Interface, pp. 495–504. In B.D. Ruben, (ed.) *Communication Yearbook 2*. New Brunswick, New Jersey, Transaction Books.

Cassidy, M. (1938) Doctor and Patient, *Lancet* I: 175–79.

Chrisman, N. (1977) The Health Seeking Process: An Approach to the Natural History of Illness. *Culture, Medicine and Psychiatry*, 1:351–77.

Cicourel, A.V. (1964) *Method and Measurement in Sociology*. New York: Free Press.

Cochrane, A.L. (1972) Effectiveness and Efficiency, Random Reflections on the Health Service. *The Rock Carling Lecture 1971*. London: Nuffield Provincial Hospitals Trust.

Cohen, J. (1968) Weighted Kappa–Nominal Scale Agreement with Provision for Scaled Disagreement or Partial Credit. *Psychological Bulletin* 70:213–19.

Commission of the European Communities (1980) *Proceedings of the International Symposium, The Role of the Physician in Health Education*. Luxembourg: European Economic Community.

Cormack, J.J.C. (1981) Prescribing (Appendix, Eleven Principles of Prescribing). In J.J.C. Cormack, M. Marinker, and D. Morrell (eds) *Teaching General Practice*. London: Kluwer Medical.

Cormack, J.J.C., Marinker, M., and Morrell, D. (eds) (1976) *Practice, A Handbook of Primary Medical Care* (updated annually). London: Kluwer Medical.

Danziger, S.K. (1978) The Uses of Expertise in Doctor–Patient Encounters During

Pregnancy. *Social Science and Medicine* 12:359–67.

Davies, J., Prendergast, S., Prout, A., and Tuckett, D.A. (1982) Health Knowledge of Schoolchildren, their Parents and Teachers. *Report of the Schools Health Education Project of the Health Education Studies Unit.* London: Health Education Council.

Davis, F. (1960) Uncertainty in Medical Prognosis, Clinical and Functional. *American Journal of Sociology* 66:41–7.

Davis, M.S. (1968) Variations in Patients' Compliance with Doctors' Advice, An Empirical Analysis of Patterns of Communication. *Journal of Public Health* 58, 274–88.

Dingwall, R. (1976) *Aspects of Illness.* London: Martin Robertson.

Drass, K.A. (1982) Negotiation and the Structure of Discourse in Medical Consultations. *Sociology of Health and Illness* 4 (3): 320–41.

Drury, V.W.M., Wade, O.L., Beeley, L., and Alesbury, P.L. (1978) *Treatment, A Handbook of Drug Therapy* (updated annually). London: Kluwer Medical.

Duff, R. and Hollingshead, A. (1968) *Sickness and Society.* New York: Harper and Row.

Egbert, L.D., Battit, G.E., Welch, C.E., and Bartlett, M.K. (1964) Reduction of Postoperative Pain by Encouragement and Instruction of Patients. *New England Journal of Medicine* 270:825–27.

Ernstene, A.C. (1957) Explaining to the Patient, A Therapeutic Tool and a Professional Obligation. *Journal of the American Medical Association* 165:1110–113.

Eisenberg, L. and Kleinman, A. (1981) *The Relevance of Social Science for Medicine.* Dordrecht: D. Reidel.

Fienberg, S.E. (1981) *The Analysis of Cross-Class Category Data.* Cambridge, Mass: MIT Press.

Fink, R., Shapiro, S., and Roester, R. (1972) Impacts of Efforts to Increase Participation in Repetitive Screenings for Early Breast Cancer Detection. *American Journal of Public Health* 62:328–36.

Flavell, J.H., Botkin, P.T., Fry, L.L., Wright, J.W., and Jones, P.E. (1968) *The Development of Role Taking and Communication Skills in Children.* New York: J. Wiley.

Fletcher, C.M. (1973) *Communication in Medicine.* Oxford: Nuffield Provincial Hospitals Trust.

Fowler, G. (1982) Practising Prevention, Smoking. *British Medical Journal* 284 (II): 1306–308.

Freemon, B., Negrete, V.F., Davis, M., and Korsch, B.M. (1971) Gaps in Doctor–Patient Communication, Doctor–Patient Interaction Analysis. *Pediatric Research* 5:298–311.

Freidson, E. (1961) *Patients' Views of Medical Practice.* New York: Russell Sage Foundation.

—— (1970a) *Profession of Medicine.* New York: Dodd Mead and Company.

—— (1970b) *Professional Dominance.* Chicago: Atherton Press.

Gallagher, E. (ed.) (1978) *The Doctor-Patient Relationship in the Changing Health Scene.* Washington, DC: Dept of Health, Education and Welfare Publ. No. (NIH) 78–183.

Garfinkel, H. (1964) Studies of the Routine Grounds of Everyday Activities. *Social Problems* 11:3.

—— (1967) *Studies in Ethnomethodology.* Englewood Cliffs, NJ: Prentice-Hall.

Goldthorpe, J.H., Payne, C., and Llewellyn, C. (1978) Trends in Class Mobility. *Sociology* 12:441–68.

Good, B. and Good, M. (1981) The Meaning of Symptoms, A Cultural Hermeneutic Model for Clinical Practice. In L. Eisenberg, and A. Kleinman (eds) *The Relevance of Social Science for Medicine.* Dordrecht: D. Reidel.

Haefner, D.P. and Kirscht, J.P. (1970) Motivational and Behavioral Effects of Modifying

Health Beliefs. *Public Health Reports* 85 (6): 478–84.

Hall, J.A., Roter, D.L., and Rand, C.S. (1981) Communication of Affect Between Patient and Physician. *Journal of Health and Social Behavior* 22:18–30.

Hart, J.T. (1976) The Middle Years. In J. Cormack, M. Marinker, and D. Morrell. *Practice, A Handbook of Primary Medical Care* (instalment 5, 4.5.01–4.5.3). London: Kluwer-Harrap Handbooks.

Harwood, A. (1981) Communicating about Disease, Clinical Implications of Divergent Concepts among Patients and Physicians. Quoted by Katon and Kleinman (1981) op cit.

Haug, M.R. and Lavin, B. (1979) Public Challenge of Physician Authority. *Medical Care* 17:844–58.

—— (1981) Practitioner or Patient – Who's in Charge? *Journal of Health and Social Behavior* 21:212–29.

Hawkins, G. (1967) *Speaking and Writing in Medicine*. Springfield, Illinois: Charles C. Thomas.

Hayes-Baucista, D.E. (1976) Modifying the Treatment, Patient Compliance, Patient Control and Medical Care. *Social Science and Medicine* 10:233–38.

Haynes, R.B., Taylor, D.W., and Sackett, D.L. (eds) (1979) *Compliance in Health Care*. Baltimore: Johns Hopkins University.

Helman, C.G. (1978) Feed a Cold, Starve a Fever – Folk Models of Infection in an English Suburban Community, and their Relation to Medical Treatment. *Culture, Medicine and Psychiatry* 2:107–37.

Helman, C.G. (1981) Disease Versus Illness in General Practice. *Journal of the Royal College of General Practitioners* 31:548.

Her Majesty's Stationery Office (1970) *Qualified Manpower Tables, Sample Census 1966, Great Britain*. London: Her Majesty's Stationery Office.

Higgins, P. (1983) Things Aren't What They Seem. Wander Lecture 1983. *Journal of the Royal Society of Medicine* 77:728–37.

Holden, H.M. (1977) The Needs and Expectations of Doctors and Patients. *Journal of the Royal College of General Practitioners* 27:277–79.

Hollingshead, A.G. and Redilich, F.C. (1958) *Social Class and Mental Illness*. New York: John Wiley.

Horder, J., Byrne, P., Freeling, P., Harris, C., Irvine, D., and Marinker, M. (1972) *The Future General Practitioner, Learning and Teaching*. London: Royal College of General Practitioners.

Horton, R. (1967) African Traditional Thought and Western Science. *Africa* 37:50–60.

Hughes, D. (1982) Control in the Medical Consultation, Organizing Talk in a Situation where Co-Participants have Differential Competence. *Sociology* 16 (3) 359–76.

Inui, T. S., Carter, W.B., Kukull, W.A. and Haigh, V.H., (1982) Outcome-Based Doctor–Patient Interaction Analysis. *Medical Care* 20:535–49.

Jackson, G. (1978) Sexual Intercourse and Angina Pectoris. *British Medical Journal*, 1 July.

Joyce, C.R.B., Caple, G., Mason, M., Reynolds, E., and Mathews, J.A. (1969) Quantitative Study of Doctor–Patient Communication. *Quarterly Journal of Medicine New Series* 38 (150): 183–94.

Kasl, S.V. and Cobb, S. (1966) Health Behavior, Illness Behavior and Sick Role Behavior. *Archives of Environmental Health* 12:246–66.

Katon, W. and Kleinman, A. (1981) Doctor–Patient Negotiation and Other Social Science Strategies in Patient Care. In L. Eisenberg and A. Kleinman (eds) (1981) *The Rel-*

evance of Social Science for Medicine. Dordrecht: D. Reidel.

Katon, W., Kleinman, A., and Rosen, A. (1982) Depression and Stomatization: A Review. Part 1. *American Journal of Medicine* 72:127–35.

Kegeles, S.S. (1969) A Field Experiment to Attempt to Change Beliefs and Behavior of Women in an Urban Ghetto. *Journal of Health and Social Behavior* 10:115–24.

Kickbusch, I. (1981) Involvement in Health, A Social Concept of Health Education. *International Journal of Health Education* 24 (Supplement): 3–15.

King, J.B. (1982) The Impact of Patients' Beliefs on the Consultation, A Theoretical Analysis. Paper presented to the Colloquium of the Consultation. CIBA Foundation 15–19 March. London, MSD Foundation.

Kinsey, A.C., Pomeroy, W.B., and Martin, C.E. (1949) *Sexual Behavior in the Human Male.* Philadelphia PA: W.B. Saunders.

Kirscht, J.P. (1974) Research Related to the Modification of Health Beliefs. *Health Education Monographs* 2 (4) 455–69.

Kirscht, J.P. and Rosenstock, I.M. (1977) Patient Adherence to Antihypertensive Medical Regimens. *Journal of Community Health* 3:115–24.

Kirscht, J.P., Becker, M.H., Haefner, D.P., and Maiman, L.A. (1978) Effects of Threatening Communications and Mothers' Health Beliefs on Weight Change in Obese Children. *Journal of Behavioral Medicine* 1:147–57.

Kleinman, A. (1975) Explanatory Models in Health Care Relationships. *National Council for International Health, Health of the Family.* Washington, DC: National Council for International Health.

—— (1980) *Patients and Healers in the Context of Culture.* Berkeley, CA: University of California Press.

Kleinman, A., Eisenberg, L., and Good, B. (1978) Culture, Illness and Care, Clinical Lessons from Anthropologic and Cross-Cultural Research. *Annals of Internal Medicine* 88:251–58.

Komrad, M.S., (1983) A Defence of Medical Paternalism: Maximising Patients' Autonomy. *Journal of Medical Ethics* 9:38–44.

Korsch, B.M., Gozzi, E.K., and Francis, V. (1968) Gaps in Doctor-Patient Communications, Doctor–Patient Interaction and Patient Satisfaction. *Pediatrics* 42: 855.

Larsen, K.M. and Smith, C.K. (1981) Assessment of Non-Verbal Communication in the Patient–Physician Interview. *Journal of Family Practice* 12:481–88.

Lazare, A., Eisenthal, S., and Wasserman, L. (1975) The Customer Approach to Patienthood, Attending to Patient Requests in a Walk-In Clinic. *Archives General Psychiatry* 32:555–58.

Leventhal, H. (1971) Fear Appeals and Persuasion: the differentiation of a Motivational Construct. *American Journal of Public Health* 61:1208–224.

Leventhal, H., Hochbaum, G., and Rosenstock, I.M. (1960) Epidemic Impact on the General Population in Two Cities, The Impact of Asian Influenza on Community Life, A Study in Five Cities. *Public Health Service Publication 766.* Washington DC: Government Printing Office.

Lever, A.F. (1977) Medicine Under Challenge, The Role of Medicine. *The Lancet* I (Feb 12): 351–55.

Ley P. (1976) Towards Better Doctor–Patient Communications. In A.E. Bennett (ed.) *Communications Between Doctors and Patients.* Oxford: Oxford University Press.

—— (1977) Communicating with the Patient. In J.C. Coleman (ed.) *Introductory Psychology.*

London: Routledge and Kegan Paul.

—— (1979) Memory for Medical Information. *British Journal of Social and Clinical Psychology.* 18:245–55.

Ley, P., Bradshaw, P.W., Eaves, D., and Walker, C.M., (1973) A Method for Increasing Patients' Recall of Information Presented by Doctors. *Psychological Medicine* 3:217–20.

Ley, P. and Spelman, M.S. (1965) Communications in an Out-patient Setting. *British Journal of Social and Clinical Psychology* 4:114–16.

—— (1967) *Communicating with the Patient.* London: Staple Press.

Ley, P., Whitworth, M.A., Skilbeck, C.E., Woodward, R., Pinsent, R.J.H.F., Pike, L.A., Clarkson, M.E., and Clark, P.B. (1976) Improving Doctor–Patient Communication in General Practice. *Journal of the Royal College of General Practitioners* 26:720–24.

Locker, D. (1981) *Symptoms and Illness, The Cognitive Organization of Disorder.* London: Tavistock.

Lorber, J. (1975) Good Patients and Problem Patients, Conformity and Deviance in a General Hospital. *Journal of Health and Social Behavior* 16:213–24.

Lucas, S. (1978) *Health Education in General Practice, An Analysis of Information and Advice Given by Doctors in Consultations with Elderly Patients.* Mimeograph Report. London: Health Education Council.

MacLeod, J. (1977) *Davidson's Principles and Practice of Medicine* (12th edn). Edinburgh: Churchill Livingstone.

Mahler, H. (1975) Health – A Demystification of Medical Technology. *The Lancet* II: 829–33.

—— (1981) The Meaning of 'Health Care for All by the Year 2000'. *World Health Organisation Forum* 2 (1): 5–22.

Maiman, L.A., Becker, M.H., Kirscht, J.P., Haefner, D.P., and Drachman, R.H. (1977) Scales for Measuring Health Belief Model Dimensions, A Test of Predictive Value, Internal Consistency and Relationship among Beliefs. *Health Education Monographs* 5:215–30.

Marinker, M. (1970) Truce. In M. Balint, J. Hunt, D. Joyce, M. Marinker, and J. Woodcock *Treatment or Diagnosis.* London: Tavistock.

—— (1981) 2010. *Journal of the Royal College of General Practitioners* 31:540–47.

Mason, S., and Swash, M. (1980) *Hutchinson's Clinical Methods* (17th edn). London: Bailliere Tindall.

McCall, G., and Simmonds, J.L. (1966) *Identities and Interactions.* New York: Free Press.

McHugh, P. (1968) *Defining the Situation, The Organization of Meaning in Social Interaction.* Indianapolis: Bobbs-Merrill.

McKeown, T. (1976) *The Role of Medicine, Dream, Mirage or Nemesis?* Oxford: Nuffield Provincial Hospitals Trust/Basil Blackwell.

McKinlay, J.B. (1973) Social Networks, Lay Consultations and Help-Seeking Behavior. *Social Forces* 53:275–92.

Metcalfe, D., (1982) Flexible Doctoring. *The Health Services* 23:20.

Morrell, D., Gage, H.C., and Robinson, N.R. (1970) Patterns of Demand in General Practice. *Journal of the Royal College of General Practitioners* 19:331.

Murray, J.A.H., Bradley, H., Craigie, W.A., and Onions, C.T. (1933) *The Oxford English Dictionary.* Oxford: Oxford University Press.

Ogionwo, W. (1973) Socio-psychological Factors in Health Behavior, An Experimental Study on Methods and Attitude Change. *International Journal of Health Education* 16:1–16.

Oliver, M.F. (1981) The Role of the Physician in Health Education, *Health Bulletin* 39

(5): 296–28.

Parsons, T. (1937) *The Structure of Social Action, A Study in Social Theory with Special Reference to a Group of Recent European Writers*. Paperback edition 1968. New York: Free Press.

—— (1951) *The Social System*. New York: Free Press.

—— (1978) Epilogue. In E. Gallagher (ed.) *The Doctor-Patient Relationship in the Changing Health Scene*. Washington, DC. Dept of Health Education and Welfare Publ. No. (NIH) 78–183.

Pendleton, D. (1982a) *Doctor-Patient Communication*. D.Phil Thesis. Department of Experimental Psychology. Oxford: University of Oxford.

—— (1982b) The Communication of Medical Information, What is given and what is remembered. Paper presented to the Colloquium on the Consultation. CIBA Foundation 18 and 19 March. London: MSD Foundation.

Pendleton, D.A. and Bochner, S., (1980) The Communication of Medical Information in General Practice Consultations as a Function of Patients' Social Class. *Social Science and Medicine* 14a:669–73.

Pendleton, D.A., Schofield, T., Tate, P., and Havelock, P. (1984) *The Consultation, An Approach to Learning and Teaching*. Oxford: Oxford University Press.

Phillips, A. and Rakusen, J. (1978) *Our Bodies Ourselves* (revised edition of that originally published in 1971 in the USA by the Boston Women's Health Collective). London: Penguin Books.

Pike, L.A. (1969) Health Education in General Practice. *Journal of the Royal College of General Practitioners* 17:133–34.

Pridham, K.F. and Hansen, M.F. (1980) An Observational Methodology for the study of Interactive Clinical Problem-Solving Behavior in Primary Care Settings. *Medical Care* 18:360–75.

Richardson, S.A., Dohrenwend, B.S., and Klein, D. (1965) *Interviewing, Its Forms and Functions*. New York: Basic Books.

Robertson, G. (1981) Informed Consent to Medical Treatment. *The Law Quarterly Review* 97:102–26.

Robinson, D. (1971) *The Process of Becoming Ill*. London: Routledge and Kegan Paul.

Rogers, P.L., Scherer, K.R., and Rosenthal, R. (1971) Content-Filtering Human Speech, A Simple Electronic System. *Behavior Research Methods and Instrumentation* 3:16–18.

Rosengren, W. R. and De Vault, S. (1964) The Sociology of Time and Space in an Obstetrical Hospital. In E. Freidson (ed.) *The Hospital in Modern Society*. New York: Free Press.

Rosengren, W.R. and Lefton, E. (1969) *Hospitals and Patients*. New York: Atherton.

Rosenstock, I.M. (1966) Why People Use Health Services. *Millbank Memorial Fund Quarterly* 44 (2): 94–127.

Roter, D.L. (1977) *Patient Participation in the Patient-Provider Interaction, the effects of patient question asking on the quality of interaction, satisfaction and compliance*. PhD Thesis. Baltimore: School of Hygiene and Public Health, Johns Hopkins University.

Royal College of General Practitioners (1976) *The Education of Patients and Public by General Practitioners in the Seventies*. Report of the Education Study Group. London: Royal College of General Practitioners.

—— (1981) *Health and Prevention in Primary Care* (Report Number 18). *Prevention of Arterial Disease in General Practice* (Report Number 19). *Prevention of Psychiatric Disorders in General Practice* (Report Number 20). London: Royal College of General Practitioners.

Royal College of Physicians (1971) *Smoking and Health Now*. London: Pitman Medical.
Royal Commission on Medical Education (1968) Report. London: Her Majesty's Stationery Office.
Russell, M.A.H., Wilson, C., Taylor, C., and Baker, C.D. (1979) Effect of General Practitioners' Advice Against Smoking. *British Medical Journal* 2:231–35.
Sackett, D.L. and Snow, J.C. (1979) The Magnitude of Compliance and Non-Compliance. In R.B. Haynes, D.W. Taylor, and D.L. Sackett (eds) (1979) *Compliance in Health Care*. Baltimore: Johns Hopkins University.
Schutz, A. (1953) Concept and Theory Formation in the Social Sciences. In A. Schutz, (1973) *Collected Papers* Volume 1. The Hague: Martinus Nijhoff.
Sharrock, W. (1979) Portraying the Professional Relationship. In D.E. Anderson (ed.) *Health Education in Practice*. London: Croom Helm.
Silverman, D. (1981) The Child as a Social Object, Down's Syndrome Children in a Pediatric Cardiology Clinic. *Sociology of Health and Illness* 3:254–74.
Skipper, J.K. (1965) Communication and the Hospitalized Patient. In J.K. Skipper and R.C. Leonard *Social Interaction and Patient Care*. Philadelphia: J.B. Lippincott.
Skipper, J.K. and Leonard, R.C. (1968) Children, Stress and Hospitalization. *Journal of Social Health and Behavior* 9:275–86.
Slack, W.V. (1977) Points of View, The Patient's Right to Decide. *The Lancet* (II): 240.
Smail, S.A. (1982) Opportunities for Prevention, the Consultation. *British Medical Journal* 284:874–75.
Stiles, W.B., Putman, S.M., Wolf, M.H., and James, S.A. (1979) Interaction Exchange Structure and Patient Satisfaction with Medical Interviews. *Medical Care* 17:667–79.
Stimson, G.V. (1978) Interaction Between Patients and General Practitioners in the United Kingdom. In E. Gallagher (ed.) *The Doctor-Patient Relationship in the Changing Health Scene*. Washington DC: Dept. of Health, Education and Welfare Publ. No. (NIH) 78-183.
Stimson, G.V. and Webb, B. (1975) *Going to see the Doctor*. London: Routledge and Kegan Paul.
Strauss, A., and Schatzman, L. (1960) Cross-Class Interviewing. In R. Adams and J. Preiss (eds) *Human Organization Research*. Homewood, Ill.: Dorsey Press.
Suchman, E.A. (1967) Preventive Health Behavior, A Model for Research on Community Health Campaigns. *Journal of Health and Social Behavior* 8:197–209.
Svarstad, B. (1974) *The Doctor-Patient Encounter, An observational study of communication and outcome*. Doctoral Dissertation. Madison: Dept. of Sociology, University of Wisconsin.
Szasz, T.S. and Hollender, M.H. (1956) A Contribution to the Philosophy of Medicine, *A.M.A. Archives of Internal Medicine* 97:585–92.
Tagliacozzo, D.L. and Mauksch, H.O. (1958) The Patient's View of the Patient's Role. In E.G. Jaco (ed.) *Patients' Physicians and Illness*. New York: Free Press.
Tash, R.H., O'Shea, R.M., and Cohen, L.K. (1969) Testing a Preventive-Symptomatic Theory of Dental Health Behavior. *American Journal of Public Health* 59:514–21.
Tuckett, D.A. (1970) *Why People Go To Psychiatrists*. M.Sc. Thesis. Bedford College, University of London.
—— (ed.) (1976) *An Introduction to Medical Sociology*. London: Tavistock.
—— (1978) Do Doctors' Expectations Bear any Relationship to Patients' Lifestyles? *Mims Magazine* 2:159–65.
Tuckett, D.A., and Williams, A.J., (1984) Approaches to the Measurement of Explanation and Information-Giving in Medical Consultations, A Review of Empirical Studies.

Social Science and Medicine 18 (7): 571–80.

Voysey, M. (1975) *A Constant Burden*. London: Routledge and Kegan Paul.

Wadsworth, M. and Robinson, D. (eds) (1976) *Studies in Everyday Medical Life*. London: Martin Robertson.

Waitzkin, H. and Stoeckle, J.D. (1976) Information Control and the Micro-Politics of Health Care, Summary of an Ongoing Research Project. *Social Science and Medicine* 10:263–76.

Wallen, J., Waitzkin, H. and Stoeckle, J.D. (1979) Physician Stereotypes About Female Health and Illness, A Study of Patient's Sex and the Informative Process During Medical Interviews. *Women and Health* 4 (2): 135–46.

Wallston, B.S. and Wallston, K.A. (1978) Locus of Control and Health: A Review of the Literature. *Health Education Monographs* 6 (2):107.

Walt, F. (1971) The Role of the General Practitioner in Health Education. *Journal of the Royal College of General Practitioners* 21:479–84.

Walton, J., Duncan, A.S., Fletcher, C.M., Freeling, P., Hawkins, C., Kessel, N., and McCall, I. (1980) *Talking With Patients, A Teaching Approach*. London: Nuffield Provincial Hospitals Trust.

Webb, B. and Stimson, G.V. (1976) People's Accounts of Medical Encounters. In M. Wadsworth and D. Robinson (eds) *Studies in Everyday Medical Life*. London: Martin Robertson.

West, P. (1976) The Physician and the Management of Childhood Epilepsy. In M. Wadsworth and D. Robinson (eds) *Studies in Everyday Medical Life*. London: Martin Robertson.

World Health Organisation (1978) Alma-Ata 1978, Primary Health Care. *Report of the International Conference on Primary Care*. Geneva, World Health Organisation.

WONCA (1979) ICHPPC-2 *International Classification of Health Problems in Primary Care* (1979 Revision). Prepared by the World Organization of National Colleges, Academies, and Academic Associations of General Practitioners/Family Physicians (WONCA). Oxford, Oxford University Press.

Zola, I.K. (1972) The Concept of Trouble and Sources of Medical Assistance. *Social Science and Medicine* 6:673–79.

—— (1973) Pathways to the Doctor – From Person to Patient. *Social Science and Medicine* 7:677–89.

—— (1981) Culture, Meaning and Negotiation – Structural Constraint in the Doctor-Patient Relationship, The Case of Non-Compliance. In L. Eisenberg and A. Kleinman (eds) *The Relevance of Social Science for Medicine*. Dordrecht: D. Reidel.

PATIENT INDEX